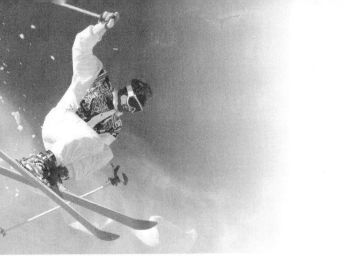

INTRODUCTION TO EXERCISE SCIENCE

Editor

Stanley P. Brown, Ph.D., F.A.C.S.M.

Associate Professor of Physical Therapy

Director of Research

Director, Laboratory of Applied Physiology

Southwest Baptist University

Bolivar, Missouri

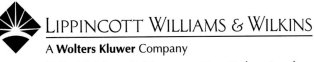

LIPPINCOTT WILLIAMS & WILKINS

A **Wolters Kluwer** Company

Philadelphia • Baltimore • New York • London
Buenos Aires • Hong Kong • Sydney • Tokyo

Editor: Peter Darcy
Managing Editor: Linda S. Napora
Developmental Editor: Nancy Peterson
Marketing Manager: Christen DeMarco
Production Editor: Jennifer D. Weir

351 West Camden Street
Baltimore, Maryland 21201-2436 USA

530 Walnut Street
Philadelphia, Pennsylvania 19106-3621 USA

The publisher is not responsible (as a matter of product liability, negligence, or otherwise) for any injury resulting from any material contained herein. This publication contains information relating to general principles of medical care which should not be construed as specific instructions for individual patients. Manufacturers' product information and package inserts should be reviewed for current information, including contraindications, dosages, and precautions.

Library of Congress Cataloging-in-Publication Data
Introduction to exercise science / editor, Stanley P. Brown.
      p. cm.
   Includes index.
   ISBN 0-683-30280-9
      1. Exercise. 2. Sports sciences. I. Brown, Stanley P.

QP301 .I652 2000
613.7'1--dc21

00-041955

The publishers have made every effort to trace the copyright holders for borrowed material. If they have inadvertently overlooked any, they will be pleased to make the necessary arrangements at the first opportunity.

To purchase additional copies of this book call our customer service department at **(800) 638-3030** or fax orders to **(301) 824-7390**. International customers should call **(301) 714-2324**.

Visit Lippincott Williams & Wilkins on the Internet: **http://www.lww.com**. Lippincott Williams & Wilkins customer service representatives are available from 8:30 am to 6:00 pm, EST, Monday through Friday, for telephone access.

00 01 02 03 04
1 2 3 4 5 6 7 8 9 10

To the four ladies in my life:
Yvonne, my wife,
and
Joanna, Elizabeth, and Ruth, our daughters,
who constantly teach me things about myself.

PREFACE

Exercise science is a well-respected academic discipline that integrates the knowledge bases of a number of other academic disciplines. Within the field of exercise science one can easily find the content of anatomy, biochemistry, epidemiology, molecular biology, physics, physiology, and psychology, to name just a few. These important parent disciplines provide the conceptual framework within which the scientific bases for movement during exercise, sport performance, and other forms of physical activity are studied. As a broad and eclectic discipline, exercise science, in many ways, reflects society's current fascination with sports and the recognized importance of exercise in the maintenance of health. Because of these trends, exercise science has affected society in a number of important ways, ranging from its influence on our understanding of the physiology, biochemistry, psychology, and biomechanics of exercise and sports performance to the advocacy of exercise in the prevention of lifestyle-related disease in the general population.

Because of its reliance on many basic sciences, graduates of exercise science programs often fail to have an appreciation of the broad nature of the discipline as a whole and of its development. For example, it is not uncommon to find exercise science academic programs that lack course work in one or more of the representative subdisciplines of the field. Although one may find many outstanding textbooks designed for courses covering each of the subdisciplines of exercise science, there is no comprehensive text focusing on exercise science at the introductory level. *Introduction to Exercise Science* fills that void.

This book is intended for exercise scientists, kinesiologists, physical educators, physical therapists, and other allied health specialists interested in a broad-based introduction to exercise science. This book is also conceived as a companion to one-semester undergraduate foundation courses in exercise science; it is designed to provide the student in such courses with current understanding of the broad nature of the field, its development, and the scope of its content.

Introduction to Exercise Science is divided into three parts. Part One ("The Discipline") contains two sections that survey the development of exercise science. Section 1 ("Historical and Cultural Aspects") contains two chapters, one providing an overview of the history of exercise science, and the other a discussion of how exercise science has affected society. Section 2 ("Professional Activities") contains five chapters surveying issues and trends regarding the ongoing professional development of exercise science. Specifically, this section investigates avenues students may take in their own professional development by describing the major exercise science certifications, job activities, and employment settings available to the exercise science major. The section includes a timely discussion of trends that describe the current state of flux of many of the issues regarding exercise science education, certification, licensure, practice, and the relationship of exercise science to healthcare professions such as physical therapy and nursing. A chapter on administrative concerns with descriptions of sports and fitness management and sports marketing rounds out the section.

Part Two ("Exercise Science Subdisciplines") contains five sections that provide a comprehensive examination of the subdisciplines of exercise science. Sections 3 to 7 present descriptions of each of the subdisciplines. The 11 chapters of these sections are grouped according to the knowledge base that provides those subdisciplines with their theoretical framework. The rationale for this approach is that exercise science is an umbrella term under which the different knowledge bases operate. Each chapter is written in a complimentary fashion, and the goal of the sections is to mold a complex and multifaceted field into a cohesive unit so that the student can have an appreciation of exercise science as a single discipline rather than a collection of unrelated disciplines. An effort was made to give a comprehensive description of the subdiscipline while maintaining a focus on the undergraduate exercise science student. However, enough science content is provided to make the book an attractive reference source for professionals and students in any of the allied health fields; key areas of research affecting our understanding of exercise and sports performance are addressed.

Part Three ("Future Development") concludes the text. Section 8 ("Exercise Science in the Twenty-First Century") provides commentary on the future development of exercise science, including a discussion on how the basic sciences, medicine, and new technology continue to affect exercise science.

Because the book is a companion for academic courses, there are some design features that will enhance learning. Each chapter begins with a topical outline and learning objectives. Key terms are set in boldface print at first occurrence, and all key terms are defined in the "Glossary." The concepts in the text are presented in a style appropriate to the readership. Illustrations and tables help clarify information for the reader. Most chapters include boxes, sidelights, and practical applications that highlight important conceptual material; numerous case studies are also included. Each chapter ends with a chapter summary, review questions, references, and suggested readings. Appendix B provides a complete list of the review questions along with the answers.

Recognizing that exercise science is a rapidly evolving discipline, I have made every attempt to ensure that parts one and two present information that was current at the time of printing. However, as with any rapidly evolving field, our knowledge is expanding and the book will need to be updated in future editions. I believe this text will serve a particular need for a comprehensive description of exercise science. I welcome your comments. Your input will be a valued factor for future editions.

Stanley P. Brown, Editor

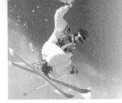

ACKNOWLEDGMENTS

First, I wish to thank my colleagues who contributed to this text. Without their expertise, there would have been no book. Writing a textbook is never undertaken as a sole project, but only during the course of the many other activities university professors do during the day. Yet, a work of this magnitude must, at some point, consume a large amount of one's time. It is with that realization that I acknowledge Dr. Dorothy Hash, Chair, Department of Physical Therapy at Southwest Baptist University for supporting me through the completion of this project.

In addition, I thank the publishing team at Lippincott Williams & Wilkins for their outstanding contributions during the text development and production processes. A special thanks is extended to Nancy Peterson who provided keen insight, endless support, and encouragement.

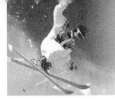

CONTRIBUTORS

John G. Alvarez, Ph.D.
Assistant Professor
Division of Health, Physical Education, and
    Recreation
Delta State University
Cleveland, Mississippi

Randy W. Brynar, Ed.D.
Associate Professor
Division of Exercise Physiology
West Virginia University
Morgantown, West Virginia

Ronald J. Byrd, Ph.D.
Professor
Department of Kinesiology and Health
    Science
Louisiana State University—Shreveport
Shreveport, Louisiana

Kathleen M. Cahill, M.S., A.T.C.
Health Enhancements
Germantown, Tennessee

Joy T. DeSensi, Ed.D.
Professor
Department of Educational Administration
    and Cultural Studies
The University of Tennessee
Knoxville, Tennessee

J. Larry Durstine, Ph.D., F.A.C.S.M.,
    F.A.A.C.V.P.R.
Professor and Director
Clinical Exercise Programs
Department of Exercise Science
School of Public Health
The University of South Carolina
Columbia, South Carolina

Shannon J. FitzGerald, Ph.D.
Department of Epidemiology
Graduate School of Public Health
The University of Pittsburgh
Pittsburgh, Pennsylvania

Mark A. Guadagnoli, Ph.D.
Associate Professor and Director
Motor Behavior Laboratory
Department of Kinesiology
University of Nevada, Las Vegas
Las Vegas, Nevada

W. Guyton Hornsby, Jr, Ph.D.
Associate Professor
Division of Exercise Physiology
West Virginia University
Morgantown, West Virginia

Benjamin F. Johnson, Ed.D.
Associate Professor and Director
Biomechanics and Ergonomics Laboratory
Department of Kinesiology and Health
Georgia State University
Atlanta, Georgia

Leonard Kravitz, Ph.D.
Assistant Professor
Division of Physical Performance and
    Development
The University of New Mexico
Albuquerque, New Mexico

Richard B. Kreider, Ph.D., F.A.C.S.M.
Professor and Director
Exercise & Sport Nutrition Laboratory
Department of Human Movement Sciences
    and Education
The University of Memphis
Memphis, Tennessee

Andrea M. Kriska, Ph.D., F.A.C.S.M.
Associate Professor
Department of Epidemiology
Graduate School of Public Health
University of Pittsburgh
Pittsburgh, Pennsylvania

Barney F. Leveau, Ph.D., P.T.
Professor
Department of Physical Therapy
Alabama State University
Montgomery, Alabama

Brian C. Lyons, Ph.D.
Assistant Professor
Department of Physical Education
Rockford College
Rockford, Illinois

Joan Paul, Ed.D.
Professor Emeritus
Department of Educational Administration
    and Cultural Studies
The University of Tennessee
Knoxville, Tennessee

Mark A. Pereira, Ph.D.
Instructor
Department of Pediatrics
Harvard Medical School
Boston, Massachusetts

Steven J. Petruzzello, Ph.D., F.A.C.S.M.
Associate Professor and Director
Exercise Psychophysiology Laboratory
Department of Kinesiology
University of Illinois at Urbana—Champaign
Urbana, Illinois

James M. Rankin, Ph.D., A.T.C.
Associate Professor and Program Director
Athletic Training Education
Department of Health Promotion and Human
  Performance
The University of Toledo
Toledo, Ohio

Synthia Sydnor, Ph.D.
Associate Professor
Department of Kinesiology
University of Illinois at Urbana—Champaign
Urbana, Illinois

Walter R. Thompson, Ph.D., F.A.C.S.M.
Professor and Director
Center for Sports Medicine, Science, and
  Technology
Department of Kinesiology and Health
Georgia State University
Atlanta, Georgia

Stella L. Volpe, Ph.D., F.A.C.S.M.
Associate Professor and Director
Center for Nutrition in Sport and Human
  Performance
Department of Nutrition
University of Massachusetts
Amherst, Massachusetts

Kirk L. Wakefield, Ph.D.
Associate Professor of Marketing
Department of Management and Marketing
The University of Mississippi
Oxford, Mississippi

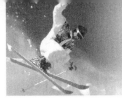

CONTENTS

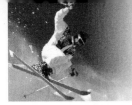

COMPREHENSIVE CONTENTS

INTRODUCTION TO EXERCISE SCIENCE

THE DISCIPLINE

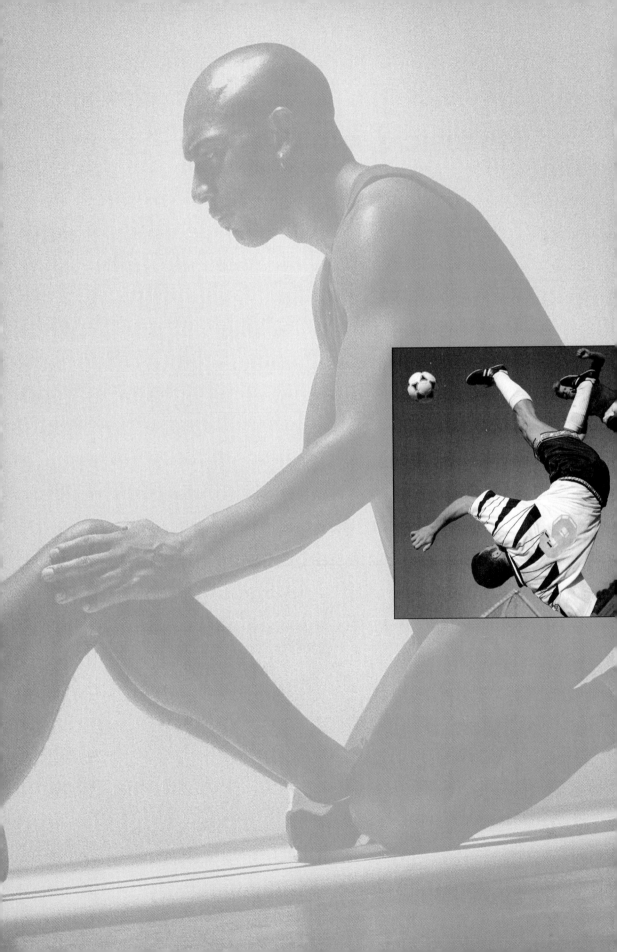

HISTORICAL AND CULTURAL ASPECTS

The ability to move is basic to our nature. Our culture, science, art, and communication and many other fields of human endeavor are inextricably woven together with our ability to move. Throughout history, cultures have explored the science and art of movement, often giving it legendary significance. In this first section, we explore how exercise science as an academic discipline came to be (Chapter 1) and the effect it has had on our culture (Chapter 2).

Chapter 1 first describes the differences between exercise science and its sister discipline, physical education, and then gives a brief historical treatment of the development of exercise science as an academic discipline.

Chapter 2 introduces significant key themes and the vocabulary of cultural study and provides readers with examples of how they are theoretically applied to the cultural study of exercise. Chapter 2 also describes important, radical changes that exercise and society have undergone since about 1990.

As we enter the new millennium, the science of movement—exercise science—will continue to develop, expand, and become ever more significant to the human experience.

1

The Emergence of Exercise Science

RONALD J. BYRD AND STANLEY P. BROWN

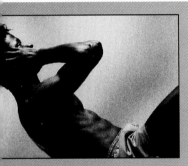

Objectives

1. Describe the relationship between exercise science, its subdisciplines, and the body of knowledge.
2. Describe the relationship between physical education and exercise science.
3. Describe the contributions of scientists to the development of the foundations of the exercise sciences.
4. Explain how World War II affected the exercise sciences.
5. Identify the events that precipitated the emergence of the subdisciplines in physical education departments.
6. Explain the need for increased interdisciplinary research.
7. Identify and discuss the roles of individuals who have made important contributions to the exercise sciences.

In the 1960s, **physical education** was challenged by those in and out of the field to become a well-respected academic discipline. Since then, a tremendous amount of change occurred in physical education, the result being the emergence of a field of study that is different from the discipline of physical education, yet keeping a vital connection to it. The new discipline, **exercise science,** is the subject of this book. In this chapter we examine exercise science and explore its emergence from the field of physical education. Students discover very early that the discipline of exercise science, although one field of study, comprises many separate subdisciplines, each having a unique role to play within the larger field of exercise science.

THE FIELD OF EXERCISE SCIENCE
Definition of Discipline and Subdiscipline

To have an appreciation for the field as a whole, students of exercise science need to grasp the relationship between *discipline* and *subdiscipline*. A discipline is defined as an organized, formal body of knowledge. Typically, most disciplines are discrete—that is, the topic is limited to a particular subject matter. For example, mathematics, biology, and chemistry are discrete subjects with their own body of knowledge. This is not so easily said of exercise science. Although in its broadest sense exercise science is the study of movement, it uses many other disciplines of science, including mathematics, chemistry, and biology, in this endeavor.

> *An academic discipline is an organized body of knowledge collectively embraced in a formal course of learning. The acquisition of such knowledge is assumed to be an adequate and worthy objective as such, without any demonstration or requirement of practical application. The content is theoretical and scholarly as distinguished from technical and professional.* —*Franklin Henry*

The study of movement is what distinguishes the discipline of exercise science from its parent academic disciplines. To study movement, exercise science uses specific principles from its many parent disciplines and, through rigorous scientific inquiry, attempts to describe and expand its body of knowledge. This process has led to a virtual explosion of the knowledge base of exercise science. Although the body of knowledge of exercise science is movement, describing and expanding our understanding of it require the totality of those subdisciplines that make up exercise science. In this respect, exercise science differs from other academic disciplines in that it is composed of subdisciplines that have as parent disciplines many of the "hard" and "soft" sciences. The subdisciplines, therefore, are the science components of exercise science within which the body of knowledge (movement) is described, studied, and expanded. The relationships among exercise science, the subdisciplines, and the body of knowledge are illustrated in Figure 1.1. Through the subdisciplines, movement is explored by scientific inquiry from every conceivable vantage point. The rest of this text is devoted to presenting the subdisciplines and their interrelationships within the academic discipline of exercise science (see Part 2).

The Sciences of Exercise Science

The term *exercise science* refers to the application of science to the phenomenon of **exercise.** This text treats exercise as being inclusive of all human movement, including random or infrequent movement, work, habitual activity, training done for fitness or health, dance, sports, and leisure activities of all sorts. Any movement that can be imagined can be studied or described, using one or more of the subdisciplines of exercise science. The phrase *application of science* in the definition is rather vague. Certainly there are many branches of science that can be applied to exercise. Some of the traditional and most historically relevant foundational sciences that serve as parent disciplines for the sciences of exercise science are biology, chemistry,

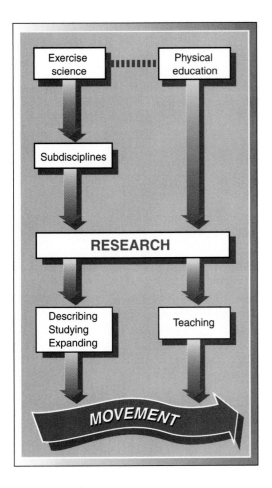

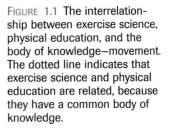

FIGURE 1.1 The interrelationship between exercise science, physical education, and the body of knowledge—movement. The dotted line indicates that exercise science and physical education are related, because they have a common body of knowledge.

physics, and psychology. Psychologic applications led to development of **motor behavior** (Chapter 16) and **exercise and sports psychology** (Chapter 15), physics was used in exploring the mechanics of movement **(biomechanics),** and biology and chemistry were the foundations of **exercise physiology** (Chapter 8). Interdisciplinary research among the subdisciplines of exercise science is becoming increasingly common, and it is clear that the supporting sciences for the different subdisciplines are not unique in their applications. For example, physics is used in explaining the dynamics of cardiovascular function in exercise physiology, biomechanics occasionally borrows from neuromuscular function, and motor behavior specialists have adapted **dynamical systems theory** from physics to measure galvanic skin response and heart rates.

Only the major foundational subdisciplines of exercise science (motor behavior, exercise and sports psychology, biomechanics, and exercise physiology) are presented for an historical overview in this Chapter. Table 1.1 places these and the rest of the subdisciplines in the approximate time frame of their emergence as distinct branches of exercise science. Note that the table provides a time reference for the subdisciplines that are not treated in detail in this chapter. The subdisciplines are presented with their academic foundations, important contributors, and major events and work that coincided with and established their emergence. The historical overview in this chapter focuses on exercise science within the United States. Without doubt, the foundations were laid mostly by scientists from abroad; but from the emergence of the various subdisciplines (mostly in the 1960s and 1970s) to the present, exercise science in the United States has been the standard of excellence for the world. Table 1.2 identifies current key leaders and other prominent scientists by subdiscipline.

| Table 1.1. | THE EMERGENCE OF THE SUBDISCIPLINES OF EXERCISE SCIENCE, THEIR ACADEMIC FOUNDATION, AND IMPORTANT CONTRIBUTORS |

Sub-discipline[a]	Time Period[b]	Academic Foundation	Key Contributors[c]	Key U.S. Events and Important Work
Exercise physiology	1940s–1960s	Chemistry, physiology	Thomas Cureton, David B. Dill, S. M. Horvath	Harvard Fatigue Laboratory closed; *Journal of Applied Physiology* established; ACSM founded
Sports nutrition	1980s	Biochemistry, nutrition	Melvin Williams, David Lamb	Studies investigating contribution of nutrition to athletic performance; nutrition and human performance texts
Physical activity epidemiology	1980s	Mathematics, statistics, research methodology	Steve Blair, Ralph Paffenbarger	Studies establishing physical inactivity as a disease risk factor
Clinical exercise physiology	1970s	Physiology, pathophysiology	Roy Shephard, John Holloszy	Exercise training as a rehabilitative agent for several patient populations
Clinical biomechanics	1980s	Physics, mathematics, anatomy	John Basmajian, Peter Cavanaugh, David Winter	Orthotics; diabetic foot ailments; posture and balance; locomotion; electromyography
Sports biomechanics	1960s	Physics, mathematics	James Hay, John Cooper, Richard Nelson	Movement analysis with sports applications
Athletic training	1950s	Anatomy	Robert Behnke, William E. Newell	Accreditation; education
Exercise and sports psychology	1960s	Psychology	Rainer Martens, Daniel Landers	Incorporation of NASPSPA; applied research using scientific psychology as a model
Motor behavior	1960s	Psychology, neuroscience	Franklin Henry, Anna Espenschade, G. Lawrence Rarick	Memory drum theory; publication of major textbooks on motor development
Sports history	1970s	History	Marvin Eyler, Guy Lewis	Completion of seminal dissertations
Sports Sociology	1970s	Sociology	Gerald Kenyon, George Sage	Treatises on the sociology of sports; major textbooks

[a]Listed in the order in which they are presented in Part 2 of the book.
[b]Refers to the decade(s) when the subdiscipline emerged as distinct entity within exercise science and/or physical education. Note that an earlier "foundations" period exists for each subdiscipline.
[c]This list is necessarily short and is not intended to be inclusive; significant contributions have been made by other scientists, many of whom are discussed in the text.
ACSM, American College of Sports Medicine; *NASPSPA,* North American Society for the Psychology of Sport and Physical Activity.

Figure 1.2 depicts the various subdisciplines of exercise science with reference to their underlying knowledge bases. The subdisciplines often overlap, because in many instances they use similar scientific methods to study human movement. Many of the subdisciplines of exercise science have further split into distinct subdisciplines. For example, as exercise physiology matured into a subdiscipline it splintered into a number of different areas, with **sports nutrition** (Chapter 9) being a major spin-off subdiscipline. In addition, the health and fitness aspects of exercise science have spawned two distinct subdisciplines: **clinical exercise physiology** (Chapter 11) and **physical activity epidemiology** (Chapter 10). The symbiotic relationships and common knowledge base among **clinical biomechanics** (Chapter 12), **sports biomechanics** (Chapter 13), and **athletic training** (Chapter 14) led to a combined historical treatment in this chapter. Two of the subdisciplines of exercise science study movement within an historical and social context. These are **sports history** (Chapter 17) and **sports sociology** (Chapter 18).

We consider these subdisciplines to be the major areas of exercise science that have emerged since the 1960s or 1970s. Certainly there is room for argument that other subdisciplines exist. However, it is our contention that the subdisciplines listed here are the most viable ones. Other possible subdisciplines are listed in Box 1.1. Of the eight listed, two (sports physiology and exercise biochemistry) are important areas within exercise physiology. The other six are not considered viable candidates for inclusion as subdisciplines of exercise science because they are outside the realm of the science disciplines—that is, either the hard sciences or the social sciences (see Sidelight 1.1). Sports philosophy and sports literature can be subsumed within the hu-

Table 1.2.   **CURRENT PROMINENT EXERCISE SCIENTISTS AND THEIR SUBDISCIPLINE AREAS[a]**

Subdiscipline	Current Key Leaders (Institution)	Other Prominent Scientists (Institution)
Exercise physiology	Jack H. Wilmore (Texas A&M University) Russell R. Pate (University of South Carolina)	Scott Powers (University of Florida) William Kraemer (Ball State University)
Sports nutrition	Pricilla Clarkson (University of Massachusetts) Mike Sherman (Ohio State University)	John Ivy (University of Texas) Stella Volpe (University of Massachusetts)
Physical activity epidemiology	Steve Blair (Institute for Aerobics Research) Carl Casperson (Centers for Disease Control and Prevention)	Barbara Ainsworth (University of South Carolina) Andra Kriska (University of Pittsburgh)
Clinical exercise physiology	Barry Franklin (Wayne State University) William Herbert (Virginia Polytechnic Institute and State University)	Larry Durstine (University of South Carolina) Carl Foster (University of Wisconsin, LaCrosse)
Sports biomechanics	Robert J. Gregor (Georgia Institute of Technology)	Rafael E. Bahamonde (Indiana University, Purdue University, Indianapolis) Michael E. Feltner (Pepperdine University)
Clinical biomechanics	Peter Cavanough (Pennsylvania State University) Carlos J. DeLuca (Boston University)	James J. Collins (Boston University) J. J. Crisco (Brown University)
Athletic training	Kenneth E. Knight (Brigham Young University)	Chris Ingersoll (Indiana State University) David Perrin (University of Virginia)
Exercise and sports psychology	Rod K. Dishman (University of Georgia) William P. Morgan (University of Wisconsin)	Edward McAuley (University of Illinois) W. Jack Rejeski (Wake Forest University)
Motor behavior	Waneen Spirduso (University of Texas) Robert Singer (University of Florida)	Richard Magill (Louisiana State University)
Sports history	Roberta Park (University of California, Berkeley)	Nancy Stuna (University of Maryland)
Sports sociology	Jay Coakley (University of Colorado, Colorado Springs) Susan Birrell (University of Iowa)	Jan Harris (California State University, Los Angeles)

[a]Note that this list is necessarily short and is not intended to be inclusive; many other prominent scientists are working within each subdiscipline.

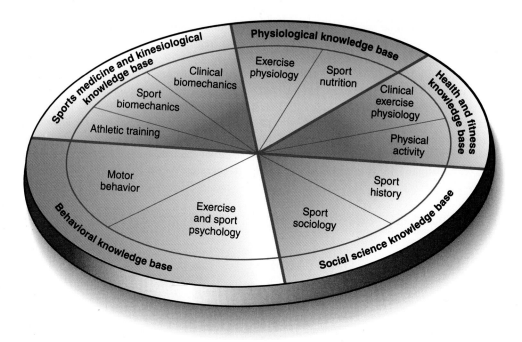

FIGURE 1.2 The sciences of exercise science and their related knowledge bases in the study of movement.

manities that bear their name. Sports art is subsumed under the umbrella of the fine arts. Sports management is an important content area for the exercise science student and is presented in Chapter 6. These four fields along with adapted physical education may also be included under physical education and thus are outside of the scope of this text. Last, an argument is made below that **sports pedagogy** (physical education) is a distinct sister discipline of exercise science, but not a subdiscipline.

A New Name or a New Discipline

Before turning to history to discover the beginnings of exercise science, a proper understanding of exercise science must start with an understanding of its relationship to physical education. Has physical education evolved into exercise science or has exercise science emerged out of physical education? This question is one that continues to foster debate among members of both dis-

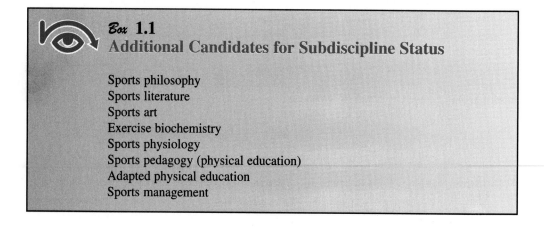

Box **1.1**
Additional Candidates for Subdiscipline Status

Sports philosophy
Sports literature
Sports art
Exercise biochemistry
Sports physiology
Sports pedagogy (physical education)
Adapted physical education
Sports management

ciplines. Over the years, this debate has focused on finding a new name for physical education, because an obvious evolution is considered to have occurred. We present exercise science as a distinct discipline, separate from the discipline of physical education. Although there is some sentiment for a reclassification of physical education as a separate subdiscipline of exercise science, there is ample evidence that they are largely autonomous. Physical education (the term *sports pedagogy* is now coming into vogue among practitioners advocating it as a subdiscipline of exercise science) remains a discipline, and its purpose is to investigate how the teaching process can be used most effectively to acquire movement skills. Although this is the focus of physical education, it remains outside of the scope of exercise science. Even though exercise science emerged out of physical education, and physical education continues to benefit from the research conducted in several of the exercise science subdisciplines (most notably motor behavior and sports psychology), exercise science today can at best be viewed as being a sister discipline of physical education. Both disciplines are, however, concerned with movement (see Sidelight 1.2); Figure 1.1 illustrates this relationship. Note that the body of knowledge for both disciplines is movement, but physical education conducts research in the pedagogical area (research in teacher education and in teaching physical education), whereas exercise science conducts research on many fronts—the subdisciplines. The rest of this chapter provides students with a more in-depth overview of the historical development of exercise science. In addition, students are referred to Practical Application 1.1.

▶▶ Sidelight 1.1

ACADEMIC SUBJECTS AND THE PROCESS OF SCIENCE

College students may sometimes be perplexed with the way universities are set up administratively and why university subjects are arranged in academic units the way they are. The underlying reason for the way a university is organized has much to do with how the courses students take are separated. Basically, the subject matter in a comprehensive university is divided into the following areas: *(a)* natural sciences, *(b)* social sciences, *(c)* humanities, *(d)* fine arts, and *(e)* the professional schools (e.g., law, medicine, education, business, engineering, and journalism). Although this listing may not be complete and the words and phrases used to designate specific areas often change, all comprehensive universities are arranged into similar units. This is important when considering what may be included as an academic subdiscipline under exercise science. The word *science* is important because whether a subject is considered a science, a humanity, or a fine art says a great deal about its content and how it approaches the body of knowledge. Although movement, as a realm of human experience, may be explored from the standpoint of the fine arts and humanities, it does so far differently from that of scientific enquiry, which uses a specific process and particular tools to discover why and how we move.

The *process* of science refers to how researchers go about seeking to expand the knowledge base (i.e., what we know about movement). They may do this through **empirical** experimentation, by which the **inductive** process has the potential to further establish a theory or to reject the theory. Scientists may also expand the knowledge base by **deductive** means—that is, proceeding first from the standpoint of the theory. The tools of science refer to the methods used to treat the data and how experiments are conducted. Part 2 of this text examines some of the specific ways each subdiscipline examines or studies movement.

➤➤ Sidelight 1.2

COMPARING THE DISCIPLINES

The distinction between physical education and exercise science can best be seen by comparing representative research journals of the two disciplines. For instance, recent issues of the *Journal of Teaching in Physical Education* contained articles on class management, student socialization, teacher preparation, supervision of student teachers, instructional behavior, and faculty profiles. *Medicine and Science in Sports and Exercise* is the official journal of the American College of Sports Medicine and includes research reports and reviews from many of the subdisciplines of exercise science. Recent issues contained articles on physical activity and its relation to cancer risk (physical activity epidemiology), endurance performance and selenium supplementation (sports nutrition), prediction of maximal oxygen consumption in children and young adults (exercise physiology), and psychophysiologic stress response and body fatness (sports and exercise psychology). Although both disciplines are concerned with movement, their dissimilarities relegate them to the familial status of siblings at best. When compared in this manner, the differences between the two disciplines become apparent. Exercise science expands the movement knowledge base by drawing on the many *parent* foundational sciences of the subdisciplines. Physical education, however, seeks to develop better strategies to teach movement. One discipline is mainly concerned with research in pedagogy, whereas the other is mainly concerned with expanding our understanding, through scientific enquiry, of how and why we move.

Practical Application 1.1

CHOOSING A SPECIALTY

As you begin your academic career in exercise science, you will no doubt come to the realization that many of the areas identified as subdisciplines in this text require specialization. This is particularly true if you wish to pursue a graduate degree. Although most undergraduate (bachelor of science) programs in exercise science do not require specialized attention to particular subdisciplines, you should, nevertheless, start to think about your career alternatives early in your academic program so you can identify appropriate minor fields that will likely advance you in your career path. The earlier you can choose a career path within exercise science, the more time you will have for academic and professional training and specialization. For instance, students who may eventually want to enter management after a few years on the job will do good to minor in management and marketing as an undergraduate. Nutrition is a natural minor for exercise science students wishing to advance in careers that rely mostly on the health and fitness and physiologic knowledge bases. Individuals interested in sports psychology should minor in psychology. If you want to specialize in biomechanics, you should take extra mathematics and physics classes. Chapter 5 explores many other possible options, and Chapter 4 details exercise science certification programs you may want to pursue.

HISTORICAL PERSPECTIVE

This section presents a brief overview of the history of exercise science, with particular attention paid to the subdisciplines of biomechanics, motor behavior, and exercise physiology. Although this discussion presents a particular historical snapshot, students should realize that these and the other subdisciplines are continuing to evolve, with each producing unique contributions to society.

Exercise Scientists

Who were the early exercise scientists? The answer to this question would be different at different points in time. One could argue for an almost limitless number of starting points, because history is replete with anecdotal information on the study of human movement. As early as about 450 B.C., Greek scholars (including Plato, Aristotle, Socrates, Archimedes, and Galen) examined physical activity in a scientific fashion. During the Renaissance, Leonardo da Vinci, Galileo, and others had an analytic interest in human physical activity. One could argue that the initial scientific focus on exercise in the twentieth century was promoted by engineers, physicians, psychologists, physicists, biologists, and chemists who just happened to be interested in sports or in human movement in general. Certainly, leaders in physical education must be considered in the context of exercise science. Many pioneers in physical education came from medical backgrounds and were interested in scientific applications related to health. Compared to the early contributions of basic scientists to exercise science, early research by individuals with professional preparation in physical education may seem less robust by scientific standards; however, these contributions were important. A typical example of the type of work done both by pedagogically trained physical educators and by medical doctors was the anthropometric measurements (i.e., body dimensions, such as height, weight, and girth measures) that were popular just before and after the end of the nineteenth century. When World Wars I and II led to research on physical fitness as related to military performance, little of the sophisticated research done was by physical educators. The same was true of perceptual motor research stimulated by demands of aviator training in World War II. Other important areas were ergonomics in the design of military equipment and the application of biomechanical principles by engineers rather than by physical educators. Most physical educators in the first two or three decades of the twentieth century were largely concerned with K to 12 curriculum development.

Effects of Technology

Development of technology has had a profound effect on all of the subdisciplines of exercise science. In the earliest days of exercise science, much measurement was made possible by researchers who invented and developed prototypical devices for obtaining the desired data (Fig. 1.3). It was not then possible to simply shop around for vendors of sophisticated equipment for research purposes. Interfacing with computers was out of the question; they weren't available (Fig. 1.4). Extrapolating the exponential rise in technological capabilities that has taken place over the past century gives rise to expectations that whatever can be imagined can one day be accomplished. It can be readily observed that the science fiction of today has frequently become the technology of tomorrow; and there is no reason to think that this does not apply to exercise science as well.

Physical Educators as an Emerging Force

The outlook for the discipline of physical education began to change in the late 1960s as a result of events described by Swanson and Massengale (1). Earlier physical education doctoral curricula required students to take little, if any, science course work. Generalist preparation was the

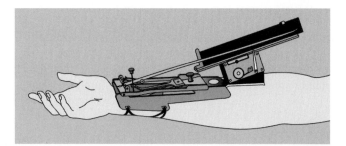

FIGURE 1.3 Marey's advanced sphygmograph (here used to record pulse tracing) was a forerunner of modern cardiovascular instrumentation. Reprinted by permission from McArdle WD, Katch FI, Katch VL. Exercise physiology: energy, nutrition, and human performance. 4th ed. Baltimore, MD: Williams & Wilkins, 1996.

rule, and graduates went on to teach a wide variety of classes. Largely a result of Conant's (2) 1963 criticism of teacher education and recommendation for eliminating graduate physical education, however, there was serious examination of existent curricula. Henry (3), a pioneer in motor behavior and respected leader in physical education, concurred and led an introspective movement that resulted in strengthening curricular requirements and producing specialists in subdisciplines who were well prepared to enter the arena of research and scholarship.

> ⚬⚯ *Conant's 1963 recommendation that graduate physical education be abolished led to reforms that resulted in the emergence of the many subdisciplines of exercise science.*

It is interesting that, although specialization worked well (as evidenced by the large body of research literature published by physical education faculty members after 1966), an atten-

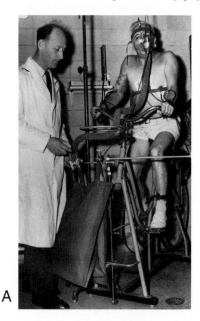

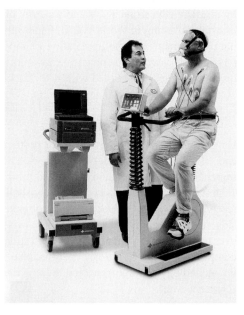

A   B

FIGURE 1.4 **A,** Respiratory gases are collected into Douglas bags, and oxygen consumption and carbon dioxide production are calculated later. Reprinted by permission from McArdle WD, Katch FI, Katch VL. Exercise physiology: energy, nutrition, and human performance. 4th ed. Baltimore, MD: Williams & Wilkins, 1996. **B,** Using current technology, oxygen consumption values are provided online during the test. See Chapter 8 for a discussion of these terms. Courtesy of SensorMedics, a subsidiary of Thermo Electronics (Yorba Linda, CA).

dant problem accompanied this success. Before 1966, exercise science classes were often taught by **generalists;** afterward, it became increasingly likely that new doctoral graduates, who were well-trained **specialists,** would have to teach courses for which they were ill-prepared if they assumed positions in smaller universities. This led to some discomfort among faculty as a result of philosophical differences between traditional generalists and the new wave of specialists.

The preceding material is generic to exercise science, but there are specific events and individuals within each of the subdisciplines that must be considered. Although arbitrary delineations between periods of development are used for each subdiscipline, it is important to keep in mind that such markers are almost never precise but rather serve a useful purpose in only a general sense (Table 1.1). Biomechanics, motor behavior, and exercise physiology all have rich histories; each is briefly treated in the remainder of this chapter.

Biomechanics

Examination of the history of biomechanics should lead to some understanding of the current disagreement over use of the terms *biomechanics* and **kinesiology.** Early in the history of exercise science, the term kinesiology was used in a rather general way to mean, from the Latin roots, "the study of movement." In later years, a commonly taught undergraduate class that dealt with anatomical applications was called kinesiology. That particular course is now more precisely titled **anatomic kinesiology** and is sometimes part of a class called biomechanics. If that isn't confusing enough, kinesiology is a term frequently used to describe the entire field of what once was almost universally called physical education. Because a wide variety of titles are used for departments that house the exercise sciences, the historically relevant phrase "physical education" will be used throughout this chapter. Chapter 7 presents some additional titles academic departments have recently chosen.

Foundations: To 1900

The latter part of the nineteenth century marked two critical events: the establishment of the basic understanding of neuromuscular function that would later lead to the development of electromyography and the first use of motion pictures for the analysis of movement. Although the horse was the original model for motion picture study in the 1880s, cinematography became one of the most important tools for human movement analysis by the middle of the twentieth century.

Research during this period was largely descriptive, and anthropometry dominated. Three medical doctors made noteworthy contributions. Edward Hitchcock Jr., who received an appointment as professor in the first department of hygiene and physical education in the United States from 1861 to 1911, was noted for his anthropometric work on students at Amherst. He and his father collaborated on one of the first anatomy and physiology textbooks to be geared to college physical education. Concurrently, H. O. Bowditch (dean of the Harvard Medical School) contributed significantly in describing anthropometric differences across time in children aged 5 to 16 years.

In 1879, Dudley Sargent began a long career at Harvard University as assistant professor of physical training and director of the Hemenway Gymnasium. Besides his anthropometric measurements, he did important early work in the measurement of various aspects of physical fitness, probably the best known of which is the Sargent jump. He also taught a course in applied anatomy in the Department of Anatomy, Physiology, and Physical Training at Harvard University just before the turn of the twentieth century (4). This was perhaps a precursor to later biomechanics courses.

Pre-Emergence (Kinesiology): 1900 to 1966

After the turn of the twentieth century, the term *kinesiology* appears with increasing frequency in the literature. The first half of the century was marked by widespread development of undergraduate physical education classes in kinesiology, initially aimed at developing an understanding of the relationship between anatomy and movement, today's version of anatomic kinesiology. Not solely the domain of physical education, kinesiology became important in orthopedic medicine and in the allied health fields of physical and occupational therapy.

Before the age of specialization, researchers in kinesiology such as T. K. Cureton, who established in 1948 the Physical Fitness Research Laboratory at the University of Illinois, frequently published research articles involving psychomotor measurement, fitness, and exercise physiology. Anthropometric measurement continued, but technical sophistication was increasing and cinematography was becoming increasingly common. Articles published in the 1930s dealt with biomechanics and procedures for cinematographic analysis (5–7). Technological advances were impressive. Adaptation of the stroboscope for movement analysis, Adrian's (8) work with electromyography, and Karpovich and Wilklow's (9) electrogoniometer provided new avenues for research. A relevant landmark publication in 1962 was Basmajian's work based on electromyography (a technique that measures the electrical activity of muscle) (10). Textbooks during this period moved from anatomic kinesiology to treatment that included aspects of mechanics. Bunn's (11) *Scientific Principles of Coaching* was a focused view of mechanics in sports from an engineer's perspective. Although not clearly delineated, the kinesiology period gave way to the biomechanics period as a result of increased attention to mechanics along with the advent of doctoral-level specialty training for biomechanics in departments of physical education.

The Subdiscipline (Biomechanics): 1966 to Present

Three significant events occurred early in the modern period: The *Journal of Biomechanics* was first published in 1968, the International Seminar on Biomechanics was held in the United States for the first time in 1973, and the American Society of Biomechanics was established in 1976. Probably as important as any other single event was the publication of guidelines and standards for classes in undergraduate kinesiology (12). This document outlined prerequisites in anatomy and mathematics, listed competencies in anatomic and mechanical considerations, noted expectations for applications, listed laboratory and equipment needs, and recommended that specialists teach undergraduate kinesiology classes. Although still not universally adopted, these recommendations have had a strong and positive influence on the profession. By 1978, doctoral programs in biomechanics were available at Indiana University, Pennsylvania State University, Purdue University, University of Iowa, University of Illinois, University of Maryland, University of Massachusetts, University of Oregon, University of Wisconsin, and Washington State University. Leaders of and graduates from these programs set the pace for subsequent development.

Advances in instrumentation continued during this period, but a 1973 report by Adrian (13) was limited to cinematographic, electromyographic, and electrogoniometric techniques. Subsequently, high-speed cameras, strain gauges, and force plates were in ever-increasing use. When small computers and interfaces became available and cost-effective, it was possible to collect and treat data in a fraction of the time previously required. Videotaping, three-dimensional cinematography, and real-time computer analysis have combined to facilitate even greater productivity (see Fig. 1.5).

Much of the research during this period was directed at techniques of data collection and analysis, but there was no lack of attention to modeling, basic research, and increasingly interdisciplinary work. More recently, the subdiscipline of clinical biomechanics applied principles of mechanics to the clinical setting in studying such things as locomotion, bone modeling, and shoe design. Currently, motor behavior specialists are joining exercise physiologists in using measurement techniques that were previously the domain of biomechanics. With increasing sophistication in professional preparation and available technologies, there appears to be a trend toward more interdisciplinary work among these previously disparate groups of exercise scientists.

Motor Behavior

Motor behavior encompasses **motor control, motor learning,** and **motor development.** Although exercise and sports psychology is recognized as a separate subdiscipline of exercise science, its own emergence as a subdiscipline was closely tied to events leading to the emergence

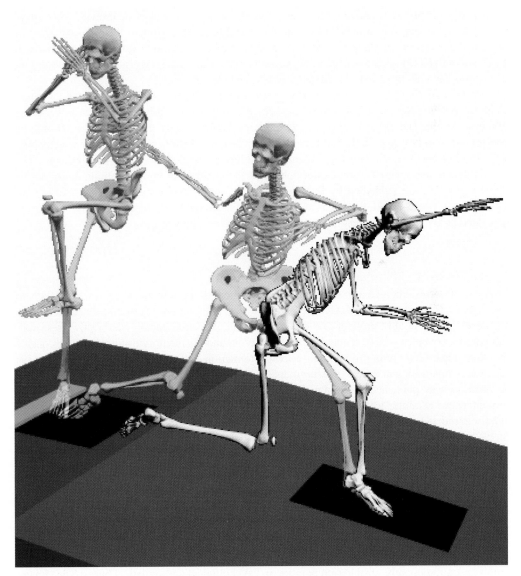

FIGURE 1.5 A linked computer and video system measured, analyzed, and displayed three-dimensional kinematics of baseball pitchers. Five 200-Hz cameras captured retroreflective markers and a incremented pitching mound collected ground reaction forces. Kinematics were determined from marker positions, and kinetics were determined from kinematics and estimated inertial properties. Computer-animated models of the musculoskeletal system helped scientists visualize the results. See Chapters 12 and 13 for discussions of movement kinematics and kinetics. Courtesy of Biomechanics Laboratory, Johns Hopkins University (Baltimore, MD).

of motor behavior. In addition, because exercise and sports psychology shares a common knowledge base with motor behavior, this section suffices as an historical treatment for both subdisciplines.

Foundations: To 1945

Around the turn of the twentieth century, the stage was set for what was later to be referred to as *motor behavior* by psychologists, physiologists, and physicians who explored the neurologic bases of movement, infant development, and cognitive learning. Sherrington (14) laid the foundation for motor control in his definitive work on neurophysiology in 1906. He also coined the word **proprioception.** Scientists described early developmental stages of growth. Many psychologists were involved in developing the theoretical bases of cognitive learning that were to become the points of departure for subsequent applications to the motor (movement) domain. In 1927 Thorndike (15) departed from other psychologists' approaches by using motor learning in developing his Law of Effect, which dealt with knowledge of results.

A seminal event that had only a temporary effect was the establishment of Coleman Griffith's Athletic Research Laboratory in 1925, which was used to investigate various aspects of motor learning and exercise and sports psychology. Unfortunately, this venture was short lived and produced only a few published records. Nevertheless, Griffith, a professor of psychology, was ahead of his time, teaching classes and publishing in exercise and sports psychology.

Although there were several earlier published anecdotal descriptions of infant motor development, norms were published by Bayley (16) in 1936 and by Gesell and Armatruda (17) in 1941. During World War II, there was an explosion of motor behavior research by psychologists, prompted by the sudden interest in the training of pilots for the war effort.

Pre-Emergence: 1945 to 1966

Physical educators emerged as a force in the development of motor behavior during the 1940s to 1960s. Anna Espenschade, H. H. Clarke, Ruth Glassow, and Laurence Rarick were active in motor development in this product-oriented period that produced mostly descriptive research. Franklin Henry emerged as a leader in motor behavior, and his memory drum theory was one of the first departures from product to process orientation (18). In the 1960s, Cratty's (19) *Movement Behavior and Motor Learning* and Bilodeau and Biodeau's (20) *Principles of Skill Acquisition* were published and had a strong influence on subsequent work by physical educators interested in motor learning. Exercise and sports psychology was not yet established as a subdiscipline, but Lawther's (21) book *The Psychology of Coaching* was a landmark publication in 1951.

The Subdiscipline: 1966 to Present

As exercise science subdisciplines mature, research typically changes from descriptive (product orientation) to more sophisticated approaches that examine and attempt to explain cause, usually by experimental methods (process orientation). A change occurred in the study of motor behavior in the mid-1960s that was tied to increased specialization in graduate physical education programs and, subsequently, stronger preparation in psychological and statistical bases. The change in orientation was described by Clark (22) as follows:

> The beginning of the Process-Oriented period saw research in motor development primarily consisting of descriptions of motor performance in children. Twenty years into the Process-Oriented period, motor development research has moved from the description of children's motor performance to explanations about its causes.

Physical education graduate programs had come of age, and their alumnae were increasingly in the forefront of scholarly work in motor behavior. Comparison of historical reviews dealing with motor skill acquisition by Irion (20) in 1969 and Adams (23) in 1987 reveal a striking increase in scholarly contributions by physical education motor behavior specialists across time.

A series of theories emerged, each of which was subjected to scholarly examination by a new breed of motor behaviorists. These motor behaviorists began to analyze early motor behavior work that was based on theories of learning proposed by psychologists and Adams's proposed closed-loop theory (developed in 1971). Schmidt's schema theory (submitted in 1975) stimulated research for more than a decade; but since the middle 1980s, application of dynamical systems theory has held a dominant position. The application of both chaos theory and dynamical systems from physics is another example of the current trend toward increasing interdisciplinary nature of the science of motor behavior.

Motor development and motor learning texts were published in 1967 and 1968 that were influential for decades. Robert Singer was only one of many motor behavior specialists during the early stages of its development who was active in more than one of the subdisciplines. As the subdisciplines matured, this became more the exception than the rule. Today, leading scholars are likely to be more focused in their study.

The North American Society for the Psychology of Sport and Physical Activity (NASPSPA) was established in 1967 with Arthur Slater-Hammel as its first president. Richard Schmidt's establishment of the *Journal of Motor Behavior* in 1969 provided a new specialized outlet for scholarly work in motor behavior and was one of the era's most important landmarks.

Two volumes edited by George Stelmach that dealt with motor control and information processing were arguably among the most important contributions to motor behavior literature in the 1970s (24,25). Lawrence Rarick (26) and Robert Malina (27) published influential texts on growth and development during this period, and the *Journal of Sports Psychology* was established in 1979, with Dan Landers as the first editor. The first edition (1982) of the motor learning text by Richard Schmidt (28) was frequently adopted by college professors teaching in this area and remains influential today.

Exercise and sport psychology continued its rapid development, with the founding of the Association for Advancement of Sport Psychology in 1985 and the establishment of a new journal, *The Sport Psychologist,* in 1987 with Dan Gould and Glyn Roberts as editors. Rainer Martens, an outstanding exercise and sports psychology scholar, provided much-needed visibility to motor behavior (and other subdisciplines) through his work as a publisher (Human Kinetics). During this same time, psychologists became increasingly interested in exercise and sports psychology and the opportunity for consulting; in 1986, exercise and sports psychology was established as a division within the American Psychological Association. Competition between psychologists and exercise and sports psychologists with physical education roots led to a territorial conflict that is still active. Individuals from both groups have been involved with Olympic, university, and professional teams. Among the more visible from physical education have been Dan Landers and Rainer Martens with Olympic sports and Jack Lewellyn with the 1990s Atlanta Braves.

In 1989, the December issue of *Quest* focused on the direction for motor development. Clark and Whitall (22) emphasized the importance of understanding motor control and motor learning by those studying motor development. Others, from a slightly different perspective, recommended that motor development should logically be studied as a focus within areas of motor control and motor learning (29). Both views lend credence to the critical nature of the interrelationships and interdependence among the different components of motor behavior. In the same issue of *Quest,* both Roberton (30) and VanSant (31) speak to the importance of viewing motor development in the context of life span, rather than continuing to focus only on the child and adolescent. The work of Spirduso at the University of Texas has been influential in this regard; she has been a powerful force in motor control and motor learning for many years and has extended that particular expertise to the study of motor behavior in aging populations.

Specialization within the different areas of motor behavior initially led to a degree of isolation among the areas of control, learning, and development. It later became apparent that commonalities and interdependencies could lead to new perspectives and greater depth of understanding. Thomas (32) stated: "The sub-areas of motor behavior—motor control, motor learning, and motor development—appear increasingly to overlap in research focus. Both the cognitive and dynamical-systems views of motor skill performance and acquisition are influencing this common interest." Further, maturation of motor behavior has been accompanied by increasing interaction with other disciplines, such as physiology, psychology, and physics. The marriage of motor behavior to biomechanics—applying cinematography, kinematics, and electromyography to motor behavior problems—is an example of a trend in the 1990s that is expected to continue.

Exercise Physiology

Although the history presented here admittedly deals with the development of exercise science in the United States, contributions from abroad have been especially important for exercise physiology. Åstrand's textbooks and his regular attendance and participation in American College of Sports Medicine (ACSM) meetings make him perhaps one of the most obviously influential scientists. A few other researchers whose work has been immensely important to the development of exercise physiology in this country are listed in Table 1.3.

Foundations: To 1945

Attention has been given to health, fitness, anatomy, and physiology by physicians and other scholars at least as far back as the Golden Age of Greece. However, the foundation of exercise physiology was not laid until the latter part of the nineteenth century. Among numerous journal articles and books dealing with various aspects of physiology published during that period, two books by Flint (33,34) dealt specifically with aspects of exercise physiology. Shortly thereafter, the first exercise physiology course was taught by George Wells Fitz in the short-lived (1892 to 1900) Department of Anatomy, Physiology, and Physical Training at Harvard University (4).

Bainbridge's (35) 1919 *Physiology of Muscular Exercise* was updated by Bock and Dill (36) in 1928. Dill (37) later commented, "We think now of 1925 as a remote period in exercise physiology, but I was astonished recently to count over 400 references in our 1928 edition of Bainbridge." About that same time, A. V. Hill's (38) important work, *Muscular Movement in Man,* was published, followed by Schneider's (39) and McCurdy and Larson's (40) physical education-based texts on exercise physiology in the 1930s. *Research Quarterly* contained a few articles related to exercise physiology in the 1930s, and physical educators Steinhaus (41) and Hellebrandt (42) contributed important exercise physiology reviews in prestigious physiology journals during this foundational period.

> ⚷   *The exercise physiology course taught by George Wells Fitz, M.D., was part of a science-based physical education curriculum. This course included experimental investigation and 6 hr per week of laboratory study. Its prerequisites included a course in general physiology (or its equivalent) at the medical school.*

Laboratories devoted to exercise physiology in the context of physical education were set up in two institutions in which YMCA fitness directors were trained. Arthur Steinhaus at George Williams College in 1923 and James McCurdy at Springfield College in 1927 directed these early ventures. In later years, Peter Karpovich would be extremely productive in further research and development at Springfield.

Henderson's brainchild, the Harvard Fatigue Laboratory, was established in 1927 and flourished until its closure in 1947. David Bruce Dill was director during that period, entering as a

Table 1.3.	**FOREIGN CONTRIBUTORS TO THE DEVELOPMENT OF EXERCISE PHYSIOLOGY IN AMERICA**
R. J. Shephard (University of Toronto; Canada)	Erling Asmussen (University of Copenhagen; Denmark)
Martti Karvonen (Institute of Occupational Health; Finland)	L. Brauer (University of Cologne; Germany)
Lars Hermansen (Institute of Work Physiology; Norway)	Ernst Jokl (Witwatersrand Technical College; South Africa)
R. Margaria (University of Milan; Italy)	Bengt Saltin (Karolinska Institute Medical School; Sweden)

chemist and exiting as one of the world's outstanding figures in exercise physiology. The effect of the Harvard Fatigue Laboratory and Dill can hardly be overestimated. The laboratory made two important contributions during World War II: research was done that directly related to military personnel performance, and several scientists left the laboratory to work in other centers that were involved in military-related research. After a precipitous loss of federal funding after World War II, a reluctant decision was made to close the laboratory. Dill (37) noted: "I do not consider it to have been an irreparable loss to physiology. Successful organisms have a way of reaching maturity, declining, and dying, but not without perpetuating their kind." The reader is referred to Dill's (37) 1967 article, which details how this procreation occurred and how graduates of the Harvard Fatigue Laboratory established their own laboratories across the country and around the world and continued the work of exercise physiology in their own spheres of influence. Box 1.2 provides a brief listing of the kinds of research projects conducted at the Harvard Fatigue Laboratory.

Pre-Emergence: 1945 to 1966

In 1948, Morehouse and Miller (43) and Schneider and Karpovich (44) produced two excellent texts on exercise physiology. The same year, Cureton established the Physical Fitness Research Laboratory. Many individuals, programs, and laboratories can trace their roots back to Cureton and the University of Illinois. Cureton was an early leader in terms of his contributions to the understanding of physical fitness and its relationship to exercise physiology and to the emergence of exercise physiology as a subdiscipline.

Among a group of 11 individuals responsible for founding the ACSM in 1954 were physical educators Karpovich, Larson, and Steinhaus. The other founders, representatives of medicine and physiology, understood the importance of physical education's relationship to **sports medicine.** In the early stages, ACSM's focus was on athletics, injuries, fitness, and physiology. Only

Box **1.2**

Sample Research Topics Conducted in the Harvard Fatigue Laboratory: 1927 to 1947

Maximal oxygen uptake
Oxygen debt
Work at altitude
Harvard Step Test
Oxygen saturation during exercise
Maximal heart rate
Aging and exercise

later did diversification cover the range of exercise sciences, with a strong emphasis on exercise physiology. It is interesting that in ACSM's founding year the 10th International Congress on Sports Medicine was held in Luxembourg, the first meeting having been in Amsterdam in 1928 (45). ACSM met a long-overdue need in the United States.

Although most scholarly work in exercise physiology through the foundation and pre-emergence periods was still being done by scientists outside the realm of physical education, there was increasing recognition of the importance of exercise physiology in undergraduate and graduate physical education programs. Two additional textbooks were published in the early 1960s by Johnson (46) and Jokl (47). Johnson's was an edited volume that saw frequent use as a graduate reference, but there was no text really suitable for graduate study at that time. It was not a coincidence that in 1963 Conant (2) wrote in regard to graduate physical education that departments

> should cancel graduate programs in this area. If the physical education teacher wishes to enter into a research career in the field of physiology of exercise and related subjects, he should use the graduate years to build…a knowledge of the physiological sciences that will enable him to stand on equal footing with the undergraduate major in these sciences.

As the pre-emergence period came to an end, Conant's advice was followed, and exercise physiology developed into a subdiscipline within the field of physical education and became increasingly more respectable.

The Subdiscipline: 1966 to Present

Franklin Henry (3), generally identified with motor behavior but who also published in exercise physiology, met Conant's challenge, urging the profession to strengthen graduate academic preparation. The result was a widespread move toward requiring graduate students with a major or emphasis in exercise physiology to take graduate courses (and undergraduate prerequisites, when appropriate) in departments of physiology, anatomy, and chemistry. Three obvious effects were

- With increased rigor, doctoral programs changed from 2 to 3 years in residence to 4 to 5 years.
- Graduates were able to compete on a more equal footing, publishing in sophisticated refereed journals and earning the respect of scientists outside of physical education.
- For the first time, a group of individuals was clearly defined as exercise physiologists.

No longer was exercise physiology the exclusive domain of individuals trained in physiology, biochemistry, or medicine who just happened to have an interest in exercise as a means of furthering their understanding of other disciplines. Exercise physiology had reached maturity. This process was not instantaneous, but evolved gradually after the initial reform to the present state of professional preparation.

Several increasingly sophisticated texts on exercise physiology, some clearly suitable for graduate study, were published in the 1960s and 1970s. The first edition of Åstrand and Rodahl's (48) text found wide acceptance by graduate faculties. ACSM first published *Medicine and Science in Sports* in 1969. Although the journal's intended sports medicine audience was wide-ranging and interdisciplinary, a strong exercise physiology emphasis evolved.

Steve Horvath's prestigious Institute of Environmental Stress at the University of California, Santa Barbara offered postdoctoral opportunities to several of the new breed of exercise physiology doctoral graduates. Students were exposed to an interdisciplinary institute reminiscent in many ways of the Harvard Fatigue Laboratory, at which Horvath studied under Dill more than 20 years earlier. Horvath's expertise, as was true of many of the early scientists who contributed to exercise physiology, was not easily defined. Although he was trained as a physiologist, his interests in exercise, environmental stressors, and aging led him to do research on a wide variety of questions.

First- and second-generation exercise physiologists after the closure of the Harvard Fatigue Laboratory were instrumental in developing the first generation of well-trained exercise physiologists from physical education backgrounds. The influence of schools associated with the Big Ten Athletic Conference was perhaps greatest, but the movement was nationwide, and many physical education leaders not necessarily trained in any of the exercise sciences saw the need for specialization and thus led curriculum revisions at their institutions.

Scholarly productivity by the new specialists has been truly remarkable. In 1996, a computer search using *exercise* and *exertion* as keywords revealed that from a base of about 1000 citations in 1966 (roughly the onset of the modern era of exercise physiology), the number jumped to just over 1700 in 1976 and soared to well over 3000 in 1986 (4). The same study projected a plateau in scholarly output around 2000. Certainly there is no evidence that all of the increased research productivity has been from exercise physiologists, but few would argue that their contributions have not been great.

Two primary factors that led to the exponential increase in scholarly publications in the exercise sciences were an increase in the number of graduating doctoral specialists after 1966 and the technological advances that facilitated research.

ACSM's *Medicine and Science in Sports* (retitled *Medicine and Science in Sports and Exercise* in 1980) was an important forum for exercise physiology papers. The interdisciplinary nature of the organization and journal notwithstanding, national and regional annual meetings of the ACSM have been and continue to be among the most important such gatherings for exercise physiologists with roots in physical education. ACSM's manual on standardization of professional preparation for individuals interested in exercise leadership on several levels, along with guidelines for testing and prescription (now in its sixth edition), has been an important contribution to institutions, which have responded to the need for undergraduate and graduate training of students interested in corporate fitness, clinical exercise physiology, and related areas.

New employment opportunities emerged in the early 1970s and increased into the 1990s, reviving many university physical education programs that had experienced decreased interest in traditional undergraduate and master's teacher education degrees. Concurrently, it became common for individuals with generic physical education degrees to call themselves exercise physiologists and to compete well in a market in which employers were somewhat naive. In an attempt at quality control in Louisiana, legislation specified rigorous requirements for licensure as a clinical exercise physiologist, and the first such license was granted in January 1996, a strong indication of the state of maturity of this subdiscipline of exercise science.

SUMMARY POINTS

- Exercise science consists of the subdisciplines of exercise physiology, sports nutrition, physical activity epidemiology, clinical exercise physiology, clinical biomechanics, sports biomechanics, athletic training, exercise and sports psychology, motor behavior, sports history, and sports sociology.
- These exercise sciences rest on a foundation built throughout recorded history by philosophers, physicians, psychologists, engineers, physicists, biologists, chemists, and physical educators, relatively few of whom were citizens of the United States.
- Contributions by citizen-scientists and by physical educators commenced about the end of the nineteenth century.
- After the reform in graduate physical education that began after 1966, physical educators became the new and respected exercise scientists, yet physical education continues as a distinct discipline.
- The modern trend toward more interdisciplinary research allows researchers to solve problems that were impossible to address via a single-discipline approach.

- Finely focused, process-oriented research provides solutions to more basic questions.
- Exercise science continues to meet needs of coaches, trainers, and teachers through applied research and development.

REVIEW QUESTIONS

1. List the subdisciplines of exercise science.
2. What are the major areas of motor behavior? What is the major focus of each?
3. What events precipitated the reforms that let to specializations in graduate physical education programs?
4. Describe how individuals outside of physical education played such an important part in establishing the foundation on which the exercise sciences would later be developed.
5. How did World Wars I and II affect the exercise sciences?
6. Give a hypothetical example of an interdisciplinary approach to a research problem.
7. List six individuals who have been important to exercise science in a historical sense, giving a very brief description of the contribution of each.
8. What is the relationship between exercise science, its subdisciplines, and the body of knowledge?
9. How are physical education and exercise science related?

References

1. Swanson RA, Massengale JD. Exercise and sport science in 20th century America. In: JD Massengale, RA Swanson, eds. The history of exercise and sport science. Champaign, IL: Human Kinetics, 1997:1–14.
2. Conant JB. The education of American teachers. New York: McGraw-Hill, 1963.
3. Henry FM. Physical education—an academic discipline. In: Proceedings of the annual meeting of the National College Physical Education Association for Men. Washington, DC: AAHPER, 1964:6–9.
4. McArdle WD, Katch FI, Katch VL. Exercise physiology: energy, nutrition, and human performance. 4th ed. Baltimore, MD: Williams & Wilkins, 1996:xxx.
5. Fenn WO. A cinematographic study of sprinters. Sci Monthly 1931;32:346–354.
6. Fenn WO. Mechanical energy expenditure in sprint running as measured by moving pictures. Am J Physiol 1929;90:343–344.
7. Glassow RB, Broer MR. A convenient apparatus for the study of motion picture films. Res Q 1938;9:41–49.
8. Adrian ED. Interpretation of the electromyogram. Lancet 1925;2:1229–1233.
9. Karpovich PV, Wilklow LB. A goniometric study of the human foot in standing and walking. US Armed Forces Med J 1959;10:885–903.
10. Basmajian JV. Muscles alive: their functions revealed by electromyography. Baltimore, MD: Williams & Wilkins, 1962.
11. Bunn JW. Scientific principles of coaching. Englewood Cliffs, NJ: Prentice Hall, 1955.
12. Kinesiology Academy. Guidelines and standards for undergraduate kinesiology. J Health Physical Educ Recreat 1980;51:19–21.
13. Adrian MJ. Cinematographic, electromyographic, and electrogoniometric techniques for analyzing human movement. In: J. Wilmore, ed. Exercise and sport science reviews. Vol. 1. New York: Academic, 1973:339–363.
14. Sherrington CS. The integrative action of the nervous system. New Haven, CT: Yale University Press, 1906.
15. Thorndike EL. The law of effect. Am J Psychol 1927;39:212–222.
16. Bayley N. The California infant scale of motor development. Berkeley: University of California Press, 1936.
17. Gesell A, Armatruda CS. Developmental diagnosis: normal and abnormal child development, clinical methods, and practical applications. New York: Hoeber, 1941.
18. Henry FM, Rogers DE. Increased response latency for complicated movements and a "memory drum" theory of neuromotor reaction. Res Q 1960;31:448–458.
19. Cratty BJ. Movement behavior and motor learning. Philadelphia: Lea & Febiger, 1964.
20. Irion AL. Historical introduction. In: EA Bilodeau, IM Bilodeau, eds. Principles of skill acquisition. New York: Academic, 1969:1–31.

21. Lawther JD. The psychology of coaching. Englewood Cliffs, NJ: Prentice Hall, 1951.
22. Clark JE, Whitall J. What is motor development? The lessons of history. Quest 1989;41:183–202.
23. Adams JA. Historical review and appraisal of research on the learning, retention, and transfer of human motor skills. Psychol Bull 1987;101:41–74.
24. Stelmach GE, ed. Motor control: issues and trends. New York: Academic Press, 1976.
25. Stelmach GE, ed. Information processing in motor control and learning. New York: Academic Press, 1978.
26. Rarick GL. Physical activity: human growth and development. New York: Academic Press, 1973.
27. Malina RM. Growth and development: the first twenty years. Minneapolis: Burgess, 1975.
28. Schmidt RA. Motor control and learning. Champaign, IL: Human Kinetics, 1982.
29. Thomas JR, Thomas KT. What is motor development: where does it belong? Quest 1989;41:203–212.
30. Roberton MA. Motor development: recognizing our roots, charting our future. Quest 1989;41:213–223.
31. VanSant AF. A life span concept of motor development. Quest 1989;41:224–234.
32. Thomas JR. Motor behavior. In: JD Massengale, RA Swanson, eds. The history of exercise and sport science. Champaign, IL: Human Kinetics, 1997:203–292.
33. Flint A Jr. On the physiological effects of severe and protracted muscular exercise; with special reference to its influence upon the excretion of nitrogen. New York: Appleton-Century-Crofts, 1871.
34. Flint A Jr. On the source of muscular power. New York: Appleton-Century-Crofts, 1878.
35. Bainbridge FA. The physiology of muscular exercise. London: Longmans, Green, 1919.
36. Bock A, Dill DB. The physiology of muscular exercise. 3rd ed. London: Longmans, Green, 1931.
37. Dill DB. The Harvard Fatigue Laboratory: its development, contributions, and demise. Circ Res 1967;20–21(suppl 1):161–170.
38. Hill AV. Muscular movement in man. New York: McGraw-Hill, 1927.
39. Schneider EC. Physiology of muscular activity. Philadelphia: Saunders, 1931.
40. McCurdy JH, Larson LA. Physiology of exercise. Philadelphia: Lea & Febiger, 1939.
41. Steinhaus AH. Chronic effects of exercise. Physiol Rev 1933;19:103–147.
42. Hellebrandt FA. Exercise. Ann Rev Physiol 1940;2:411–432.
43. Morehouse LE, Miller AT Jr. Physiology of exercise. St. Louis: Mosby, 1948.
44. Schneider EC, Karpovich PV. Physiology of muscular activity. 3rd ed. Philadelphia: Saunders, 1948.
45. Ryan AJ. History of the development of sport sciences and medicine. In: LA Larson, ed. Encyclopedia of sport sciences and medicine. New York: Macmillan, 1971:xxxiii–lxvii.
46. Johnson WO, ed. Science and medicine of exercise and sports. New York: Harper & Row, 1960.
47. Jokl E. Physiology of exercise. Springfield, IL: Thomas, 1964.
48. Åstrand PO, Rodahl K. Textbook of work physiology: physiological bases of exercise. New York: McGraw-Hill, 1970.

Suggested Readings

Berryman JW. Out of many, one: a history of the American College of Sports. Champaign, IL: Human Kinetics, 1995.

Dill DB. The Harvard Fatigue Laboratory: its development, contributions, and demise. Circ Res 1967;20–21(suppl 1):161–170.

Massengale JD, Swanson RA, eds. The history of exercise and sport science. Champaign, IL: Human Kinetics, 1997.

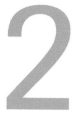

Exercise and Society

SYNTHIA SYDNOR

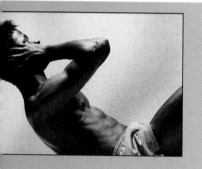

Objectives

1. Explain the key differences between the humanities/cultural studies (such as history, anthropology, cultural studies, philosophy, and sociology) perspective and that of the sciences in studying exercise.
2. Describe several creative ways of defining exercise in postmodern society.
3. Describe the following concepts: hegemony theory, binaries, postmodernity, and representations.
4. Describe how exercise is ubiquitous and why some scholars say that exercise is the foundation of civilization.

At the beginning of the third millennium, exercise, as broadly defined in Chapter 1 to encompass all human movement—including random or infrequent movement, work, habitual activity, training done for fitness or health, dance, sports, and leisure activities of all sorts—is an assumed and fundamental part of today's world. Exercise is ubiquitous, appearing everywhere, and is usually practiced in spaces and times set apart from "real" life; hence, it is also often considered to be fun. Because we consider exercise to be universal and strictly associated with leisure time, people find it difficult to approach the study of exercise from philosophical, historical, anthropologic, and sociologic standpoints. Rather than assigning any cultural significance to exercise, people generally understand exercise as an innocent pastime. Yet, when we examine our society closely, we find exercise to be tremendously influential and sometimes even attached with particular values, meanings, norms, and beliefs that may serve to dominate or harm innocent groups of people. For this precise reason, it is crucial that students of exercise science come to think deeply about the culture of exercise.

At first, the terminology in this chapter may seem very philosophical or abstract to undergraduate readers. The challenge here is to relax, be creative, and try to apply some of your own experiences with exercise to some of the ideas discussed in this chapter. Like all the sciences, the humanities/cultural studies has its own jargon and theories that take some getting used to. Stick with it! Students of exercise science must be intellectuals who understand the whole of their careers and world, not just certain formulas or behaviors in a specific area. The best scientists are also well read in the humanities, which is the perspective from which this chapter hails. Remember that you can view your world from an infinite variety of perspectives. The more perspectives we embrace, the more enriched our lives and world will be.

The age-old questions that cultural studies scholars ask about exercise and society are What is exercise? What is its origin? How does exercise reflect the society of which it is a part? How does exercise transform or change the society of which it is a part? and Is exercise unique to the condition of humanity? Although these questions are not posed explicitly, this chapter does address them. As you read, contemplate what your answers would be to these difficult questions.

Seemingly everywhere we turn we find people exercising. There no longer exist special or particular cultural *spaces* where we exercise, study exercise, represent exercise, or buy and sell exercise. All of our cultural terrain, exercise and otherwise, is postmodern space where we are **whatever** and where whatever can happen.

Whatever is a word emphasized by the Italian philosopher Agamben (1) in an important book called *The Coming Community*. The word *whatever,* used as a tool by Agamben, can be used by us to conceptualize the profound intertwining of exercise within all aspects of our society. *Whatever,* as used in this context, is a philosophical term referring to "precisely that which is neither particular nor general, neither individual nor generic" (1). This means that exercise saturates our world. If we look closely enough, and if we free our imaginations to broaden the definition of exercise, we find the whatever of exercise to extensively encode our society. Thus we may say that not only is exercise in society but exercise is society. This chapter discusses images, ideas, and practices that are linked to the whatever of exercise in postmodern (present-day) times. This chapter highlights the basic premise that to study exercise and society today is to study what it means to be human (see Box 2.1).

Much information concerning exercise and society is available today in traditional textbooks and the popular media. *Sports Illustrated, Health Today, Outside Magazine,* and *The New Yorker,* for example, confront the student of exercise science with thought-provoking ideas about human exercise. This chapter provides an overview of significant themes that are not usually included in traditional textbooks on exercise and society or in the popular media. No easy answers or formulas for understanding exercise and society are offered. Instead, this chapter magnifies the disparate complexity of the concepts of exercise and society, mirroring the idea that the world

Box 2.1
Culture and Society

In this chapter, the words *culture* and *society* are used interchangeably and are not exactly defined. In essence, culture/society is an infinite, abstract, unpredictable soup that humans live in. Culture/society may be real, virtual, fantasy, or past. As we realize when we take our individual life histories into account, culture is made up of communications surrounding myriad activities, representations, and performances in which humans engage. When culture/society is defined to magnify the complexity of human life, it can be seen that there are no absolute truths about exercise. Exercise does not necessarily make one healthy, teach good citizenship, forge world peace, erase differences, return the world to normalcy, or enrich life. If we probe deep enough into the elaborate workings of society, it is obvious that it is a mistake for exercise scientists to begin their studies by simply presuming the above truths.

today is itself disparate and complex. For example, the French philosopher Baudrillard (2) poetically wrote:

> The thousands of lone men, each running on their own account, with no thought for others, with a stereophonic fluid in their heads that oozes through their eyes…to carry on running by a sort of lymphatic flagellation till sacrificial exhaustion is reached, that is truly a sign from the beyond.

Contrast Baudrillard's phrase concerning exercise with that of Shalala (3), secretary of the U.S. Department of Health and Human Services under President Clinton: "A lot of character building is achieved when we put children in swimming pools and on playing fields." These quotations illustrate the complexity of studying exercise culturally. These two individuals have such differing tones and philosophies that the reader may easily suppose that their statements might have come from two different worlds, yet they were written in the same decade about the same topic, exercise. How do we make sense of clashing ideas about exercise and society such as are echoed in these quotations? One way to begin is to use a particular academic framework.

CULTURAL STUDIES

The ideas and concepts discussed in this chapter come from the particular framework of cultural, interpretive, philosophical, anthropologic, sociologic, and historical study of exercise and culture. Taken together, these areas encompass the field of **cultural studies.** Exercise scientists working in cultural studies have made important inroads into understanding exercise and society. Sports history (Chapter 17) and sports sociology (Chapter 18) are included in this text as the major subdisciplines of exercise science from the arena of cultural studies. Those chapters introduce the student to the basic theory and methodology in the social science content of exercise science. To understand exercise and society today, one needs to do what cultural studies scholars call "critically interpret" the world of which you are a part (see Sidelight 2.1). Instead of addressing scientific goals—such as how to prolong human life and enhance or predict athletic performance—this chapter provides an overview that will stimulate readers to recognize the culture of exercise in all its incredible fullness in society today. Exercise, what it means to us as individuals, exercise science professionals, communities, nations, and planet, is *whatever* and is always in the act of becoming at any one time. That is, exercise today is different from exercise 20 years ago or even a month ago. For example, it was once inconceivable (and deemed illegal by

►► Sidelight 2.1

CULTURAL STUDIES

In the study of exercise science and society, some scholars describe their work as cultural studies. The field of cultural studies comprises many parent disciplines, among them literary criticism, sociology, economics, political science, history, psychology, anthropology, English, and pedagogy. Some major categories of work in cultural studies include gender and sexuality, nationhood and national identity, identity politics, colonialism, aesthetics, popular culture, narrative and rhetoric, and transnational economies. To study these categories, scholars use a mixture of ideas, theories, and methodologies, creatively borrowing and combining them from parent disciplines. Generally, cultural studies are concerned with three things:

- Understanding and attempting to untangle the complex history of everyday things and institutions in culture, such as sports in a particular time and place. This type of cultural studies is termed *conjunctural analysis*.
- Identifying the dominant ideas, values, representations, groups of people, and traditions that have power in specific time periods over specific groups of people and their everyday practices. This analysis is termed *hegemony studies*. Hegemony means power or dominance of an idea, ideal, or value over other ideas, ideals, or values. Usually the power is hidden, subtle, and assumed to be the natural and received way things are done. In exercise science, such study often focuses on racism and sexism that have been ingrained in organized exercise.
- *Political action:* Those working in cultural studies not only study change but also try to make small social change. For example, while studying the subcultures of inner-city basketball, one might also launch a campaign to eliminate billboards in the vicinity that further racist beliefs about athletic success and poverty.

athletic federations and national Olympic committees) that Olympic athletes endorse products. In a famous incident in the 1970s, an Olympic skier who, in a televison interview, held up a ski in such a way that the brand name could be seen by viewers was considered to be horribly unethical, and there was great public outcry over his taboo behavior for which he was stripped of his Olympic status.

Cultural studies coax the beginning student of exercise science to be an eloquent conversationalist with a more sophisticated understanding of the place of exercise in society. The humanities and cultural studies, among other fields, give us the tools (methodologies, theories, specialized vocabularies) to enter into some of these profound conversations centering on exercise and society.

Why study exercise and society from the perspective of the humanities and cultural studies? Every human experience is enhanced by higher levels of knowledge. The more knowledge you have, the more exciting life is. The more you know, the more you can hear and see and feel. Knowledge extends and intensifies experience. There is even the saying that knowledge makes you beautiful.

Cultural studies hail from the humanities and the social sciences. Within particular branches of these major disciplinary groups (e.g., history, sociology, philosophy, and anthropology), the common tenets are to understand and discuss the condition of humanity. Scholars

(again, in cultural studies lingo) such as sexism, white hegemony, and anti-Semitism to be romanticized as fun and innocent. For example, U.S. physical educators loved the 1936 Berlin Olympic Games. They wanted to mimic the rituals initiated by Adolf Hitler's regime that they saw at the games, such as introducing the Nazi salute or the lighting of the Olympic torch in U.S. gym classes. U.S. teachers were blind to the racist and anti-Semitic undertones that these practices symbolized. Sports sociologist Hargreaves (7) points out that because exercise is generally rule governed and characterized by ritual practices and because exercise seems to be frivolous and pure, the thoughts and feelings attached to it "are not normally defined as political" (8). *Who plays? Who pays? Who works?* is a catch phrase that has long been used in the cultural study of exercise and society. To begin to interpret exercise culturally, start with these questions.

Societal Changes in Exercise

So far, some of the most important present-day vocabulary and theories specific to studying the cultural aspects of exercise, such as hegemony theory and the idea of the ever-changing meaning of exercise (which Agamben's label *whatever* designates), have been reviewed. Now we turn to another theme that dominates the cultural study of exercise: How does exercise reflect the society of which it is a part?

Postmodernism

During the 1990s, vast changes encompassed both exercise and society. Consider some of these changes in the scope and substance of exercise.

- Female participation in all aspects of exercise experienced a phenomenal growth.
- Fantasy, role-playing, and virtual-reality sports were introduced and popularized.
- Countless exercise sites were developed on the World Wide Web, including gambling, fantasy team competitions, virtual participation in real sports events, chat groups, celebrity-athlete "stalker" sites, the latest scores, recruiting, sports statistics, and exercise clothing and equipment shopping.
- Micro surgery, athletic training, and sports nutrition for exercise injuries, rehabilitation, and performance enhancement were made widely available to the public.
- Learning or participating in a sport was tied to procuring the correct equipment, training, coaching, and education.
- Mass sports tourism to special sporting sites was promoted and primitive and remote exercise sites were enjoyed via high-tech equipment and transportation (see Practical Application 2.1).
- Extreme, alternative, and noncommercial sports (e.g., snowboarding and artificial wall or rock climbing) were birthed and moved immediately into mainstream commercial society.
- Olympic Games became unapologetically professionalized and commercial; changes in nationhood (the collapse of the USSR) and political status (e.g., the fall of apartheid in South Africa) tempered international competitions.
- Snow sports experienced a great boom in participation.
- For millions, collecting sports-related items (e.g., baseball cards) became more important than playing or watching the game; a team's colors or mascot, instead of its record, attracted fans and souvenir buyers (see Box 2.2).
- Free agency and the era of mega salaries changed the face of professional sports. Sports were transnational and driven by the market economy.
- New fabrics, materials, computer design, and nutritional and training aids were counted among the causes for the unprecedented breakage of long-standing performance records.

Practical Application 2.1

EXERCISE TOURISM

The vast number of people engaged in exercise as related to travel and tourism may be one of the defining characteristics of postmodernity and is certainly a form of conspicuous consumption. Why do people travel? Cultural studies scholars have forwarded several ideas.

- Travel to championship games has set beginning and end points. These boundaries, as well as the novel locales offered by travel, intensify fun and erotic freedom, heightening the imagination. Travel to bowl games temporarily equips people with unaccustomed power to have fun and spend money.
- Activities such as climbing Mount Rainier (Washington State) offer an escape from the confinement of existing social roles and obligations. In such travel, discovery and re-creation, which are often lacking in today's lifestyles, are encountered.
- Travelers assume they gain prestige and respect from peers when they venture to authentic or remote locales. For example, like all tourists, the extreme sports traveler (kayaking, snowboarding, sky surfing, street luging, BMX biking, etc.), may seek the exotic. Like all tourists, X-athletes look for signs (or markers) that they have found the authentic, the back region, the perfect move, etc.

- Exercise machines, videos, prosthetics, and implants occasioned participants to be perceived as Cyborgs (humans, often depicted in movies and science fiction literature, who depend on mechanical devices for various physiologic or social functions).
- Exercise availability was opened to a segment of the population who were once not socially accepted as exercisers (e.g., the very young, the physically disabled, senior citizens, the poor).
- The advent of the truly mega celebrity athlete (exemplified by Michael Jordan) caused U.S. professional sports, dream teams, and celebrity athletes to be revered throughout the world.
- Exercise **couture** became high fashion, filtering globally to street wear.
- Subcultures arose whose members blended drugs, pornography, alternative music, and/or gang activity with exercise and exercise symbols.
- A manufactured nostalgia and intense public demand developed for old-time exercise, authentic exercise clothing and equipment, and old-time stadia.
- Celebrities and movie stars with no training in exercise science were heeded as exercise and health experts by the mass public.
- Enhanced technologies in photography, super-slow-motion film, and holography were developed. Reality was experienced not only directly but also through the filtered, enhanced, and distorted mediation of editors. Sports competitions of all sorts became the objects of the lens (e.g., the stands at youth games were filled with parents watching through video cameras).
- Ironic and performative sports (e.g., American Gladiators, Sumo diving, and dwarf bowling) appeared.
- The public became willing voyeurs to scandals of all sorts (murder, sexual behavior, game fixing, and drug addiction) involving athletes. Famous athletes, such as Magic Johnson, were among the celebrities who changed the public perception of AIDS when they revealed their HIV status.

- Results of research by exercise scientists showed racism and sexism in sports hiring, recruiting, and announcing and gave rise to public awareness of these issues.
- Increased speeds, thriller terrains, and new-sprung motivations for undertaking exercise contributed to neoteric exercise-related injuries. New technologies and occupations brought forth injuries such as repetitive stress syndrome and carpal-tunnel syndrome; the wrist, hand, and fingers and mouth and jaw became the objects of novel exercise strategies.

As illuminated by this long list, there is a deep intellectual change in the nature of contemporary social life taking place. Personal computing, open markets, globlization, and a learning and communication revolution are among some of the most penetrating societal transformations of our times. Advances in these realms have put us closer to being able to change the human race than ever before (9). What's more, these days, time is a scarce commodity, and our ability to create wealth seems bound not by physical limits, but by our ability to come up with new ideas. The rich are the new overworked class, and the working class is the new leisure class (9).

Indeed, there are glorious things happening in postmodern society. Some people may counter, however, that there is not much that is redemptive about our times. To take the case of exercise, we can point to the violence of sports or to the use of exercise to colonize others, as when missionaries introduce Western games (e.g., basketball) to Fourth World communities to replace "barbarian" religious practices. Sports are criticized as opiates of the masses because today more people follow sports in some way than worship or study religious texts. Sports are labeled opiates because they drug or sedate us, taking our minds off of the making of government policy or away from noticing social disaster such as local poverty or hunger. Instead of making revolutions to correct social or political ills, we obsess on the latest sports scores, collect a limited-edition baseball hat, or run an extra mile.

Box 2.2
Exercise and Collecting

Collecting things is a form of consumption; collecting is also a universal occupation of all human communities. Why do people collect exercise-related items? Some theories explain collecting as a remedy for the alienation of today's world occupants.

- Collecting brings closure for people who have a need to know that they can successfully see a project through from beginning to end.
- Collecting is a form of play, offering fun and flow experiences to collectors as they shop for, discover, create, and display their collections (note the profuse Olympic pin trading activities on the Internet and World Wide Web).
- Collecting, as do many exercise-related practices in our world, offers an artificial community for the collector. Instead of being subjected to the everyday control of the work world, the collector of things like baseball cards is empowered through controlling and owning the collection.

Baudrillard[a] says, "Our entire linear and accumulative culture would collapse if we could not stockpile the past in plain view. We need a visible past, a visible continuum, a visible myth of origin to reassure us as to our ends."

---

[a]Baudrillard J. Simulations. New York: Semiotext(e), 1983.

We can also point to how exercise is tainted with the frantic consumerism of capitalism. And exercise is certainly saturated with questions of ethics and profit sharing. Critics point out how tragic that in these technological, televisual times we are a world of sickly watchers instead of healthy doers. Critics also point out that it is wrong to make athletes (instead of poets, world leaders, scientists, or teachers) our heroes, and that the culture of sports is oppressive. Critics could say that today's society is Baudrillard's orgy, "a state of repletion and abundance where we are gorged with meaning, and it is killing us" (10,11)

A characteristic of new times that summoned the orgy metaphor lies within the nature of **consumption,** or the processes by which consumer goods and services are created, acquired, purchased, and used. As we all know, consumption is frenzied in postmodernity. We really need only shelter, food, and basic necessities to live and be happy; but in postmodernity, as we go about our everyday lives, we are subtly educated by many sources in **consumptivity,** learning how to consume more than we need. First, we become aware at a very young age that we have purchasing power, or the ability to consume. Second, through advertisements, values, and beliefs important to us and through everyday socialization, we are educated to desire things we don't really need and to buy the right brand. Third, we are socialized by a multitude of cultural beliefs and marketing about how to consume; our passions are educated and our tastes are refined. Through easy travel, enhanced communication, and the Internet, we have the whole world to shop.

Global shopping is the term used by postmodernists to refer to the mass occupation with consumerism.

What we don't know is if these changes and increased consumptivity are unique to our times or if there is nothing really new about how humans exist in the world. Whatever the exact origin of the characteristics of our age, **postmodernism** is a broad, vague label for a time period, literary form, or artistic style that is linked to changed contemporary society. In an important early article describing postmodernism, Featherstone (12) pointed out, "This word has no meaning. Use it as often as possible."

How can this term be applied to the study of exercise and society? In art and architecture, the term *postmodern* implies a fragmented, uncentered style. **Pastiche**—meaning composed of old and new and of images that would not normally be placed side by side—also defines the postmodern. In postmodern style, there is a nostalgia for designs that imitate the styles of previous work. These older designs are made fresh with new kinds of color and/or arrangement. Sports arenas being constructed today are a case in point. Full of postmodern technology and fantasy, they are designed to appear as old-time urban stadia.

Postmodern style juxtaposes images to make them seem ironical or paradoxical. The television networks MTV Sports, ESPN 2, and X-Games and the advertisements produced by companies such as Pepsi-Cola and Nike provide examples of exercise presented in postmodern style. On these screens, video artists create fragmented, blurred, gorgeously colored, and musically choreographed rushes of sports scenes that provide opportunities for aesthetic experiences for viewers in living rooms, bars, prisons, and malls. Photography, videography, literature, and cinematography (in journalism, television, film, personal computing, music videos, and advertising) are as much sites of exercise in postmodern times as are the traditional sites, such as the biomechanics laboratory or football field.

If we loosen our imaginations we observe that exercise in society today is everywhere a fragmented, uncentered, often simulated, and sometimes ironic/paradoxical pastiche. On any one day, we may look out the window to see a female senior citizen in-line skate down the street, turn on CNN to hear of space shuttle astronauts performing experiments on rats to learn about weightlessness on human muscular activity for a future trip to Mars, go to a game emporium to enter a virtual sword-fighting contest, drop by church to participate in gospel aerobics, visit a university exercise science department to see researchers studying the movement of honey bees circling a hive and using chaos theory to apply what they learn to understanding defensive moves in a soccer game, and enter a store to purchase a T-shirt with the representation of our favorite professional athlete emblazoned on it (see Box 2.3).

Representations are abstractions existing outside of the mind that are represented in ways that are thought to be accurate and true. Sometimes representations are actual objects; sometimes representations are ideas. Representations can be ephemeral (short lived) or of long endurance. For instance, the shoes that you decide to purchase are representations of your taste; a city's baseball stadium is a representation of the environment in which it is proper to play competitive baseball. The American flag is a representation that is symbolic of its country.

Consumptivity plays a crucial role in creating influential representations that we come to desire and purchase. Cultural studies point out that history and tradition also play large roles in the selection and creation of representations. It is fascinating to cultural studies scholars that sometimes an age-old history or tradition (and the representations that it spawns) is actually an invented or selected tradition that has a not-so-ancient or enduring origin. That is, representations do not necessarily represent reality: Reality is elevated and sometimes eliminated from representations in our times.

A case in point is the Olympic torch ceremony, which many believe hails from ancient Greek tradition. The ancient Greeks never had an Olympic flame, nor did they have altar-lighting ceremonies to celebrate the opening and closing of their contests. The modern ritual was invented to be ancient Greek. It first was choreographed in the 1932 Los Angeles Games, and then was magnified by the organizers of the 1936 Berlin Games, who sought to glorify Nazi achievements in part by linking themselves to the ancient Greeks (13). The term *imperialist nostalgia* is used to designate the intense emotions that onlookers feel when watching things like the Olympic torch flame (14). Paradoxically, in imperialist nostalgia, people mourn the passing of

---

 Box **2.3**
Postmodern Style Terms

- *Kitsch:* cheap, mass-produced, tacky souvenir-type items such as 5K run T-shirts, baseball caps, team mascot memorabilia, sports and Olympic collector items, sports figure key chains and dolls, humorous and prankish golf and other exercise equipment.
- *Simulacra:* copies of something for which there are no originals; they implode or proliferate in postmodern society and often become abstractly stylized, yet are still commonly recognized by the community. For example, Michael Jordan's image is found on everything from underwear, french fries, and shoes to sports drinks; other examples include the Nike symbol, Air Jordan, and Mickey Mouse)
- *Hyper-reality:* the perfect environment of simulacra. Disneyland is an example offered by Italian philosopher Eco,[a] "Within its magic enclosure, it is fantasy that is absolutely reproduced. . . . What is falsified is our will to buy. . . . When there is a fake. . . the public is meant to admire the perfection of the fake. Disneyland tells us that technology can give us more reality than nature can." Exercise-related examples are exercise clubs, professional sports arena-mall-food courts, the Superbowl, NCAA college football bowl games and other championship games, Olympic games and festivals, sports halls of fame and museums, video sports, exercise videos and CDs, Nike Town, sports statuary, and MTV Sports.

[a]Eco U. Travels in hyperreality. New York: Harcourt Brace Jovanovich, 1983.

what they themselves have changed or destroyed. "Imperialist nostalgia uses a pose of 'innocent yearning' both to capture people's imaginations and to conceal its complicity with often brutal domination" (14).

In the shoe example given above, the Nike corporation has produced many advertisements that reconstruct for viewers desires, needs, knowledge, and even imperialist nostalgia surrounding athletic shoes. Frequently, these ads showcase incredible spaces of exercise couture (the business of designing, making, and selling fashionable clothing) by magnifying a particular version of the beauty of exercise or, in their graphics, by silently shocking us with unusual images. For example, a print advertisement of New Balance running shoes showed a full photograph of a female runner squatting to urinate as other runners approached her on the back-country trail. A Gatorade commercial shows athletes sweating and bleeding in a rainbow of colors.

The exercise advertisements are often like works of art, inspiring us to question their meanings. In turn, these representations (e.g., the shoe as represented to us by Nike) are influential in forming our ongoing representations not only of athletic shoes but of ways of being (ontology) and knowing (epistemology). By purchasing a certain shoe—say a shoe marketed to alternative music fans and skateboarders—a lifestyle, not merely a foot covering, is sold to the consumer.

EXERCISE SIGNS

Foucault (15) said that social practices force the body "to carry out tasks, to perform ceremonies, and to emit signs." In cultural studies lingo, representations such as shoes and Olympic torches are said to carry signs. *Sign* is a theoretical term used in the study of culture. Anything that is

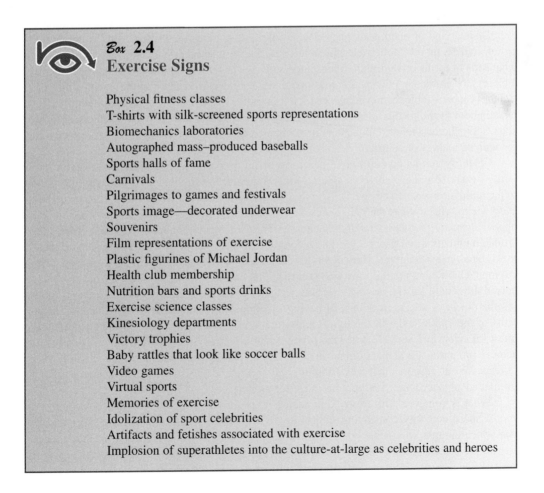

Box **2.4**
Exercise Signs

Physical fitness classes
T-shirts with silk-screened sports representations
Biomechanics laboratories
Autographed mass–produced baseballs
Sports halls of fame
Carnivals
Pilgrimages to games and festivals
Sports image—decorated underwear
Souvenirs
Film representations of exercise
Plastic figurines of Michael Jordan
Health club membership
Nutrition bars and sports drinks
Exercise science classes
Kinesiology departments
Victory trophies
Baby rattles that look like soccer balls
Video games
Virtual sports
Memories of exercise
Idolization of sport celebrities
Artifacts and fetishes associated with exercise
Implosion of superathletes into the culture-at-large as celebrities and heroes

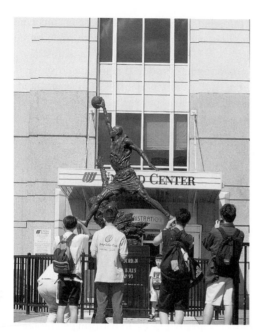

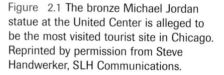

Figure 2.1 The bronze Michael Jordan statue at the United Center is alleged to be the most visited tourist site in Chicago. Reprinted by permission from Steve Handwerker, SLH Communications.

somehow culturally coded to have something to do with or to signify exercise as it was broadly defined in Chapter 1 can be called an exercise sign.

Exercise signs may encompass the things listed in Box 2.4. In cultural studies terminology, *exercise* is a kind of blank slate on which any kind of sign can be written. Thus, to study exercise in society, first we notice exercise in all of its manifestations in society, then we contemplate what sorts of ideals or values are represented and have hegemony in that exercise. Take celebrity athletes, for instance. Why is the mass population drawn to these human beings (Fig. 2.1)? Celebrity means fame; achieved recognition; notoriety; and the act of being extolled, filmed, or talked about in the media, in real time or imagined—qualities normally associated with movie stars, sports heroes, television personalities, characters, politicians, Hollywood, and the tabloids, recognized makers of culture.

Celebrity and its pursuit have a pervasive nature in postmodern society. It is significant to you, as exercise science students, that celebrity superstardom in our times is recurrently found in the realm of exercise and sports. Everyone pursues celebrity in little ways. Evidence children everywhere who want to be game-show hosts, famous athletes, fashion models, movie stars, opera singers, or members of a dream team. Evidence our acquaintances whose lives are defined around moments when they played guitar for a few seconds on stage with a famous band, saw a movie star in a restaurant, were interviewed on a news show, or made a pilgrimage to the Olympic Games and the millions who fantasize that they are Michael Jordan as they shoot baskets in the school yard. Everyone everywhere seems to harbor a fantasy of being famous, of being the object of a gaze or a lens, of having 15 minutes of fame. Andy Warhol, a famous pop artist of the 1960s said, "In the future, everyone will be famous for fifteen minutes." Why the quest for celebrity? Some forward the premise that to be famous, even for a few seconds, is to achieve immortality and that humans in all times and places quest for immortality (16). It is significant for our purposes that it is often through exercise, with its promise to keep one younger even at an advanced age, that humans quest for immortality.

What is going on with exercise in society in postmodern times? Why the obsession with sports, sports celebrity, consuming, collecting, feeling nostalgic, and enhancing performance toward once-thought impossible boundaries? One philosopher of our times observed that these activities are indicative of a "desire for desire" (17). Humans of the developed world search for meaning to life, finding answers in their religions, occupations, families, and sometimes in their exercise. But in postmodernity, many people are alienated from family, close friends, and religion, as everything seems to "spiral blindly toward oblivion" (13,18). So to forget their own troubles, they become eager voyeurs to intimate stories about others far removed from them. Following sports or participating in exercise provides a dramatic story of winning and losing, growth and descent, surprising endings, and a cast of fascinating unique players. People may gather an artificially constructed community around them made up of fellow exercisers or baseball card collectors or by closely following their favorite team (19). Although material collections of sport memorabilia rarely make one wealthy, consuming such items lends the owner cultural capital or prestige within his or her peer group. In consuming exercise in its conspicuous forms, in little daily ways, the consumer/exerciser makes history and participates in the making of history.

EXERCISE IS SOCIETY

At the beginning of this chapter, it was noted that exercise is not only a great influence on society but is society itself. The phrase *Exercise is society* speaks first to the idea that to be human is to move, to exercise. It also connotes the idea that although extraordinary changes have taken place in the scope and substance of exercise and society, particularly in the realms of the technological and medical, in essence, there remain universal similarities in how and why humans engage in exercise in society. Albeit, the exercise may be slow, forced, disabled, or minimal; as our bodies move individually and in concert with other bodies, we create momentous institutions such as community, religion, law, theater, war, society, culture, nations, and economy. In his classic work *Homo Ludens: A Study of the Play Element in Culture,* Huizinga (20) recognized that playful exercise forms the main bases of civilization. He observed that "law and order, commerce and profit, craft and art, poetry, wisdom and science" are all "rooted in the primeval soil of play."

Furthermore, in *Keeping Together in Time: Dance and Human Drill in Human History,* McNeill (21) contends that humans of all times need communities to guide their lives and give them meaning and that keeping together in time, or "moving rhythmically while giving voice together is the surest, most speedy and efficacious way of creating and sustaining communities that our species has ever hit upon." *Moving rhythmically together* refers to dancing, military drill, exercise, song, playground activities, any type of sports competition, and any ritualized work activity (e.g., hamburger assembly at a McDonald's restaurant), in other words: exercise. McNeill says that keeping together in time provides large, complex human societies with "kinesthetic undergirding," which continually "defines, and refines who we are and with whom we share a common identity."

Perhaps the exercise that saturates all aspects of postmodern society is rooted in much earlier times. It is only the speed, size, and form of human activity in postmodern society that differ from premodern and modern times. "To be human" has not changed its essence, it continues to mean that we work first at basic necessities of life. When the necessities are sufficient, we spend our time working, gathering, exchanging, communicating, playing, re-creating, inventing, gossiping, competing, idolizing heroes, and exercising. Our systems of economic and cultural exchange have produced extravagant excesses and marvelous elaboration of these basic human activities, but at their core, they remain the same.

We can discuss exercise and society among ourselves and also with people outside of our practice of exercise science. This may mean handing over, or at the least, sharing, our work with storytellers, dancers, transnational corporations, street people, athletes, advertisers and virtual players, among many others, who often are already doing better jobs at studying exercise than we are in the academy. In opening our conversations to the world, we hope to deepen and extend to new dimensions the meaning of life and exercise for each of us.

SUMMARY POINTS

- Exercise is ubiquitous (everywhere). Furthermore, it is the basis for the greatest institutions of human society.
- Society and exercise since 1990 have undergone momentous change. This change is reflected in the postmodern changes in culture that we are all experiencing.
- The vocabularies and theories of cultural studies and postmodernism are useful frameworks for studying exercise and society.
- Exercise science students are obligated to become eloquent conversationalists concerning exercise and society; they can begin this project by discerning specific kinds of hegemony inherent in exercise.

REVIEW QUESTIONS

1. What are some differences between modern and postmodern exercise? Identify some additional differences that are not discussed in this chapter. Provide some critical analysis of the differences between modern and postmodern exercise.
2. Identify a binary that is associated with the broad understanding of exercise. Be creative and discuss which part of the binary is subtly considered to be deviant and, if applicable, point out how a part or parts of the binary are made the subject of social policy or how it has been subordinated by society's values about that particular binary.
3. What are some of the sociologic reasons forwarded by scholars for why people feel nostalgic for and are obsessed with collecting exercise-related things?
4. Why do some scholars say that exercise is the foundation of civilization?
5. What are some of the main ideas of cultural studies? Give specific exercise-related examples.
6. Characterize some styles of postmodernity. Provide examples from exercise and sports screened specifically on television, film, video, and video gaming, articulating how these exemplify particular postmodern style.

References

1. Agamben G. The coming community. Minneapolis: University of Minnesota Press, 1993.
2. Baudrillard J. America. New York: Verso, 1988.
3. Miracle AW Jr, Rees CR. Lessons of the locker room: the myth of school sports. Amherst, NY: Prometheus, 1995.
4. Gorn EJ, Oriard M. Taking sports seriously. Chronic Higher Educ 1995;41:A52.
5. Comaroff J, Comaroff J. From revelation to revolution. Chicago: University of Chicago Press, 1991.
6. Virilio P. Open sky. London: Verso, 1997.
7. Hargreaves J. Sport, power and culture: a social and historical analysis of popular sports in Britain. London: Polity Press, 1986.
8. Brownell S. Training the body for China: sports in the moral order of the People's Republic. Chicago: University of Chicago Press, 1995.
9. Romer P. Change is good. Wired Mag 1998;1:199–202.
10. Baudrillard J. The ecstasy of communication. New York: Semiotext(e), 1998.
11. Rinehart E. Players all: performances in contemporary sport. Bloomington: Indiana University Press, 1998.
12. Featherstone M. In pursuit of the postmodern: an introduction. Theory Culture Society 1988;5:195–215.
13. Slowikowski S. Burning desire: nostalgia, ritual and the sport-festival flame ceremony. Sociol Sport J 1991;8:239–257.
14. Rosaldo R. Culture and truth: the remaking of social analysis. Boston: Beacon, 1993.
15. Foucault M. Discipline and punish: the birth of the prison. New York: Pantheon, 1978.

16. Slowikowski S, Loy JW. Ancient athletic motifs and the modern Olympic Games: an analysis of rituals and representations. In: AG Ingham and JW Loy, eds. Sport in social development: traditions, transitions and transformations. Champaign, IL: Human Kinetics, 1993:21–50.

17. Stewart S. On longing: narratives of the gigantic, the souvenir, the collection. Baltimore: Johns Hopkins University Press, 1984.

18. Cassell J, Jenkins H, eds. From Barbie to Mortal Kombat: gender and computer games. Cambridge, MA: MIT Press, 1999.

19. Fiske J. Sporting spectacles: the body visible. In: Fiske J, ed. Power plays, power works. New York: Verso, 1993:81–93.

20. Huizinga J. Homo ludens: a study of the play element in culture. Boston: Beacon, 1950.

21. McNeill WH. Keeping together in time: dance and drill in human history. Cambridge, MA: Harvard University Press, 1995.

Suggested Readings

Andrews DL. Deconstructing Michael Jordan: reconstructing postindustrial America. Sociol Sport J 1996;4:315–318.

Berger AA, ed. The postmodern presence: readings on postmodernism in American culture and society. Walnut Creek, CA: Alta Mira, 1998.

Cole CL, King S. Representing black masculinity and urban possibilities: racism, realism and hoop dreams. In: G Rail, J Harvey, eds. Sport and postmodern times. Buffalo: State University of New York Press, 1998:4986.

Hoberman J. Mortal engines: the science of performance and the dehumanization of sport. New York: Free Press, 1994.

Howe S. Sick: a cultural history of snowboarding. New York: St. Martin's. 1998.

Miracle AW Jr, Rees CR. Lessons of the locker room: the myth of school sports. Amherst, NY: Prometheus, 1995.

Rinehart, E. Players all: performances in contemporary sport. Bloomington: Indiana University Press, 1998.

Ryan J. Little girls in pretty boxes: the making and breaking of elite gymnasts and figure skaters. New York: Warner, 1995.

Springwood CF. From Cooperstown to Dyersville: a geography of baseball nostalgia. Boulder, CO: Westwood, 1995.

Sydnor S, Kohn NH. "How do you warm up for a stretch class?" Sub/in/di/verting hegemonic shoves toward sport. In: G Rail, J Harvey, eds. Sport in postmodern times. Buffalo: State University of New York Press, 1998:21–31.

PROFESSIONAL ACTIVITIES

The old adage "With time comes change" certainly rings true with respect to the last three decades of the twentieth century. In that time, the field of exercise science emerged from physical education after Conant's call for the abolition of graduate study in physical education and Henry's response to this provocation with his seminal paper challenging the field to rise to the occasion by becoming academically respectable. Since the late 1980s, new subdisciplines have emerged and the number of students entering exercise science has increased dramatically.

These changes have come with expanded opportunities that await students upon graduation. In the previous section, we learned how exercise science came to be and about its effect on society. In this section, we examine the current status of the discipline of exercise science by surveying the range of activities students engage in today. We start this discussion by examining in Chapter 3 the many organizations that have emerged as an outgrowth of this burgeoning field. A number of these organizations offer certifications to exercise science students in an attempt to increase students' professional standing among the general population (explored in Chapter 4). Chapter 5 investigates the myriad employment prospects available to exercise science students. Chapter 6 contains information important to exercise science students interested in management and marketing. Finally, Chapter 7 concludes the section with a timely discussion on important professional issues within exercise science.

3
Professional Organizations

STANLEY P. BROWN AND JOHN G. ALVAREZ

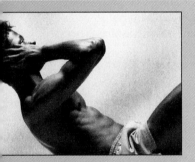

Objectives

1. Identify the leading exercise science professional organizations.
2. Identify the distinguishing features of leading exercise science organizations.
3. Name two exercise science organizations with a scholarly mission and two without such a mission.
4. List several government agencies with close ties to exercise science.
5. Explain how belonging to a professional organization can help your career and support professional growth.

As exercise science emerged as a separate discipline from physical education, the number of exercise science **professional organizations** has grown. The great increase in the number of organizations devoted to various aspects of exercise science is largely owing to the expansion of the fitness industry and the trend toward specialization as the subdisciplines of exercise science matured and others developed. A consequence of specialization is the formation of associations organized around common goals for the purpose of self-regulation. As we will see in this section of the book, professional organizations play an important role in the life of any discipline (see Sidelight 3.1) (1).

The main objective of any professional organization is to advance the agenda of its constituent members. Today, most of the subdisciplines of exercise science have a professional organization that meets the needs of its members. Although the major professional organizations committed to movement as a body of knowledge maintain important roles in the professional lives of individuals studying human movement, the advent of specialized organizations within most subdisciplines has been a significant factor in the development of the field of exercise science (see A Case in Point 3.1).

This chapter examines exercise science professional organizations by briefly describing their roles and activities. Because of the large number of these organizations worldwide, the focus is on national organizations. Therefore, this chapter distinguishes leading U.S. professional organizations specific to the exercise science subdisciplines from other organizations that are international in scope or generic to the entire field of exercise science. Three distinguishing factors are used for this purpose:

- The organization has been in existence for at least 10 years.
- The organization has research-based conferences.
- The organization is a leading advocate for the subdiscipline it represents.

Organizations selected as leading professional organizations for particular subdisciplines must meet all three of these requirements to be classified as such. Professional organizations not meeting these requirements are described in "Other Exercise Science Organizations" and in "Professional Organizations with an Interest in Exercise Science." The 10-year criterion ensures that the leading organizations have at least a minimum amount of historical precedence. That is, these organizations have been in existence long enough to have garnered a substantial amount of recognition from professionals within a particular subdiscipline.

The second criterion—research-based conferences—distinguishes major exercise science professional organizations from associations whose missions do not include a substantial amount of scholarship. Last, the leading exercise science organizations listed are recognized as the professional voice in the U.S. for the subdiscipline.

This chapter also describes other professional organizations that have a substantial interest in exercise science as well as the important offices of the U.S. Department of Health and Human Services (DHHS) that have goals tied to exercise science. Many other organizations with either strong or weak ties to exercise science exist; however, those discussed here are the most significant.

EXERCISE SCIENCE PROFESSIONAL ORGANIZATIONS

One of the criteria for professional status is that the discipline has a representative organization (see Chapter 7). Exercise science, being an eclectic and diverse field, consists of several subdisciplines, some of which are making strides toward being recognized as professions in their own right. Because not all of the 11 subdisciplines of exercise science have yet to develop their own professional organization, eight organizations are identified in this section as representative organizations for their respective subdiscipline. The American College of Sports Medicine (ACSM) and the National Strength and Conditioning Association (NSCA) are classified as umbrella organizations, and the other six are classified as specific subdiscipline organizations.

►► Sidelight 3.1

PROFESSIONAL ORGANIZATIONS AND PROFESSIONALISM

Professionalism refers to the positive feelings and support people have for their chosen careers.[a] Such organizations are important for bringing a sense of professionalism to individual members. It's hard to have one without the other. This definition of professionalism relays an emotional quality, a feeling of belonging. This is an important function of professional organizations. As Baker and Wade[a] mention, membership in an organization helps individuals develop solidarity, unity, and a professional consciousness. These three affective outcomes of belonging provide support for the member. The importance of membership in a professional organization can be seen by the following benefits members can expect.

- Members experience personal growth by participating in annual national and regional conferences. Participation is usually in the form of committee work and giving and attending professional presentations, which afford an opportunity to exchange ideas.
- Members receive the organization's publications.
- Members' interests may be protected as the organization fulfills its role as an advocate when problems affecting the personal and professional welfare of its members arise.
- Focus groups within organizations offer members a sense of personal identity.
- Members have the opportunity to become involved in the organization's political activity by working for legislation and effective public policies and funding.
- Members have voting rights that ensure participation in the future direction of the organization and the profession.
- Members may take advantage of the organization's placement services.
- Members are often aided in gaining employment by networking within the organization.

Students and young professionals usually find many kinds of rewards when they become involved and committed to an organization.

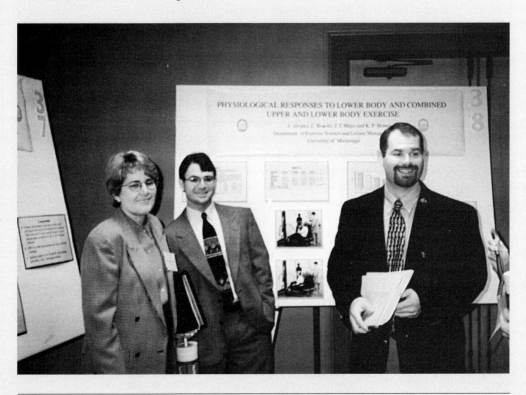

[a]Baker JAW, Wade MG. What is a profession? In MG Wade, JAW Baker, eds. Introduction to kinesiology: the science and practice of physical activity. Madison, WI: Brown & Benchmark, 1995:122–129.

A Case in Point 3.1

TO BELONG OR NOT TO BELONG

Exercise science professionals often belong to several organizations, often an umbrella organization and several specific subdiscipline associations. The question of how many organizations to belong to at any given time is a hard one to answer. Although membership dues to single organizations are often nominal, when several membership dues are added together the possibility of becoming "dues poor" is very real. The trick is to select the organizations that most closely fit your needs and interests. Some exercise physiologists, for example, are also members of the American Physiological Society in addition to their main organization, usually the American College of Sports Medicine. Most individuals weigh the benefits and costs of membership before making a decision.

These eight organizations widely vary in national exposure, membership size, and membership categories. However, all the organizations are characterized by the three criteria previously described. Each of them is widely accepted by a large cross segment of exercise science professionals. Although other organizations may be just as important to exercise science professionals, the organizations identified in this section are strongly tied to particular subdisciplines in the United States.

Important distinctions can be drawn between umbrella organizations (e.g., the American Alliance for Health, Physical Education, Recreation and Dance, ACSM, and NSCA) and organizations that are distinctly related to particular subdisciplines of exercise science. The members of umbrella organizations usually exhibit a diverse number of occupations (or job titles) and level of education (or types of degrees held). For example, the ACSM lists approximately 50 different occupations and 30 different degrees in its membership demographics. In contrast, organizations that represent only a single subdiscipline list fewer than 10 occupations and degrees. Umbrella organizations also tend to be much larger (although not necessarily so), owing to the opportunity for involvement of a wider cross segment of exercise science professionals. For instance, the ACSM has approximately 17,000 members, whereas the American Society of Biomechanics (ASB) has approximately 800 members. A notable exception to this is the National Athletic Trainers' Association (NATA), which boasts a membership of over 23,000. See Box 3.1 for the addresses of the leading exercise science organizations.

Box 3.1
Addresses of Leading Exercise Science Organizations

ACSM: 401 West Michigan St., Indianapolis, IN 46202-3233;
www.acsm.org
NSCA: 1955 North Union Blvd., Colorado Springs, CO 80909;
www.nsca-lift.org/menu.htm
AACVPR: 7611 Elmwood Ave., Suite 201, Middleton, WI 53562;
www.aacvpr.org/
ASB: asb-biomech.org/
NATA: 2952 Stemmons Frwy, Dallas, TX 75247; www.nata.org
NASPSPA: grove.ufl.edu/~naspspa/
NASSH: nassh.org/index1.html
NASSS: playlab.uconn.edu/nasss.html

Exercise Science Umbrella Organizations

The term *exercise science* is viewed in this text as the umbrella term that encompasses a range of interests in fields as widely divergent as motor behavior and sports nutrition. Most people today would agree that *exercise science* has largely supplanted *sports medicine* as the all-inclusive umbrella term for the discipline that engages in the scientific study of movement. This is because exercise science has come to have a broad meaning, whereas sports medicine has taken on a narrow focus pertaining to the medical aspects of athletic injury and the kinesiologic knowledge base (see section V) (2). The sections in part two of the text show how the many subdisciplines of exercise science are ordered (although overlapping somewhat) along the lines of distinct knowledge bases (see Fig. 1.2).

The analogy of the umbrella is also useful when considering exercise science professional organizations. The ACSM and NSCA are major exercise science umbrella organizations, whereas the American Alliance for Health, Physical Education, Recreation and Dance (AAHPERD) is the major physical education umbrella organization. Umbrella organizations are eclectic and diverse. ACSM and NSCA have broad appeal to a wide variety of professionals across the various subdisciplines (and knowledge bases) within exercise science.

American College of Sports Medicine

The ACSM is a national organization with a diverse membership (Fig. 3.1). As an umbrella organization, its membership is composed of most, if not all, of the exercise science subdisciplines. The ACSM is organized by geographic location into 12 regional chapters (Alaska, Central States, Greater New York, Mid-Atlantic, Midwest, New England, Northland, Northwest, Rocky Mountain, Southeast, Southwest, and Texas). It was founded in 1954 and continues to have as its primary concern the improvement of the health and well-being of all people (3).

> ⚷ *ACSM's mission statement: Promotes and integrates scientific research, education, and practical applications of sports medicine and exercise science to maintain and enhance physical performance, fitness, health, and quality of life.*

The ACSM's mission is accomplished through a strategic plan that includes activity in the areas of education, scientific research, and health promotion (see Box 3.2). As an outgrowth of its mission, the ACSM publishes two of the leading exercise science publications in the world. Its official journal is *Medicine and Science in Sports and Exercise,* which is published monthly and contains leading exercise science research. *Exercise and Sport Sciences Reviews* contains up-to-date review articles on pertinent issues in exercise science and is published annually. The ACSM also publishes *ACSM's Health & Fitness Journal,* which includes practical information

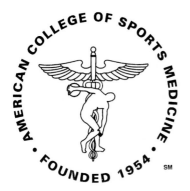

FIGURE 3.1 Seal of the American College of Sports Medicine.

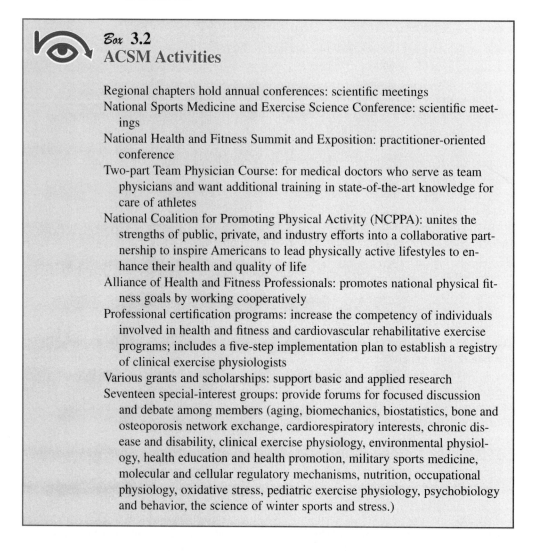

Box **3.2**
ACSM Activities

Regional chapters hold annual conferences: scientific meetings

National Sports Medicine and Exercise Science Conference: scientific meetings

National Health and Fitness Summit and Exposition: practitioner-oriented conference

Two-part Team Physician Course: for medical doctors who serve as team physicians and want additional training in state-of-the-art knowledge for care of athletes

National Coalition for Promoting Physical Activity (NCPPA): unites the strengths of public, private, and industry efforts into a collaborative partnership to inspire Americans to lead physically active lifestyles to enhance their health and quality of life

Alliance of Health and Fitness Professionals: promotes national physical fitness goals by working cooperatively

Professional certification programs: increase the competency of individuals involved in health and fitness and cardiovascular rehabilitative exercise programs; includes a five-step implementation plan to establish a registry of clinical exercise physiologists

Various grants and scholarships: support basic and applied research

Seventeen special-interest groups: provide forums for focused discussion and debate among members (aging, biomechanics, biostatistics, bone and osteoporosis network exchange, cardiorespiratory interests, chronic disease and disability, clinical exercise physiology, environmental physiology, health education and health promotion, military sports medicine, molecular and cellular regulatory mechanisms, nutrition, occupational physiology, oxidative stress, pediatric exercise physiology, psychobiology and behavior, the science of winter sports and stress.)

about everything from nutrition and exercise breakthroughs to the latest management issues; it is designed specifically for the health and fitness professional.

In an effort to support research activity among its members, the ACSM foundation funds a growing list of student and academic faculty grants and scholarships. Another important activity of the ACSM is administration of professional certification programs. Chapter 4 provides details of the various ACSM certifications that exercise science students may wish to pursue. Two tracks are available: the health-fitness track and the clinical rehabilitative track.

National Strength and Conditioning Association

NSCA was founded in 1978 and is an umbrella organization that has more than 14,500 members from more than 60 countries; members include coaches, educators, researchers, physical therapists, athletic trainers, and physicians (Fig. 3.2). Its purpose is to provide a platform for professional dialogue related to the development of strength for athletic performance and fitness.

NSCA's mission statement: As a non-profit, worldwide authority on strength and conditioning for improved physical performance, NSCA creates and disseminates related knowledge and enhances the careers of its members.

NSCA publishes *Strength and Conditioning,* a bimonthly, 80-page practitioner's journal that contains practical information and articles profiling resistance training, sports medicine and science, and issues facing the strength and conditioning professional; *Journal of Strength and Conditioning Research,* a quarterly publication that features original research addressing optimal physical performance through applied exercise science; and *NSCA Bulletin,* a bimonthly, 16-page newsletter. NSCA has established several competitive grants for its membership—the NSCA Challenge Scholarship, Student Research Grant Program, and Strength and Conditioning Professional Scholarship—which are available to members to assist them in some aspects of their career in the field of strength and conditioning. The Certified Strength and Conditioning Specialist (CSCS) certification was established in 1985 and the Certified Personal Trainer examination was established in 1993 (see Chapter 4). NSCA is considered the leader in the development of certifications for professionals in the field of strength and conditioning.

Specific Subdiscipline Organizations

The six organizations discussed in this section have been identified as specific subdiscipline organizations associated with particular exercise science subdisciplines:

American Association of Cardiovascular and Pulmonary Rehabilitation: clinical exercise physiology.

American Society of Biomechanics: clinical biomechanics and sport biomechanics.

National Athletic Trainers' Association: athletic training.

North American Society for the Psychology of Sport and Physical Activity: exercise and sports psychology and motor behavior.

North American Society for Sport History: sports history.

North American Society for the Sociology of Sport: sports sociology

The only two subdisciplines of exercise science without a specific professional organization at this time are sports nutrition and physical activity epidemiology. Sports nutrition practitioners are usually nutritionists with an interest in sports performance or exercise and fitness. They are usually associated with the American Dietetic Association (ADtA) and the Sports, Cardiovascular and Wellness Nutritionists (SCAN). The ADtA's sports dietetic practice group is discussed later in this chapter. A large percentage of researchers in sports nutrition are exercise physiologists who regard the ACSM as their main professional organization.

Physical activity epidemiology may be the newest of the subdisciplines. These professionals are usually public health epidemiologists or exercise science professionals with a research interest in physical activity and public health. The professional organization for public health epidemiologists is the American College of Epidemiology (ACEP), discussed later in this chapter. Exercise scientists with an interest in epidemiology usually regard the ACSM as their main professional organization.

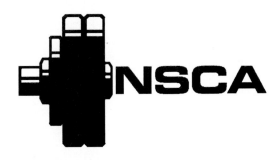

FIGURE 3.2 Logo of the National Strength and Conditioning Association

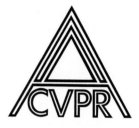

FIGURE 3.3 Logo of the American Association of Cardiovascular and Pulmonary Rehabilitation.

American Association of Cardiovascular and Pulmonary Rehabilitation

The American Association of Cardiovascular and Pulmonary Rehabilitation (AACVPR) was founded in 1988 to provide for the professional needs of those entering the growing field of cardiopulmonary rehabilitation (Fig. 3.3). Of all the subdisciplines of exercise science, this organization is most closely aligned with clinical exercise physiology (see Chapter 11) and is considered the leading professional organization of clinical exercise physiologists. AACVPR also serves allied health professionals with a primary or secondary interest in cardiopulmonary rehabilitation. Table 3.1 lists the different types of health professionals that make up the membership of AACVPR. As can be seen, 60% of the membership is composed of allied health and medical professionals. Nurses are the largest membership category, and clinical exercise physiologists are the second largest (24%). The diversity of AACVPR's membership is the result of the multifaceted nature of the cardiopulmonary rehabilitative process. This membership reflects the use of a team approach in rehabilitating the cardiac patient. Almost 70% of the members lists their employer as a hospital or private practice, which attests to the fact that AACVPR is heavily oriented toward the practitioner. However, the organization also has a strong research component at its national conferences.

AACVPR's mission statement: The AACVPR is the catalyst for visibility and communication in professional education, standards, guidelines and certification through innovative resource development. Our mission is to continually improve our products and services to meet our customer's needs, allowing us to prosper and become the preeminent association of cardiovascular and pulmonary rehabilitation professionals.

Table 3.1	AMERICAN ASSOCIATION OF CARDIOVASCULAR AND PULMONARY REHABILITATION MEMBERSHIP[a]	
Category		**Percent of Total Membership**
Cardiovascular and pulmonary nurses		40.2
Clinical exercise physiologists and exercise specialists		23.7
Other (students, unknown)		15.8
Respiratory therapists		8.7
Cardiovascular and pulmonary physicians		6.0
Cardiopulmonary physical therapists		4.4
Behavioral scientists		0.6
Nutritionists and dietitians		0.5
Vocational rehabilitation counselors		0.1

[a]October 19, 1997 statistics.

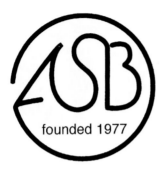

FIGURE 3.4 Seal of the American Society of Biomechanics.

Based on AACVPR's mission statement, the guiding principles for the organization are as follows:

- Quality and integrity are never compromised;
- Customers are the focus of everything we do;
- Creating and maintaining constancy of purpose is an ongoing responsibility;
- Stewardship and creative risk taking are compatible;
- Creating and cultivating productive partnerships and alliances help position AACVPR in an ever-changing health care industry; and
- Creating and maintaining a learning environment help maintain our freshness and keep us on the cutting edge.

The AACVPR publishes an official bimonthly journal: *Journal of Cardiopulmonary Rehabilitation.* Scientific meetings are held annually as one national conference and several regionally affiliated conferences.

American Society of Biomechanics

The ASB was founded in 1977 to meet the needs of biomechanists desiring a more direct platform for the exchange of ideas in biomechanics (Fig. 3.4). Membership breakdown for the ASB is as follows: engineering and applied physics (52%), exercise and sports sciences (16%), health sciences (15%), ergonomics and human factors (8%), and biologic sciences (7%).

ASB's mission statement: The purpose of the Society is to provide a forum for the exchange of information and ideas among researchers in biomechanics.

The official ASB organ is the *Journal of Biomechanics,* a monthly publication that includes reports of original, substantial findings using the principles of mechanics to explore biologic problems. The audience for the journal reflects the membership of the ASB and includes occupational groups such as orthopedic surgeons, rheologists, dentists, biomedical engineers, mechanical engineers, physiologists, physical therapists, applied physicists, plastic surgeons, materials scientists, and metallurgists. One national meeting is held yearly. A joint meeting of the ASB and the Canadian Society of Biomechanics, called the North American Congress on Biomechanics, is held approximately every 6 years.

National Athletic Trainers' Association

NATA was founded in 1950, the decade that saw the emergence of athletic training as a subdiscipline of exercise science (Fig. 3.5). Perhaps the most well established of the subdisciplines, athletic training was recognized by the American Medical Association (AMA) in 1990 as an allied health profession. NATA, therefore, serves an important function for this professional group.

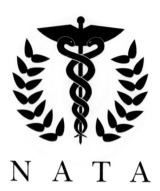

FIGURE 3.5 Logo of the National
Athletic Trainers' Association.

N A T A

Nearly 100 universities and colleges offer NATA-approved curricula for the education of athletic trainers.

🔑   *NATA's mission statement: NATA is dedicated to improving the health and well-being of athletes worldwide. The Association is committed to the advancement, encouragement and improvement of the athletic training profession.*

The official publication of NATA is the *Journal of Athletic Training,* which publishes papers on athletic injury prevention, evaluation, management, and rehabilitation; administration of athletic training facilities and programs; and athletic health care counseling and education. The journal is published quarterly.

The membership of NATA represents a broad cross section of health care and sports medicine professionals and includes certified athletic trainers, physical therapists, team physicians, orthopedic surgeons, family physicians, dentists, and other allied health professionals and manufacturers of athletic training materials and equipment. Chapter 4 gives details of the certification process operated by the NATA Board of Certification (NATABOC), which was incorporated in 1989 and sets the standard for the profession and encourages continuing education. NATA-certified members are employed in a variety of occupational settings: clinics (34%); colleges and universities (25%); high schools (20%); industrial, corporate, and private business (15%); hospitals (5%); and professional sports (3%).

North American Society for the Psychology of Sport and Physical Activity

The North American Society for the Psychology of Sport and Physical Activity (NASPSPA) was recognized by the International Society of Sport Psychology in 1966 and held its first annual meeting in 1967, the year it was officially incorporated (Fig. 3.6). It is the oldest organization in America concerned with the psychological aspects of sports and physical activity. The four main subareas within the organization are motor development, motor learning, motor control, and exercise and sports psychology.

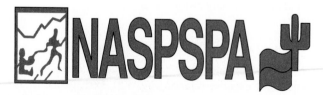

Figure 3.6 Logo of the North American Society for
Psychology of Sport and Physical Activity.

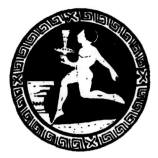

FIGURE 3.7 Seal of the North American Society for Sport History.

NASPSPA's mission statement: The NASPSPA promotes scientific research and relations within the behavioral sciences with an application to sport psychology, motor learning, control and development through meetings, investigations, and other activities.

The current membership makeup of NASPSPA is primarily individuals with doctoral degrees specializing in one or more of the areas listed above. Most of the membership is employed in the university setting; the clinical setting is a minor occupational outlet for NASPSPA's members. The organization publishes the *Journal of Sport and Exercise Psychology* and the *Journal of Motor Behavior* as well as guidelines for psychological testing within sports and other physical activity settings. The NASPSPA organizes one national conference per year.

North American Society for Sport History

The North American Society for Sport History (NASSH) was founded in 1972 and continues to be the main organization for individuals interested in sports history (Fig. 3.7). The NASSH publishes the *Journal of Sport History* (three issues per year), which promotes the study of all aspects of the history of sports. The NASSH affords its members the opportunity to be involved in concentrated discussions and debate about sports history. Annual meetings are held in either the United States or Canada.

NASSH's mission statement: The purpose of the NASSH is to promote, stimulate, and encourage study and research and writing of the history of sport; and to support and cooperate with local, national, and international organizations having the same purposes. The Society conducts its activities for scholarly and literary purposes and not for pecuniary profit.

North American Society for the Sociology of Sport

The North American Society for the Sociology of Sport (NASSS) was founded in 1978 and in 1984 began the quarterly publication of the *Sociology of Sport Journal*. The purpose of the journal is to stimulate and communicate research, critical thought, and theory development on issues pertaining to the sociology of sports.

NASSS's mission statement: The North American Society for the Sociology of Sport is organized exclusively for educational purposes to promote, stimulate, and encourage the sociological study of play, games, and sport, to support and cooperate with local, national and international organizations having the same purposes, and to organize and arrange meetings and issue publications concerning the purpose of the Society. The Society shall recognize and represent all sociological paradigms for the study of play, games, and sport and will promote scholarly activity and exchange among these alternative paradigms and perspectives.

tions in this chapter. Students are encouraged to explore the World Wide Web for other exercise science organizations. In addition, students can consult the *Encyclopedia of Associations* for a comprehensive listing of all organizations in the United States.

PROFESSIONAL ORGANIZATIONS WITH AN INTEREST IN EXERCISE SCIENCE

The organizations in this section were included because the professionals who belong to them are associated with exercise science professionals.

American Alliance for Health, Physical Education, Recreation and Dance

AAHPERD is the major umbrella organization of the physical education discipline. The organization was founded in 1885 and consists of six national associations (see Box 3.3). It is also organized by geographic location, with six regional districts that work together to promote healthy lifestyles and to ensure effective programs in the fields of health, physical education, recreation, and dance.

The total membership of AAPHERD is 25,000. Because of the eclectic nature of the organization, its membership is diverse in its characteristics but still includes a significant number of individuals interested in particular areas of exercise science. As such, AAHPERD plays a significant role in the dissemination of research in the exercise science subdisciplines.

State, regional, and national annual conferences are one means through which professional exchange takes place within AAHPERD. Activities at these meetings include research presentations, workshops, seminars, and sessions regarding professional advocacy. Several sessions provide opportunities for student involvement, including special programs, activities, and job placement. Each national association under the AAHPERD umbrella has its own journal, newsletter, and fact sheets.

Members of AAHPERD automatically become members of two AAHPERD associations of their choice. The National Association for Sport and Physical Education (NASPE), which is probably more closely affiliated with the various subdisciplines of exercise science than any other AAHPERD association, has a membership of 18,000 professionals and is divided into nine academies. NASPE has its own professional journals: *Journal of Physical Education, Recreation and Dance* and *Strategies*. It has also developed national standards concerning physical activity and professional development. As a national association, NASPE awards research grants of $7,500 to $10,000 to the members of its academies. See Box 3.4 for the World Wide Web addresses of organizations and agencies with an interest in exercise science.

Box **3.3**

American Alliance for Health, Physical Education, Recreation, and Dance's National Associations

American Association for Active Lifestyles and Fitness (AAALF)
American Association for Health Education (AAHE)
American Association for Leisure and Recreation (AALR)
National Association for Girls and Women in Sport (NAGWS)
National Association for Sport and Physical Education (NASPE)
National Dance Association (NDA)

Box **3.4**
URLs of Exerc
and Important

AAASP: www.aaasp
AAHPERD: www.aah
AAKPE: www.aakpe.c
ACE: www.acefitness.c
ACEP: acepidemiology.
ACS: www.cancer.org
AdbA: www.diabetes.org
AdtA: www.eatright.org
AEA: aeawave.com/
AFAA: www.afaa.com
AHA: www.amhrt.org
AMA: www.ama-assn.org/
ANA: www.nursingworld.org
APA: www.apa.org
APS: www.faseb.org/aps/
APTA: www.apta.org
ASEP: www.css.edu/users/tboone2/asep/toc.htm
AWHP: www.awhp.org/
CDC: www.cdc.gov
DHHS: www.hhs.gov
IDEA: www.ideafit.com
ISB: isb.ri.ccf.org/
ISBS: www.uni-stuttgart.de/External/isbs/
NASPEM: www.naspem.org/index.htm
NIH: www.nih.gov
NWA: www.wellnessnwi.org/nwa/
WELCOA: www.welcoa.org/

Handwritten note:
cdc.gov - CDC
hhs.gov - DHHS
aahperd.org - AAHPERD
diabetes.org - AdbA
eatright.org - AdtA *
ideafit.om - IDEA

American Cancer Society

The American Cancer Society (ACS) was founded in 1913 and is the nationwide, community-based, voluntary health organization dedicated to eliminating cancer as a major health problem by preventing cancer, saving lives, and diminishing suffering from cancer through research, education, advocacy, and service. The ACS is the largest nongovernment funder of research in the world. The society publishes four journals: *Cancer, Cancer Cytopathology, CA—A Cancer Journal for Clinicians,* and *Cancer Practice.*

American College of Epidemiology

Epidemiology has matured as a field of study in its own right since the 1970s and is no longer considered a subspecialty of medicine. A growing number of epidemiologists practice in a large variety of settings, including health agencies, hospitals, and research institutions; and a growing number of these individuals are interested in physical activity epidemiology. ACEP was formally organized in 1979 to develop criteria for professional recognition of epidemiologists and address their professional concerns. The college currently has approximately 750 members and serves its members through sponsorship of scientific meetings, publications, educational activities, recognizing outstanding contributions to the field, and advocating for issues pertinent to epidemiology. The official journal, *Annals of Epidemiology,* is published eight times per year.

American Diabetes Association

The American Diabetes Association (ADbA) was founded in 1940. Its mission is to prevent and cure diabetes and to improve the lives of all people affected by diabetes. The ADbA funds research; publishes scientific findings; and provides information and other services to people with diabetes, the families of diabetes patients, health care professionals, and the public. *Diabetes,* the ADbA's premier research journal, publishes original research about the physiology and pathophysiology of diabetes. The organization also publishes several journals for clinicians and professionals in diabetes education.

American Dietetic Association

The ADtA was founded in Cleveland, Ohio, in 1917. It presently has about 70,000 members and is the largest group of nutrition professionals in the nation. Approximately 75% of its members are registered dietitians. Membership categories include clinical and community dietetics professionals, food service managers, educators, researchers, dietetic technicians, and students. There are 28 ADtA practice and special-interest areas (dietetic practice groups) that members can choose to join. A dietetic practice group is a professional interest group for members who wish to network within their area of interest and/or practice. Examples include SCAN, Public Health Nutrition, Gerontological Nutritionists, and Diabetes Care and Education.

The mission of the ADtA is to serve the public through the promotion of optimal nutrition, health, and well-being. Its vision is to shape the food choices and affect the nutritional status of the public. The *Journal of the American Dietetic Association* is the official research publication of the organization. It contains articles across the range of research and practice issues in nutrition and dietetics, including nutritional science, medical nutrition therapy, public health nutrition, food science and biotechnology, food service systems, leadership and management, and dietetics education.

SCAN

It is important to mention SCAN, because of its close ties to the area of sports nutrition (see Chapter 9). The purpose of this dietetic practice group is to promote the role of nutrition in physical performance, cardiovascular health, wellness, and disordered eating. This mission is closely aligned with that of exercise science professionals with an interest in sports nutrition. SCAN accomplishes its goal by *(a)* publishing *PULSE,* its official (quarterly) newsletter, and its *Guide to Nutrition and Fitness Resources,* a comprehensive desktop reference for practitioners; *(b)* publishing ADtA position statements on issues related to nutrition for physical fitness and athletic performance across the lifespan; *(c)* providing awards, grants, scholarships, and stipends to its members; and *(d)* holding meetings and events (including its annual symposium) and professional development workshops on sports nutrition, eating disorders, and cardiovascular nutrition.

American Heart Association

The American Heart Association (AHA) was established in 1949 and has as its main goal to decrease death and disability caused by cardiovascular disease and stroke. The AHA has more than 26,000 members and is organized into 14 scientific councils. These councils consist of professionals from different disciplines to help yield a better understanding of the mechanisms and consequences of the cardiovascular disease process. The AHA publishes five science journals: *Arteriosclerosis, Thrombosis and Vascular Biology; Stroke; Hypertension; Circulation;* and *Circulation Research.*

American Medical Association

The AMA was founded in 1847 and is a service organization for physicians that advocates for physicians and their patients. The mission of the AMA is to promote the art and science of medicine and to better public health. To carry out its mission, the organization establishes ethical, clinical, and educational standards within the medical field. Because of its broad mission, it works closely with other professional organizations, such as the ACSM, to carry out important initiatives. The AMA meets annually, during which time committees are formed to research specific issues, to present recommendations at a hearing open to all members, and to vote on these by the elected body of the organization.

The organization's major journal is the *Journal of the American Medical Association,* which began publication in 1883. There are nine special-interest groups or sections of the AMA. These groups ensure that every physician and physician-in-training is given fair representation in the AMA House of Delegates.

American Nurses Association

The American Nurses Association (ANA) is a professional organization that represents 2.2 million nurses. It is an organization under which 53 state associations and 25 affiliated organizations work together. The mission of the ANA is to work for the improvement of health standards and availability of health care service for all people, to foster high standards for nursing, to stimulate and promote the professional development of nurses, and to advance the economic and general welfare of nurses. The membership meets twice a year at the national level; state associations meet once a year. The organization's goals include improving standards of nursing practice, advocating the professional's needs and rights for economic and work-related benefits, and lobbying Congress about healthcare issues.

The ANA's professional journal is the *American Journal of Nursing.* It gives detailed information to professionals about current issues and methods within the field. The organization sets the standards used for credentialing registered nurses within the United States.

American Physical Therapy Association

The American Physical Therapy Association (APTA) is the professional organization of physical therapists. It represents approximately 73,00 physical therapists, physical therapy assistants, and students. The goal of the APTA is to foster the advancement of physical therapy practice, education, and research. Members of APTA must either be a graduate of an accredited physical therapy program or enrolled in a physical therapy or physical therapy assistant program.

The organization disseminates information to professionals through two major publications. *Physical Therapy,* the official journal of the organization, is a scholarly, refereed journal that contributes to and documents the evolution and expansion of the scientific and professional body of knowledge related to physical therapy. *PT—Magazine of Physical Therapy* is the professional issues magazine of the APTA.

The APTA has annual national, state, and district conferences for professionals as well as an annual national student conclave. There are 52 APTA chapters in the United States, some of which are subdivided into districts based on geographic location. The APTA allows its members to maintain focus within their areas of interest by supporting 19 speciality areas, in which discussion and exchange of information can take place among physical therapists with shared interests. The APTA also offers certifications within the physical therapy profession.

American Physiological Society

The American Physiological Society (APS) was founded in 1887 and is a nonprofit scientific society devoted to fostering education, scientific research, and the dissemination of information in the physiologic sciences. The APS sponsors a number of scientific meetings each year. It publishes 14 science journals, many of which are devoted to a specific physiologic system. Among its publications is the *Journal of Applied Physiology,* which publishes research in six main areas, one of which is exercise physiology.

American Psychological Association

The American Psychological Association (APA) is the world's largest organization of psychologists. Since its founding in 1892, the APA has been working toward the advancement of psychology as a science, a profession, and a means of promoting human welfare. The APA's membership includes researchers, educators, clinicians, consultants, and students. The APA has specialized divisions in 50 areas of psychology as well as state, U.S. territorial, and Canadian provincial associations. Division 47, Exercise and Sport Psychology, brings together psychologists and exercise scientists interested in research, teaching, and service in this area. The APA Running Psychologists is an affiliated group of Division 47. The division sponsors preconvention workshops at the APA annual convention. *The Exercise and Sport Psychology Newsletter* is published three times a year.

MAJOR GOVERNMENT AGENCIES WITH AN INTEREST IN EXERCISE SCIENCE

Exercise has been recognized as a major factor in preventive health. This realization has led to major initiatives on the part of government at all levels, but especially by agencies of the federal government. It is, therefore, important that students of exercise science be aware of these agencies, including their interrelationships and structure. This section highlights the U.S. government agencies that are most important in advancing the public health agenda of increasing the activity level of the population.

U.S. Department of Health and Human Services

Figure 3.8 shows the organizational chart for the DHHS, which is the federal government's principal agency for protecting the health of all Americans and providing essential human services. It has more than 57,500 employees, and its budget for fiscal year 1998 was $359 billion. This budget supports more than 300 programs, which cover a wide spectrum of activities. Some of these activities are highlighted in Box 3.5.

The DHHS is the largest grant-making agency in the federal government, providing some 60,000 grants per year. It is organized into 11 agencies, or operating divisions. The DHHS's mission is to enhance the health and well-being of Americans by providing for effective health and human services and fostering strong, sustained advances in the sciences underlying medicine, public health, and social services. The DHHS has established six goals that support and carry out its mission. The mission and goals of the DHHS were formulated under a plan adopted to guide the department in performance management. The DHHS has identified strategic objectives by which to accomplish each goal. For instance, goal number 1 is associated with the exercise science discipline, but only strategic objective 1.3—improve the diet and the level of physical activity of Americans—is directly tied to the objectives of many of the subdisciplines of exercise science (4–6). Although all of the agencies of the DHHS are involved in the health care of the nation's population, some are especially important to the discipline of exercise science. Refer to Box 3.4 for federal government URLs.

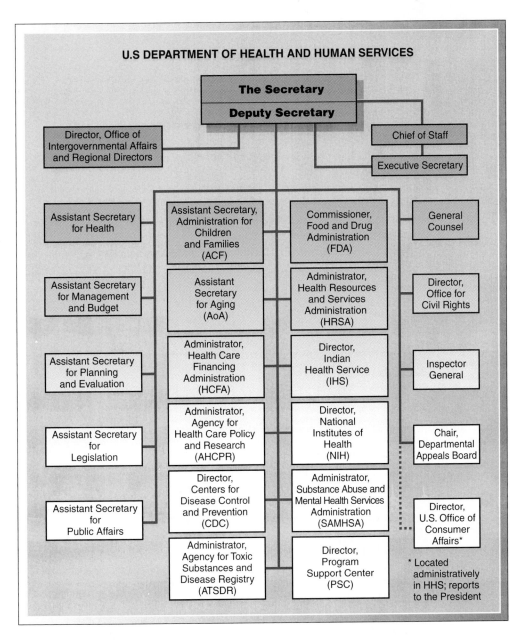

FIGURE 3.8 Organizational chart of the U.S. Department of Health and Human Services.

National Institutes of Health

The National Institutes of Health (NIH) is the world's premier medical research organization, supporting some 30,000 research projects nationwide in diseases such as cancer, Alzheimer disease, diabetes, arthritis, heart ailments, and AIDS. Within the organizational structure of the NIH there are 24 separate institutes, centers, and divisions (see Box 3.6). Its budget of $13.6 billion (for fiscal year 1998) is the third largest for a DHHS agency. NIH's mission is to uncover new knowledge that will lead to better health for everyone. To accomplish this, it funds research in every state; 81% of its financial investment is made through grants and contracts supporting re-

Box 3.5
DHHS Activities

Medical and social science research
Preventing the outbreak of infectious disease, including immunization
    services
Ensuring food and drug safety
Medicare (health insurance for elderly and disabled Americans) and
    Medicaid (health insurance for low-income people)
Financial assistance for low-income families
Child support enforcement
Improving maternal and infant health
Head Start (preschool education and services)
Preventing child abuse and domestic violence
Substance abuse treatment and prevention
Services for older Americans, including home-delivered meals

Box 3.6
NIH—Institutes, Centers, and Divisions

Center for Information Technology (CIT)
Center for Scientific Review (CSR)
John E. Fogarty International Center (FIC)
National Cancer Institute (NCI)
National Center for Research Resources (NCRR)
National Eye Institute (NEI)
National Heart, Lung, and Blood Institute (NHLBI)
National Human Genome Research Institute (NHGRI)
National Institute of Allergy and Infectious Diseases (NIAID)
National Institute of Arthritis and Musculoskeletal and Skin Diseases
    (NIAMS)
National Institute of Child Health and Human Development (NICHD)
National Institute of Dental Research (NIDR)
National Institute of Diabetes and Digestive and Kidney Diseases (NIDDK)
National Institute of Environmental Health Sciences (NIEHS)
National Institute of General Medical Sciences (NIGMS)
National Institute of Mental Health (NIMH)
National Institute of Neurological Disorders and Stroke (NINDS)
National Institute of Nursing Research (NINR)
National Institute on Aging (NIA)
National Institute on Alcohol Abuse and Alcoholism (NIAAA)
National Institute on Deafness and Other Communication Disorders
    (NIDCD)
National Institute on Drug Abuse (NIDA)
National Library of Medicine (NLM)
Warren Grant Magnuson Clinical Center (CC)

search and training in more than 1700 research institutions throughout the United States and abroad. Many of the scientific studies carried out under the auspices of one of the sections of the NIH are devoted to researching a problem in some area of exercise science.

Centers for Disease Control and Prevention

The mission of the Centers for Disease Control and Prevention (CDC) is to promote health and quality of life by preventing and controlling disease, injury, and disability. In accomplishing this mission, some of the activities of the CDC are to monitor health, detect and investigate health problems, conduct research to enhance prevention, develop and advocate sound public health policies, implement prevention strategies, promote healthy behaviors, foster safe and healthful environments, and provide leadership and training. Box 3.7 lists the centers, offices, and an institute that are incorporated in the CDC. The CDC's National Center for Chronic Disease Prevention and Health Promotion (Fig. 3.9) is most closely tied to the discipline of exercise science through its Division of Nutrition and Physical Activity. Its fourfold mission is to prevent death and disability from chronic diseases; promote maternal, infant, and adolescent health; promote healthy personal behaviors; and accomplish these goals in partnership with health and education agencies, major voluntary associations, the private sector, and other federal agencies.

Office of Public Health and Science

The Office of Public Health and Science (OPHS) is under the direction of the assistant secretary for health, who serves as the DHHS secretary's senior adviser for public health and science. The OPHS serves as the focal point for leadership and coordination across the DHHS in public health and science, provides direction to program offices within the OPHS, and provides advice and

---

𝓑ox 3.7
The CDC's Centers, Offices, and Institute

Office of the Director
Freedom of Information Act Office
Information Resources Management Office
Management Analysis and Services Office
Office of Communication, Division of Media Relations
Office of Health and Safety
Office of Women's Health
Technology Transfer Office
National Center for Chronic Disease Prevention and Health Promotion
National Center for Environmental Health
Office of Genetics and Disease Prevention
National Center for Health Statistics
National Center for HIV, STD, and TB Prevention
National Center for Infectious Diseases
National Center for Injury Prevention and Control
National Institute for Occupational Safety and Health
Epidemiology Program Office
International Health Program Office
Public Health Practice Program Office
National Immunization Program

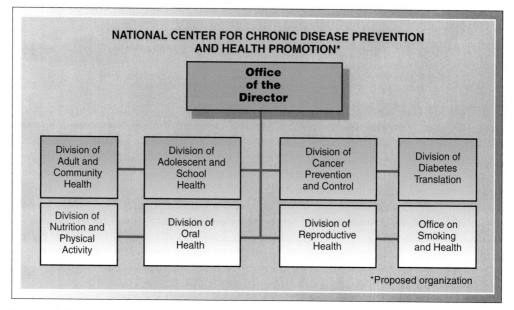

FIGURE 3.9 Organizational chart of the National Center for Chronic Disease Prevention and Health Promotion.

counsel on public health and science issues to the DHHS secretary. Figure 3.10 presents the various components of the OPHS. The following three areas within the OPHS are especially important for the exercise science discipline.

Office of Disease Prevention and Health Promotion

The mission of the Office of Disease Prevention and Health Promotion (ODPHP) is to provide national leadership in improving the health of the population of the United States through prevention of premature death, disease, and disability. Its major functions are to *(a)* establish and manage national health promotion and disease prevention goals and objectives to improve health and reduce risks to health; *(b)* convene and coordinate operating divisions and agencies of the DHHS, other federal agencies, national nonprofit voluntary and professional associations, state and local agencies, and organizations to achieve measurable improvements in health and to reduce risks to health; *(c)* provide a source of expertise on public health and science in areas related to prevention, public health, and primary health care; *(d)* provide one-stop shopping for consumer health information resources within the public and private sectors; and *(e)* define significant areas of opportunity for initiatives involving multiple agencies to improve the health of the public. Recently, the ODPHP was active in tracking the progress of Healthy People 2000, disseminating information about the status of its objectives and initiatives, and applying its objectives to a broad constituency. The organization has also been developing plans and revising the framework for a prevention agenda for the first decade of the twenty-first century.

Office of the Surgeon General

The mission of the surgeon general is to protect and advance the health of the nation by educating the public, advocating for effective disease prevention and health promotion programs and activities, and providing a highly recognized symbol of national commitment to protecting and improving the public's health. The surgeon general accomplishes this mission by *(a)* providing leadership in promoting disease prevention and health to the American public through special DHHS health initiatives (e.g., its tobacco and HIV prevention efforts), *(b)* articulating scientifically based health policy analysis and advice to the President of the United States and the secretary of the DHHS, *(c)* administering the Public Health Service Commission Corps in ongoing and emergency response activities, and *(d)* elevating the quality of public health practice in the professional disciplines.

President's Council on Physical Fitness and Sports

The mission of the President's Council on Physical Fitness and Sports (PCPFS) is to coordinate and promote opportunities in physical activity, fitness, and sports for all Americans. The PCPFS accomplishes this mission by promoting community and school physical activity and fitness programs and by providing information to the public about the importance of physical activity and fitness. Recently, The PCPFS lead the Healthy People 2000 priority area on physical activity and exercise and prepared and disseminated the first *Surgeon General's Report on Physical Activity and Health* (6), in collaboration with the CDC.

SUMMARY POINTS

- The eight leading exercise science professional organizations are American College of Sports Medicine, American Association of Cardiovascular and Pulmonary Rehabilitation, American Society of Biomechanics, National Athletic Trainers' Association, National Strength and Conditioning Association, North American Society for the Psychology of Sport and Physical Activity, North American Society for Sport History, and North American Society for the Sociology of Sport.
- Distinguishing features of the leading exercise science organizations are 10 years of existence, recognition by professionals in the subdisciplines, and a scholarly mission.
- Many other organizations and government agencies have direct or indirect ties to the academic discipline of exercise science.

REVIEW QUESTIONS

1. List the eight leading exercise science professional organizations.
2. Briefly explain why membership in a professional organization is important for professional growth.
3. List two organizations with and two without a scholarly mission.

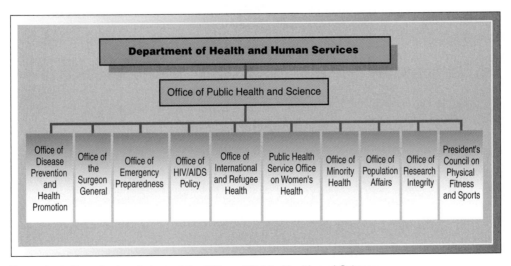

FIGURE 3.10 Organizational chart of the Office of Public Health and Science.

References

1. Baker JAW, Wade MG. What is a profession? In MG Wade, JAW Baker, eds. Introduction to kinesiology: the science and practice of physical activity. Madison, WI: Brown & Benchmark, 1995:122–129.
2. Lamb DR. The sports medicine umbrella. Sports Med Bull 1984;19:8–9.
3. Tate CA. Is anyone listening: how do we make the mission live? Sports Med Bull 1998;33:3.
4. U.S. Department of Health and Human Services. The surgeon general's report on nutrition and health. Washington, DC: GPO, 1988.
5. National Research Council. Diet and health: implications for reducing chronic disease risk. Washington, DC: National Academy, 1989.
6. U.S. Department of Health and Human Services. The surgeon general's report on physical activity and health. Washington, DC: GPO, 1996.

Suggested Reading

Abernethy B, Kippers V, Mackinnon L, Neal RJ. The biophysical foundations of human movement. Champaign, IL: Human Kinetics, 1997.

4

Exercise Science and Fitness Certifications

RICHARD B. KREIDER AND KATHLEEN M. CAHILL

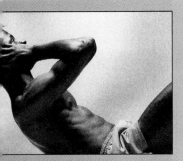

Objectives

1. Define certification and explain the purpose and rationale for pursuing certification.
2. Name the types of certifications and describe the processes involved for earning the major national certifications.
3. Explain the value of certification to professional activity.
4. Identify the allied health professions most closely affiliated with exercise science.

Preventive health and fitness, rehabilitation, and sports medicine services require a multidisciplinary team approach that includes individuals in exercise science, allied health, and medicine. The multifaceted scope of practice required of individuals in exercise science can be complicated by inconsistencies in the amount of experience and educational background. As a result, employers offer varying salaries, job titles, job duties, and training requirements for employment.

As the exercise science discipline has developed and public awareness of health, fitness, and exercise has increased, more emphasis has been placed on demonstrating professional competence by requiring college degrees in exercise science and professional certifications in special areas of competence. Consequently, a number of professional organizations have developed exercise science–related certifications. These certifications have helped individuals in exercise science demonstrate knowledge and proficiency in working in the health, fitness, and clinical exercise science areas. Moreover, **certification** assists the employer by identifying levels of expertise among candidates for employment; providing a rationale for advancement; and enhancing confidence among consumers, clients, and/or patients in the organization. In short, certification is an important part of professional preparation for careers in exercise science (see Box 4.1). This chapter provides an overview of the role of certification in exercise science, defines certification, and describes the typical process of certification. In addition, the purpose and rationale behind pursuing certification are discussed, and recommendations are given for which certifications are appropriate for the various fields of practice.

OVERVIEW OF CERTIFICATION, LICENSURE, AND REGISTRATION

Currently, there is a national debate going on regarding the merits of certification, **licensure,** and **registration** of individuals in exercise science. Exercise science students should, therefore, become familiar with these three types of professional credentialing. The purpose of credentialing is to ensure that, within a profession or service, standards of a safe and ethical practice are being maintained. It ensures that the person has mastered the expertise, advanced knowledge, skills, and proficiency necessary to practice in a particular area of specialty, identified by the administering organization. For exercise science professionals, certification identifies professionals who possess the knowledge and competency to perform a variety of duties in health, fitness, rehabilitative, and sports medicine programs.

The present lack of regulated licensure or registration in some of the exercise science fields strongly supports the need for pursuing certifications pertinent to one's scope of practice. This will assist in ensuring quality care and protecting the health, safety, and welfare of clients in rehabilitation programs, testing facilities, and health and fitness facilities. Although some progress has been made in bringing about regulation in the field (e.g., licensed athletic trainers and clinical exercise physiologists), the benefit of certification is evident through the example of allied health professionals who have been regulated for decades but still pursue certifications to demon-

Box **4.1**
Professional Benefits of Certification

Knowledge and skills obtained from degree programs can be validated by a professional organization.

The certification process can provide direction for formal and continuing education programs.

Research and development of new clinical and applied knowledge are promoted.

Specific roles and responsibilities in exercise science practice are identified.

strate advanced knowledge and competency in specific areas of training. This, in turn, commands respect from peers and the public. In a society with an educated consumer population, college degrees, experience, certification, and continuing education are necessary to keep up with consumer demand and expectations.

In addition, certification assists employers by showing that a candidate for employment or an employee possesses the baseline skills and competency necessary for a specific job. Employers hiring exercise science professionals are increasingly aware of the need to have a college-educated, certified staff to have credibility with administrators, allied health professionals, physicians, and consumers.

Certification has increasingly become a condition of employment, retention, and/or advancement.

The personal benefits of certification include better job opportunities, credibility, expanded level of competence and qualifications, self-confidence, and greater income. Professional growth is often expanded through the association offering the certification. Member benefits include journal subscriptions, continuing education, meetings, insurance services, and networking. Consequently, certification is a valuable addition to a formal professional education (see A Case in Point 4.1).

At present, the various exercise science certifications are largely unregulated. There is currently no single national organization to establish professional standards and foster public confidence in the practice of a particular exercise science subdiscipline. The fact that there are no board-certified specialties for the subdisciplines of exercise science, with one organization governing this process, puts the profession in a precarious position in relation to other allied health fields. Although there are numerous organizations that certify individuals for an area of practice within exercise science, these different certifications require widely varying qualifications, some so minimal as to not require a college degree. Consequently, anyone with minimal qualifications can lay claim to some form of expertise in exercise science and practice his or her profession without fear of legal action. This kind of abuse is not conducive to professionalization, which requires more stringent control and rigorous credentialing. The issue of the professionalization of exercise science is taken up in Chapter 7.

Certification of programs is also a concern within exercise science. For instance, in 1998 the American Association of Cardiovascular and Pulmonary Rehabilitation (AACVPR) launched a nationwide certification for programs to enhance the quality of cardiac and pulmonary rehabilitation training.

Certification

Certification is the process by which an individual, institution, or educational program is evaluated and recognized as meeting certain predetermined standards through successful completion of a valid and reliable examination (1). Certification is usually administered by a nongovernment agency, such as a professional organization, and is a voluntary process on the part of the individual. However, as expectations among employers and government agencies increase, certification is often desired and/or required for employment in many exercise science positions.

The **certification process** is outlined in Box 4.2. The certification examination often includes both written and practical components. The written examination questions are usually multiple choice. The practical examination requires candidates to demonstrate hands-on competence in performing specific tasks. After achieving a passing grade, the candidate receives a certificate and is recognized by the certifying body as a certified member.

Certified individuals are usually required to obtain continuing education credits by attending professional meetings, taking additional courses, and/or becoming involved in the certifica-

A Case in Point 4.1

CERTIFICATION ENHANCES EMPLOYMENT OPPORTUNITIES

There are many examples of how certification directly affects employment opportunities, retention, and/or pay raises.

Who would you hire?

   Certifications often are a way for the employer to differentiate among candidates applying for a position. For example, one candidate has 5 years' experience as a personal trainer but does not have ACSM or NSCA certification or a professional degree. The second candidate is completing her undergraduate degree in exercise science, has limited experience, and is planning on taking the ACSM Health/Fitness Instructor certification examination after graduation. The third candidate is an NSCA-certified Strength and Conditioning Specialist and an ACSM-certified Health/Fitness Instructor. She just completed an internship at a comprehensive wellness center and will be graduating in a few weeks with a degree in exercise science. Who would you hire? In my experience, the person who has certification with adequate academic training typically has a greater opportunity. Therefore, the third candidate would have the best chance of being hired.

Condition for employment

   Many job announcements indicate that certification is required. Sometimes, an employer may hire individuals with the contingency that they obtain certification within the first year of employment or they will lose their positions. Candidates for certification often have to pass the certification examination to obtain or keep their position. It is not uncommon for individuals with degrees in exercise science to travel across the country to take various ACSM examinations as a prerequisite for keeping their jobs. One candidate failed the examination three times within 18 months and subsequently lost his position. Another individual obtained a degree in exercise physiology and then took a position as an exercise physiologist in a cardiopulmonary exercise program. He tried unsuccessfully to pass the examination and was not certified as an ACSM Exercise Specialist. Consequently, when the hospital sought state program certification, which required that exercise physiologists be certified as ACSM Exercise Specialists, he lost his position.

Certification affects income

   Although certification can be expensive, it often leads to better positions and/or higher pay. I have had numerous students who, upon accepting a position, were given pay raises based on their obtaining additional certifications. For example, one student had a master's degree in exercise physiology and was certified by the NSCA as a Strength and Conditioning Specialist and ACSM as a Health/Fitness Instructor. He was hired as an exercise physiologist at a comprehensive fitness/wellness facility. Once he received the ACSM certification, his salary was increased by $3000. Although this does not happen in all cases, certification often leads to greater employment opportunities and increases in salary.

------

[a]By Richard B. Kreider, a former member of the ACSM Certification Committee.
ACSM, American College of Sports Medicine; *NSCA,* National Strength and Conditioning Association.

tion organization. Certification typically costs from $30 to $600, depending on the level of certification obtained.

   In addition, some individual states have **program/facility certifications,** whereby individual programs are required to meet specific criteria related to staff and facilities to maintain their certification. Program and facility certifications can be voluntary or state regulated. For example, Massachusetts, California, Georgia, and North Carolina have published guidelines for cardiopulmonary rehabilitation programs. According to these guidelines, personnel requirements include minimal certifications such as the American College of Sports Medicine (ACSM)

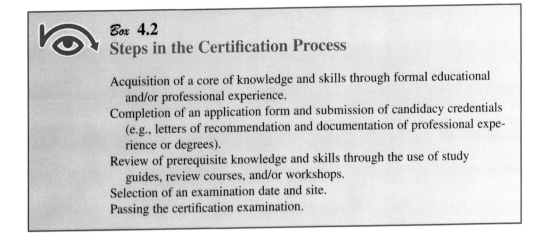

Box 4.2
Steps in the Certification Process

Acquisition of a core of knowledge and skills through formal educational and/or professional experience.

Completion of an application form and submission of candidacy credentials (e.g., letters of recommendation and documentation of professional experience or degrees).

Review of prerequisite knowledge and skills through the use of study guides, review courses, and/or workshops.

Selection of an examination date and site.

Passing the certification examination.

Exercise Specialist, the American Physical Therapy Association (APTA) Clinical Specialist, and/or Basic Life Support. In addition, organizations such as the American Heart Association (AHA), AACVPR, and ACSM have published guidelines for practice that recommend specific levels of certification for various exercise science occupations. Consequently, certification has increasingly become a requirement for many exercise science positions (see Practical Application 4.1).

Licensure

Licensure is the granting of permission by a competent authority (usually a government agency) to an organization or individual to engage in a practice or activity that would otherwise be illegal. For example, licenses are issued to general hospitals and nursing homes, medical professionals (e.g., physicians), allied health professionals (e.g., nurses, physical therapists, and occupational therapists), and individuals who produce or distribute regulated biologic products.

Practical Application 4.1
EFFECT OF NATIONAL GUIDELINES ON CERTIFICATION

Most professional groups in exercise science publish guidelines and/or recommendations of standard practice. These guidelines provide recommended standards for professional conduct, practice, and program administration. Most of these guidelines also provide job descriptions and recommendations for the level of training and certifications required for exercise science professionals to practice. Program administrators use these guidelines to develop their program; hire, retain, or advance employees; and obtain program or facility certification.

Adhering to national guidelines ensures that the program operates within the scope of practice recognized by the professional body. This, in turn, helps reduce legal liability. As long as the program and employees adhere to national guidelines and operate within the scope of practice, it is difficult to show legal negligence. Certification provides evidence that the employee has met standards established by the certifying body. Consequently, because national guidelines recommend that employees be certified, certification has increasingly become a condition of employment.

Licensure is usually granted on the basis of education and examination criteria rather than performance (1). For example, physicians take board examinations after going to medical school to obtain a legal license to practice medicine. Licensure is usually permanent, but a periodic fee, demonstration of competence, and/or continuing education may be required.

The difference between professional certification and licensure is that people who are licensed can legally practice a regulated profession, whereas people who are certified may not have legal authority to practice unless the state recognizes the certification as the licensure requirement. There is an effort among several exercise science organizations to move toward licensure for some exercise science professions (e.g., clinical exercise physiologists, athletic trainers, and health fitness instructors). The issue of licensure in exercise science is discussed further in Chapter 7.

Registration

Registration is the recording of professional qualification information relevant to government licensing regulations (1). For example, a dietitian who completes academic training and passes the American Dietetic Association (ADtA) examination becomes a Registered Dietician (RD) and, therefore, may practice as a dietitian. Registration is similar to licensure, except that the scope of practice is usually more narrow than for a licensed professional (e.g., nurse versus physician). Once a professional is registered, his or her name is listed in the organization's **registry.** A registry provides information to employers and the public about the qualifications of the listed individuals. For example, an agency may provide the names of professionals within a particular state who hold aerobics instructor certifications.

EXERCISE SCIENCE CERTIFICATIONS

The major organizations that offer exercise science-related certifications are the National Athletic Trainers' Association (NATA), the ACSM, the National Strength and Conditioning Association (NSCA), the Board of Certification in Professional Ergonomics (BCPE), and the Association for the Advancement of Applied Sport Psychology (AAASP). Only two of these organizations (NATA and NSCA) have complied with the voluntary standards set by the National Commission for Certifying Agencies (NCCA), the organization that sets the standards for organizations offering certification programs in the United States. NCCA requires that the certification program of organizations be separate from the rest of the professional body. This has led to a philosophical disagreement between the NCCA and organizations that believe a close link between the organization and its certifications is necessary for maintaining rigorous standards and that the most-qualified individuals are certified.

The aforementioned five major associations that provide certification in some aspect of exercise science are organizational members of the National Organization for Competency Assurance (NOCA; Washington, DC). NOCA's members consist of associations, certifying organizations, and government agencies that are interested in credentialing and include 164 of the approximately 1700 organizations nationwide that have certification programs. Of NOCA's members, only 34 have opted to comply with NCCA's nine standards for accreditation. This in no way, however, suggests that those not choosing to comply with NCCA standards have inferior certification programs. The NCCA standards simply ensure an objective and independent assessment of the certification. See Box 4.3 for a list of NOCA's functions.

The NCCA is the accrediting arm of NOCA. The NCCA (formerly the National Commission for Health Certifying Agencies) establishes national voluntary standards for and recognizes compliance with these standards by agencies certifying individuals in a wide range of professions and occupations. The NCCA focuses its review on issues of high-quality certification practice without limiting its review to programs in a particular field or discipline. Sidelight 4.1 examines the standards of NCCA certification. The following discussion provides informa-

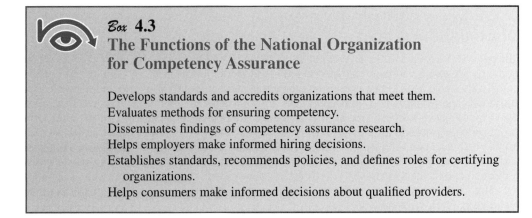

Box **4.3**
The Functions of the National Organization for Competency Assurance

Develops standards and accredits organizations that meet them.
Evaluates methods for ensuring competency.
Disseminates findings of competency assurance research.
Helps employers make informed hiring decisions.
Establishes standards, recommends policies, and defines roles for certifying organizations.
Helps consumers make informed decisions about qualified providers.

tion necessary for understanding the major exercise science certifications, contacting the organizations, and sitting for the certification examinations.

National Athletic Trainers' Association

The title of the certification received by NATA is Certified Athletic Trainer (ATC). In addition to certification, athletic trainers may be required to meet individual state licensing and regulation requirements for each state in which they practice. The title obtained in this process is Licensed Athletic Trainer (LAT).

Athletic trainers follow a defined scope of practice (see Chapter 14 for a description of athletic training as a subdiscipline of exercise science). Athletic training is recognized by the American Medical Association (AMA) as an allied health profession. It includes specialists in the prevention, recognition, management, and rehabilitation of injuries incurred by athletes. Athletic trainers administer immediate emergency care and, under the supervision of a physician, use their knowledge of each athlete's injuries and the factors influencing them to develop a treatment program based on sound medical and athletic training principles. In addition, athletic trainers are responsible for healthcare administration, education, and counseling as part of the complete healthcare team. Athletic trainers work in secondary schools, colleges and universities, professional sports, sports medicine clinics, health clubs, clinical and industrial healthcare programs, and athletic-training curriculum programs.

NATA's Board of Certification (NATABOC) is the certifying body for NATA (800-879-6282; www.nata.org). It was established to keep the professional organization (NATA) separate from the certifying agency (NATABOC). NATABOC provides a certification program for entry-level athletic trainers and continuing education standards for certified athletic trainers. It is a member of NOCA, and it uses Columbia Assessment Services (Raleigh, NC) as its testing agency for technical examination adequacy. Examination content is determined by committees of certified athletic trainers. Questions are validated and meet the specifications of the role-delineation study (2).

The prerequisites for certification are *(a)* cardiopulmonary resuscitation (CPR) or Emergency Medical Technician (EMT) certification and *(b)* proof of graduation at the baccalaureate level from an accredited college with either a Commission for the Accreditation of Allied Health Education Programs (CAAHEP)–approved athletic training education program (with 800 hr of practical experience supervised by a certified athletic trainer) or a NATA-approved internship program (with 1500 hr of practical experience supervised by a certified athletic trainer and specific course work in health, anatomy, kinesiology, human physiology, physiology of exercise, basic athletic training, advanced athletic training, therapeutic modalities and rehabilitative exercise, psychology, and nutrition). To meet these specific requirements, professional preparation

►► Sidelight 4.1

STANDARDS AND ACCREDITATION OF THE NATIONAL COMMISSION FOR CERTIFYING AGENCIES

The general headings for the nine standards of NCCA accreditation are *(a)* purpose of certification organization, *(b)* structure of certification organization, *(c)* resources of certification organization, *(d)* candidate testing mechanism(s) of certification program, *(e)* public information about the certification program, *(f)* responsibilities to applicants for certification or recertification, *(g)* responsibilities to the public and to employers of certified practitioners, *(h)* recertification program, and *(i)* criteria for maintaining accreditation. Under each of these are numerous other criteria that each certifying agency must meet to achieve accreditation. The NCCA accredits certifying agencies that meet all of its standards. These standards have been used by courts in adjudicating certification cases.

The following questions and answers were adapted from an article written by James P. Henderson, Ph.D., former NCCA chair.[a]

What can certifying agencies say about NCCA?

NCCA operates as a private, not-for-profit accrediting body within the National Organization for Competency Assurance and accredits certifying agencies in a wide variety of professions. NCCA uses a peer-review process to establish accreditation standards, evaluate compliance with these standards, and recognize organizations whose programs demonstrate compliance. NCCA serves as a resource on quality certification.

What is the meaning of NCCA accreditation in public protection?

NCCA accreditation helps inform the public in identifying professionals for a wide variety of services and professional disciplines by determining that the certifying agency operated in accordance with standards that emphasize objectivity, fairness, and competence.

What is the most effective way for accredited groups to inform the public of their accreditation?

When NCCA accredits an organization, it supplies a frameable certificate that the certifying agency can display. NCCA also provides its logo in camera-ready format so that the accredited agency can document its accreditation on certificates, Web sites, stationery, brochures, candidate guides, and other publications. It also provides a press release that can be distributed to publications within the profession. The accredited certifying agency can state that NCCA has reviewed the organization and its programs and found that it has met every accreditation standard. The accredited agency may also point out that it submits annual reports to NCCA and must undergo a re-accreditation every 5 years.

Groups that have not been accredited by NCCA often use its standards as a guideline for organizing their certifying agencies and related certification programs, even though they have not yet applied for accreditation. What can these groups say in informing the public about their use of NCCA standards?

Certifying agencies that have not been accredited by NCCA but used the standards in developing their governance, certification policies, and programs cannot suggest in any way that they adhere to NCCA standards. It is only by submitting an application and receiving accreditation that a certifying agency can claim compliance with NCCA standards. Although NCCA recognizes that many organizations use its standards and believes this is an important part of its service to the public, NCCA strongly discourages unaccredited groups from making any public statement about their use of the standards for any purpose.

What statements can be made about the legal defensibility of the certifying agency after it achieves NCCA accreditation?

NCCA believes its standards help define good certification practice that is consistent with the law and other guidelines for certification activity; however, decisions about legality are made by courts based on the issues and arguments surrounding specific circumstances that may or may not pertain to the accreditation standards. All certifying agencies, whether they are accredited or not, should follow the advice of legal counsel in establishing and implementing their certification activities.

---

[a]Adapted from Henderson JP. Marketing NCCA accreditation. *NOCA News*, May 1998; 7–8.

Does NCCA accreditation mean that NCCA has reviewed all certifying agencies within a profession and selected the best one? Does accreditation mean that the profession is more important than other professions?

NCCA reviews the governance, certification policies, and programs of all certifying agencies choosing to submit applications. It does not evaluate the standing of the profession among professions, nor does it compare certifying agencies or programs within the professions or trades. NCCA accreditation means simply that NCCA has reviewed the application and supporting documents and found that the agency has met all accreditation standards.

---

consists of an undergraduate education and experience. The NATA *Credentialing Information* booklet (2) outlines the identified knowledge, skills, and abilities required of athletic trainers. Individuals sitting for NATA certification take written and practical examinations. Once certified, there are specific continuing education requirements. NATABOC lists approved providers of continuing education and the requirements for continuing education units (CEUs), which must accomplished every 3 years to maintain certification. If continuing education is not maintained, certification will be revoked (2).

> ⚷ *Students who began college in the fall of 1999 (the graduating class of 2003) are the last group that will normally be able to receive their degree in time to complete the certification examination under the internship program.*

American College of Sports Medicine

The ACSM is the professional association that oversees certification for individuals in preventive and rehabilitative exercise programs (317-637-9200; www.acsm.org). The ACSM has two certification tracks. The clinical track includes the ACSM Exercise Specialist and Program Director certifications. The health and fitness track includes the ACSM Exercise Leader, Health/Fitness Instructor, and Health/Fitness Director certifications. The ACSM certification programs have been criticized by some professionals for focusing too much on aerobic exercise testing and training, with a perceived lack of focus on resistance training and associated evaluation of strength-fitness parameters.

The scope of practice for clinical track candidates is in clinical settings with high-risk or apparently healthy individuals or individuals with medical problems (see Box 4.4). Specifically, for special, high-risk, or populations with diagnosed diseases, the ACSM Exercise Specialist performs exercise testing, exercise prescription, exercise leadership, patient education, and counseling. The ACSM Program Director primarily functions as an administrator of preventive and rehabilitative programs in clinical settings (3).

The scope of practice for health and fitness track candidates is in corporate, commercial, or community settings with apparently healthy individuals. Specifically, the Exercise Leader often works as an aerobics instructor and/or exercise program leader. The Health/Fitness Instructor can lead group programs and perform fitness testing and health education programs (personal trainers, strength trainers). The Health/Fitness Director often serves as a health club manager and performs administrative duties for preventive or health and fitness programs (3).

ACSM is the certifying body for clinical and health and fitness certifications. The examination content and questions are determined by experts from a variety of disciplines in exercise science who function under the direction of the ACSM Committee on Certification and Education. These experts draft questions for the test item data bank that are then statistically analyzed, validated, and reviewed by a committee of psychometricians and professionals to ensure that they meet specific knowledge, skills, and abilities (KSAs). A nationwide role-delineation study then validates the KSAs.

Box 4.4
Key Points in the Scope of Practice for the Registered Clinical Exercise Physiologist (CEP)[a]

The CEP applies exercise and physical activity in clinical and pathologic situations in which exercise has been shown to provide therapeutic or functional benefits.

The CEP works with a variety of individuals, including patients with cardiovascular, pulmonary, metabolic, orthopedic, neuromuscular, inflammatory, and immunologic disorders.

The CEP applies exercise principles to groups and/or populations when delivering preventive services, especially to geriatric, obstetric, and pediatric clients.

The CEP performs the following exercise services: evaluations, prescriptions, supervision, education, and exercise outcome evaluation.

The CEP restricts his or her practice to clients who are referred by and are under the continued care of a licensed physician.

[a]American College of Sports Medicine. The ACSM registered clinical exercise physiologist: the premier clinical credential for graduate-level exercise physiologists. Am Coll Sports Med Certified News 1998;8:5.

Prerequisites for the certifications are as follows:

- *Exercise Specialists:* KSAs described in the *Guidelines for Exercise Testing and Prescription* (3); a minimum of 600 hr of practical experience in a clinical exercise program, including exercise testing; a baccalaureate degree in an allied field or the equivalent; and current basic life support certification.
- *Program Director:* KSAs described in the *Guidelines for Exercise Testing and Prescription* (3); postgraduate degree training in exercise science, medicine, or an allied health field plus 2 years of clinical experience; a minimum of 1 year of recent experience in a position of administrative authority working with a clinical exercise program; current basic life support certification; and a written recommendation from a current ACSM-certified Program Director.
- *Exercise Leader:* fitness certification from a nationally recognized organization or completed or current enrollment in exercise-related college courses at a regionally accredited college or university, or 300 hr of group exercise instruction experience.
- *Health/Fitness Instructor:* a 2-year, 4-year, or master's degree from a regionally accredited college or university in a health-related field or current enrollment in a regionally accredited college or university in a degree-granting health-related field or a minimum of 900 hr of practical experience in a fitness setting.
- *Health/Fitness Director:* A 2-year, 4-year, or master's degree from a regionally accredited college or university in a health-related field plus a minimum of 2 years or 4000 hr of experience as a fitness manager or director or current ACSM Health/Fitness Instructor certification plus 2 years or 4000 hr of experience as a fitness manager or director.

To meet these requirements, the ACSM strongly recommends specific educational degrees, training, and experience for the various levels of certification. As the level of certification increases, the depth of understanding and the knowledge base are expected to increase commensurately. Both written and practical examinations are given. ACSM-sponsored week-long workshops are conducted worldwide at more than 60 different locations. Continuing education is required for all levels of certification and must be maintained and documented every 4 years or the certification will be revoked.

National Strength and Conditioning Association

The NSCA is another professional association that offers certification to exercise science professionals (402-476-6669; www.nsca-cc.org). The NSCA offers two certifications: Certified Personal Trainer and Certified Strength and Conditioning Specialist (CSCS). Certified Personal Trainers consult and train individual clients to accommodate specific goals. They work in clients' homes, health and fitness clubs, and community centers. The CSCS is for professionals who work in commercial or community health and fitness facilities implementing safe and effective conditioning and strength training programs.

The CSCS Agency is administratively and financially independent of the NSCA and is responsible for the examinations. The agency is accredited by the NCCA. Examination content is determined by a national task analysis study conducted by the CSCS Agency and is reviewed by psychometricians and an examination service for technical assistance.

The prerequisite for becoming a Certified Personal Trainer is current CPR certification. The prerequisites for becoming a CSCS are a baccalaureate degree and current CPR certification. A role-delineation study identifies content areas, specific knowledge, and skills required. The written multiple-choice examinations include an applied section, which consists of viewing a videotape and answering multiple-choice questions. To maintain certification, CEUs must be accumulated every 3 years. A criticism of the NSCA certifications is that there is no specific degree, experience, or practical examination requirement.

Professional Ergonomists

Ergonomists are professionals who study the interaction between people and machines and investigate environmental factors that affect work. Ergonomists design or redesign workplace, social, and physical work environments; assist engineers in designing systems and machines; implement new programs; provide rehabilitation and educational training; and perform ongoing evaluation of systems. Ergonomists often work as part of a team and are responsible for developing training aids. The following certifications are available to professional ergonomists: Certified Professional Ergonomist (CPE), Certified Human Factors Professional (CHFP), and Certified Ergonomics Technologist (CET). The Board of Certified Safety Professionals (BCSP) also offers specialty examinations for Certified Ergonomists. There are four levels of practice identified by the BCPE for the ergonomics profession, depending on background, experience, capabilities, and knowledge. These levels of practice are defined and can be obtained from the BCPE.

The Board of Certification in Professional Ergonomics is the certifying body for the CPE, CHFP, and CET certifications (360-671-7601; humanics-es.com). The content of the certification examinations is determined by a group of ergonomic academicians, researchers, and practitioners functioning under the direction of the board. Questions are analyzed according to guidelines set by the National Commission for Competency Assurance (4).

Prerequisites to sitting for the examination include a master's degree in ergonomics or an equivalent life science or engineering science. Course work includes such areas as anatomy, kinesiology, biomechanics, engineering sciences, physiology, psychology, management, statistics, ergonomics, and architectural design. Candidates must also have 4 years of full-time professional practice as an ergonomist practitioner. Individuals can be certified as Associate Ergonomics Professionals or Associate Human Factors Professionals if they meet the educational degree requirement, pass the basic knowledge section of the examination, and are currently working to fulfill the required 4 years of practical experience. Associate certification is provided as a stepping stone to full certification while the professional is working toward obtaining work experience in the field (4).

Academic preparation is available through undergraduate or graduate programs in accredited colleges or universities. Human factors or ergonomics degree programs are accredited by an International Ergonomics Association (IEA) federated society, such as the Human Factors and Ergonomics Society (HFES). The extensive KSAs needed for certification are outlined in the BCPE's *Information on Certification Policies, Practices and Procedures* (4). A written examination that includes questions for scenarios in specialty areas of practice is given. Ergonomists do not have continuing education requirements.

Association for the Advancement of Applied Sport Psychology

The AAASP is the professional certifying agency for sport psychologists (215-204-8717; www.aaasponline.org/index2.html). Upon certification professionals receive the title of Certified Consultant. Prerequisites for certification include a doctoral degree and a supervised practicum in counseling at the graduate level (400 hr supervised by a licensed sport psychologist). Other prerequisites are AAASP-specified course work, experience, and training in sports psychology and exercise science (5).

Because this is a doctoral-level certification, formal education and training at the postgraduate level are required. An example of the depth of knowledge required includes, but is not limited to, course work in advanced knowledge of scientific and professional sport psychology standards, social psychology, health/exercise psychology, kinesiology, exercise physiology, motor learning and development, psychopathology, counseling, research design, statistics and psychological assessment (5).

There is no examination. The application process documents evidence that all the extensive criteria have been met, which is then reviewed by a board. No continuing education requirements exist at this time.

FITNESS CERTIFICATIONS

There are currently many organizations offering fitness certification; however, it is beyond the scope of this chapter to present a comprehensive list and a detailed description of all the fitness certifications available to exercise science students. The following organizations are the most prominent ones offering fitness certifications. Table 4.1 provides a list of recommended certifications appropriate for specific careers in exercise science.

Aerobics and Fitness Association of America

The AFAA administers the following types of certifications: Primary Aerobic Instructor Certification, Personal Trainer/Fitness Counselor Certification, Step Certification, Weight Training Certification, and Fitness Practitioner Certification (800-446-2322; www.afaa.com) (6). Aerobic instructors teach a variety of aerobics classes, including dance, high and low impact, step, and aquatic. They are responsible for the content, format, and choreography of their sessions. Personal trainers perform assessment evaluations, set up programs, help meet clients' goals, track progress, and make adjustments to their clients' programs.

The AFAA uses an independent testing and research agency to administer and score their certification examinations. The AFAA's National Fitness Testing Council consists of fitness professionals from a variety of health and fitness areas; this board is ultimately responsible for the examination content (6). The board is not certified by the NCCA. For the Primary Aerobic Instructor Certification, Personal Trainer Certification, Step Certification, and Weight Training Certification, current CPR and either previous AFAA certifications or a degree in exercise science are required. The Fitness Practitioner certification requires that individuals have a 4-year college degree, CPR certification, liability insurance, another AFAA certification, and a record of workshop attendance. They also must complete home-study course work and pass two case

Table 4.1 RECOMMENDED CERTIFICATIONS FOR EXERCISE SCIENCE OCCUPATIONS	
Occupation	**Certifications**
Fitness jobs	
Aerobic dance; group leadership	ACSM Exercise Leader; ACE; AFAA
Health or fitness instructor; personal trainer	ACSM Health/Fitness Instructor; NSCA Personal Trainer; YMCA
Strength and conditioning trainer	NSCA CSCS; ACSM Health/Fitness Instructor
Health and fitness or wellness director	ACSM Health/Fitness Director
Clinical jobs	
Sports medicine	NATA Certified Athletic Trainer; NSCA CSCS; ACSM Health/Fitness Instructor
Exercise testing and evaluation	ACSM Exercise Specialist or Program Director
Special-population rehabilitation	ACSM Exercise Specialist or Program Director
Kinesiology or biomechanics	BCPE Certified Ergonomist; NSCA CSCS
Sports psychology	AAASP Certified Consultant

studies (6). Written and practical examinations are given for all certifications except the Fitness Practitioner, which is a cumulative certification that has specific requirements (listed on previous page). To maintain any level of certification, individuals must maintain CEUs every 2 years.

American Council on Exercise

The American Council on Exercise (ACE) offers the Personal Trainer Certification, the Group Fitness Instructor Certification, and the Lifestyle and Weight Management Consultant Certification (800-825-3636; www.acefitness.org). These certificates ensure the competency of individuals leading group exercise programs, working with clients during one-on-one training, and offering preventive health and fitness counseling (7). ACE uses Columbia Assessment Services as its testing agency. The examination content is determined by a committee of experts who conducted a national job analysis that was validated by a research survey sent to 2000 fitness professionals (7).

The only prerequisite for certification is current CPR certification. Examination content and the weighting for each area of the examination are outlined for all three certifications in the *ACE Certification Guide* (7) booklet. The written examinations are multiple choice. Once certified, CEUs must be accumulated every 2 years to maintain certification. There is no practical examination, and there are no prerequisites for experience and education.

YMCA

The YMCA offers certification courses, including Working with Active Older Adults, Active Older Adult Program Director, Active Older Adult Exercise Instructor, and Active Older Adult Land/Water Exercise Instructor (800-872-9622; www.ymca.net). Aquatics courses range from Lifeguard Instructor to Special Populations Instructor and Arthritis Foundation YMCA Aquatic Program Instructor. In addition, a variety of health and fitness certification courses (e.g., Exercise Instructor, Strength Training Instructor, and Healthy Back Instructor) are available.

Many of the certification courses are designed to meet training requirements for YMCA staff. However, college credit and continuing education for other fitness organizations are also offered through these programs. Owing to the variety of courses offered, the scope of practice is suitable only for the specialty area of the individual course. The certifying body is the staff development department of the YMCA.

Prerequisites vary for each certification, but generally have age, CPR, and YMCA certification course requirements. To receive the certification, course participants must attend the number of hours indicated for each course. The certifications are course work oriented and provide practical and/or theoretical information for fitness professionals; textbooks are used for reference. There are no specific KSAs identified, because not all courses require examinations (8). Examinations are written and/or practical.

Cooper Institute for Aerobics Research

The following categories and certifications are offered by the Cooper Institute for Aerobics Research (800-635-7050; www.cooperinst.org).

- Personal training and fitness programming: Physical Fitness Specialist Certification, Master Fitness Specialist Certification, Biomechanics of Resistance Training Specialty Certification, Fitness Specialist for Older Adults Specialty Certification, and Special Populations Speciality Certification
- Dietary guidance: Nutrition Specialty Certification
- Aerobics fitness instruction: Group Exercise Leadership Certification, Indoor Cycling Specialty Certification, and Aquatics Speciality Certification
- Health promotion: Health Promotion Director Certification, Program Evaluation and Outcomes Measurement (special topic), and Helping Sedentary Adults Become Physically Active
- Public safety fitness: Police Physical Fitness Specialist Certification (offered in conjunction with the International Association of Chiefs of Police), and Master Fitness Specialist Certification

These certifications vary widely in cost, and all require registration in a workshop. For most certifications, written and practical examinations and CPR training are required. They are targeted to professionals in the healthcare and the fitness industry who wish additional credentials.

SUMMARY POINTS

- Certification is an important component in the professional development of exercise science professionals.
- Certification exceeds a professional's degree attainment, educational background, training, and licensing requirements.
- Certification allows for an individual's knowledge and skills in a specific area of practice to be evaluated and validated by a recognized professional group.
- Many programs and administrators require employees to be certified.
- Professionals who become certified are often provided greater career opportunities and income.
- Although there are many certifications offered for exercise science professionals, the primary certification organizations in exercise science are the American College of Sports Medicine, National Strength and Conditioning Association, National Athletic Trainers' Association, Board of Certification in Professional Ergonomics, YMCA, American Council on Exercise, Aerobics and Fitness Association of America , and Association for the Advancement of Applied Sport Psychology.
- Nurses, physical therapists, registered dietitians, and other certified clinicians often contribute to a multidisciplinary sports medicine team and seek exercise science academic training and/or certification.
- Professionals should look for a validated and reliable certification examination that reflects the breadth of knowledge and expertise required in their specialty area.
- The certifications administered by credible organizations are the most respected.

REVIEW QUESTIONS

1. What is professional certification?
2. What is the typical process of becoming certified?
3. What is the purpose and rationale for becoming certified?
4. What are the major professional groups that provide certification for exercise science professionals?
5. What are the recommended certifications for aerobic dance and exercise leadership, personal training and health fitness instruction, strength and conditioning training, directing health fitness and wellness programs, sports medicine, exercise testing, special population rehabilitation, kinesiology and biomechanics, and sports psychology?
6. Describe some of the benefits of certification.

References

1. Anderson K, ed. Nursing and allied health dictionary. 4th ed. St. Louis: Mosby Year Book, 1994.
2. National Athletic Trainers' Association Board of Certification. Credentialing information. Raleigh, NC: NATABOC, 1995.
3. American College of Sports Medicine. Guidelines for exercise testing and prescription. 6th ed. Baltimore: Lippincott Williams & Wilkins, 2000.
4. Board of Certification for Professional Ergonomists. Information on certification policies, practices and procedures. 3rd ed. Bellingham, WA: BCPE, 1995.
5. American Association of Applied Sports Psychology. Certification guidelines. www.aaasponline.org/consult_cert_main.html, 1997.
6. Aerobics and Fitness Association of America. AFAA certification brochure. Sherman Oaks, CA: AFAA, 1997.
7. American Council on Exercise. ACE certification guide. San Diego, CA: ACE, 1997.
8. YMCA of the USA. 1998 course catalog. Chicago, IL: YMCA, 1998.

Suggested Readings

Boland AL. Presidential address of the American Orthopaedic Society for Sports Medicine. Am J Sports Med 1996;24:712–715.

Foster C. Licensure—the quest for the holly grail? ACSM Certified News 1992;2:9.

Gillespie WJ. A model for licensure of exercise professionals. Exerc Stand Malpract Reporter 1993;7:81–86.

Otto RM, Wygand J. American College of Sports Medicine Exercise Specialist Workshop/Certification. A modality for career preparation. J Cardiopulm Rehab 1996;16:353–355.

Southard DR, Certo C, Comoss P, et al. Core competencies for cardiac rehabilitation professionals. J Cardiopulm Rehab 1994;14:87–92.

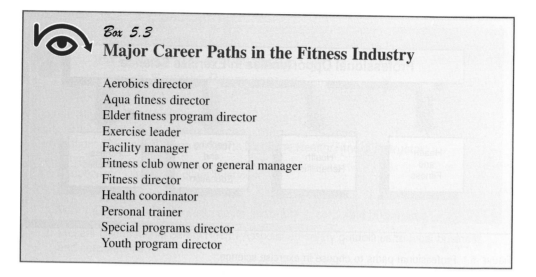

million people) will be older than 85 years (3). Already, there is a major trend developing, with elders embracing fitness to improve the quality of their lives and live longer. More and more of these active seniors have incomes that will drive the implementation of a variety of different health and fitness programs that were once restricted because of the fixed incomes of many seniors. Opportunities for working with elders can be found at community centers, hospitals, long-term care facilities, community park and recreation centers, adult education programs, older-adult communities, and health clubs. Exercise scientists should enhance their knowledge of gerontology to be most effective with this population.

YOUTH FITNESS PROGRAMS   There is a rise in obesity in today's children. But, paradoxically, an increasing number of schools are eliminating physical education opportunities for today's youth. This may be owing to a perceived lack of academic rigor of physical education by administrators who are willing to drop these programs owing to financial necessity (see Sidelight 5.1). Many of the employment opportunities for youth fitness can be found at the same centers at which the elder fitness programs are delivered. Challenges facing the exercise science professionals include the development of innovative, energetic, instructional programs for the expanding needs of youth.

AQUA FITNESS PROGRAMS   Aquatic exercise programs and interest in water fitness is on the rise. The broad appeal of water and the ability to provide a multitude of different types of programs make aquatic fitness inviting for the exercise professional. Opportunities are available at rehabilitation centers, hotels, fitness facilities, and park and recreation centers. Advanced swimming skills are generally not required to direct, teach, or lead aquatic exercise programs. Owing to the low-impact nature of this medium, aqua exercise has expanded to include programs for seniors, injury rehabilitation, cardiac rehabilitation, sedentary individuals, physically challenged individuals, individuals with land exercise limitations, and the apparently healthy population.

Club Industry

Each year, *Club Industry: The Business Magazine for Health and Fitness Facility Management* publishes a listing of the largest 100 fitness clubs and chains in North America, including phone numbers. For more information contact Club Industry, PO Box 3055, Northbrook, IL 60065 (888-291-5214). For employment opportunities contact: ACSM's *Health & Fitness Journal,* 351 West Camden St., Baltimore, MD 21201 (800-638-6423) or YMCA of the USA (800-872-9622).

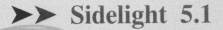

➤➤ Sidelight 5.1

HIGHLIGHTS FROM THE *SHAPE OF THE NATION REPORT*[a]

During the summer of 1997 the National Association for Sport and Physical Education conducted a survey in which physical education consultants form the department of education of each state responded to questions regarding their state's mandate for physical education at the elementary-, middle-, and secondary-school levels. Questions concerning acceptance of substitutions, time allocation, and qualification directives for teaching physical education were included. This survey followed a 1993 survey that assessed where physical education programs stood in the public school systems of the country. There is currently no federal mandate or funding targeted to physical education, despite federal actions such as Resolution 97 (1987), which encouraged state and local government and local educational agencies to provide high-quality daily physical education programs for all children in K–12; Healthy People 2000[b] objectives; the *Surgeon General's Report on Physical Activity and Health*[c]*;* and the *Guidelines for School and Community Health Programs to Promote Lifelong Physical Activity among Young People.*[d]

Here are some results of the 1997 survey:

- Major finding: most states are not living up to the recommendations of the surgeon general's report and the CDC's call to require daily physical education for all students in grades K–12.
- A total of 47 states have mandates for physical education.
- Illinois is the only state that requires daily physical education for K–12 (down from 4 states in 1993).
- Alabama and Washington require daily physical education for K–8.
- Time requirements range from 50 to 200 min per week at the elementary level and from 55 to 275 min per week at the middle-school level.
- The majority of high school students take physical education for only 1 year between grades 9 and 12.
- Of students surveyed, 25% participate in physical education daily and 25% participate in no physical education.

(continued)

[a]Data from National Association for Sport and Physical Education. Shape of the nation report: a survey of state physical education requirements. NASPE, 1998.
[b]U.S. Department of Health and Human Services. Healthy people 2000: national health promotion and disease prevention objectives. Washington, DC: GPO, 1991.
[c]U.S. Department of Health and Human Services. The surgeon general's report on physical activity and health. Washington, DC: GPO, 1996.
[d]Centers for Disease Control and Prevention. Guidelines for school and community programs to promote lifelong physical activity among young people. MMWR 1997;46:1–36.
CDC, Centers for Disease Control and Prevention.

Corporate Wellness

The initiative established by *Healthy People 2000* (1) to improve the health of all Americans through an emphasis on prevention, not just treatment, will serve as a cornerstone for the direction of corporate wellness in the twenty-first century. One important goal of this initiative is to increase the proportion (> 85%) of workplaces with 50 or more employees that offer health promotion activities. As such, private industry may become a pivotal player in helping Americans choose healthy lifestyles, offering employment opportunities for exercise science professionals.

➤ *There is a need to provide a variety of physical and cognitive interventions to lessen the negative effect of stress at the work site. The exercise scientist can work with allied health professionals in developing supportive work environments and healthy interventions.*

VIABILITY OF PHYSICAL EDUCATION IN THE UNITED STATES

Category	Number of States by Type of School		
	Secondary	Middle	Elementary
Who teaches physical education?			
Certified physical education specialists	46	38	7
Certified physical education specialists and classroom teachers	4	11	39
Classroom teachers only	–	–	4
Certified physical education specialists or physical education aides	–	1	–
How many units are required for graduation?			
1 (1 year)	19		
2 (2 years)	6		
0	3		
0.5	6		
1.5	5		
Set by local school districts	11		
Grading practices?			
Grade given and included in grade point average	34		
Grade given and not included in grade point average	1		
Inclusion of grade in grade point average set by local school districts	15		
Substitutions allowed for physical education?			
No	23		
Yes	29		

The report concluded that physical education is woefully lacking the necessary federal, state, and local support, despite the wide recognition of its positive benefits. Although every state has a good undergraduate program to prepare certified physical education teachers, the current neglect given physical education at all levels of public education means that the demand for certified physical education teachers is far lower than the supply. This, therefore, poses dim prospects for physical education graduates finding teaching jobs in most states if they do not have credentials in other subject areas.

Budgetary cutbacks, expanded hours, increased administrative duties, and workload issues contribute to on-going job stress and employee health problems. Thus there is a need to provide a variety of physical and cognitive interventions to lessen the negative effect of stress on health. Wellness programs addressing the needs of all constituents in the corporate setting may be able to positively influence the development of good health practices and supportive environments.

Exercise science professionals entering the corporate wellness arena must be prepared to implement and design programs for a melting pot workplace that reflects a broad ethnic and cultural diversity. In addition, the marketplace is becoming much more global, offering several international career opportunities in work site health promotion programs (see Practical Application 5.2). For employment opportunities in corporate wellness contact the Association for Worksite Health Promotion, 60 Revere Dr., Suite 500, Northbrook, IL 60062 (847-480-9574); Welltech International (314-995-9838); or Health Promotion Recruiters International (www.hpridirect.com).

Wellness Programs

The range of opportunities in wellness programs is extensive and depends on the training and skills of the exercise science professional. Wellness professionals can work around the world in a variety of settings, including schools, medical sites, YMCAs, YWCAs, YMHAs, Boys and Girls Clubs, community centers (religious and nonaligned), and in communities. Additional wellness opportunities can be found in colleges, long-term care facilities, recreation depart-

---

Practical Application 5.2

INTERVIEW WITH A HEALTH AND WELLNESS MANAGER—CORPORATE SERVICES

What do you like about your job?

Helping people improve the quality of their life is wonderfully gratifying. In addition, I have never been bored with my job. My job responsibilities continue to challenge me. I feel as though I am constantly learning.

What is the biggest surprise of this job?

How much organization it takes to present successful programs and classes.

What are the pros of your job?

There is so much variety to all of the classes and programs I present. I regularly work with different people, of all socioeconomic incomes, and get a chance to facilitate positive lifestyle changes. I love giving presentations on anything related to fitness, health, and wellness. Also, my salary is quite satisfactory.

What are the cons of your job?

I wish I could impress upon people how to be more proactive about making behavior changes. This change process for people is slower than I had hoped. I am so busy that I often find myself missing my workouts, which bothers me. Also, I did not have any formal business education classes and I am having to learn how to do cost–benefit analyses on the job.

---

ments, aquatic centers, health management systems, and lifestyle management organizations. For employment opportunities in wellness programs contact the National Wellness Association, PO Box 827, Stevens Point, WI 54481 (800-244-8922).

Spa Fitness

To be classified as a residential spa by the International Spa and Fitness Association (I/SPA), a facility must include a fitness and nutrition component. Residential spas involve a stay over for one or more nights. The job opportunities in residential spas include fitness director, health and fitness instructors, and personal trainers. Because participants at spas are interested in many aspects of health and fitness, professionals must have a broad understanding of exercise, health, nutrition, and weight management information and be able to explain it well to others. Students who do their internships at spas often have a competitive edge in getting employment in this area. One of the drawbacks at spas is that staff often have to work during holidays or weekends, when spa use is high. A positive aspect of the spa industry is the ability to work in a beautiful setting. For more information contact I/SPA, 546 East Main St., Lexington, KY 40508 (888-651-4772) or Fodors Healthy Escapes, 201 East Fiftieth, New York, NY 10022 (212-572-2460).

Personal Training

Personal training is enjoying a surge of growth with exercise science professionals who have made careers out of helping people improve the quality of their life through a personalized approach to exercise. With personal training, it is important to recognize some of the additional responsibilities the job entails. Success in this field includes having some essential skills necessary to run a business. Personal trainers need to be able to promote, market, and sell their services. This also requires learning how to keep business records, handle budgets, and prepare tax information.

The personal trainer must be able to teach safe and effective exercise for each client. Much of this information will be gained through some of the leadership classes taken in an exercise science curriculum. Moreover, a large part of personal training is motivating clients to adopt a lifestyle of physical activity. Practical Application 5.3 shows highlights of a personal training industry survey conducted in 1996. The survey was commissioned by IDEA. Participants in the survey were selected randomly and balanced geographically across the nation from IDEA's list of personal trainer members (totaling approximately 8000). The response rate was 48%; data were used from 736 members who classified themselves primarily as personal trainers.

Individuals in personal training are branching out and establishing working ties with allied healthcare professionals to work with symptomatic individuals. Some personal trainers have established strong working relations with physicians' offices, community hospitals, and outpatient physical therapy groups to provide physical reconditioning, muscular fitness, and cardiovascular function and flexibility programs.

Before starting a personal training business, one may choose to work for an established fitness facility with a personal training structure in place. This can be an excellent way to build a clientele and gain exposure. There are a number of good resources for personal trainers who are looking for periodical information, resources, and conventions on personal training; contact IDEA (800-999-4332) or the National Strength and Conditioning Association (402-476-6669). In addition, several texts have been written on how to start and run a personal training business (see Suggested Reading).

Health Rehabilitation

Health rehabilitation is a catch-all category for a specialization of exercise science professionals working with people who have special needs or are at higher health risks. Special intervention training is required for working with individuals with neurologic, orthopedic, muscular, and cardiorespiratory deficiencies as well as seriously deconditioned and disabled individuals. The fuel for this interest in health rehabilitation stems from the apparent mission of the medical community to emphasize disease prevention and wellness through physical activity. Allied health fields in which the exercise science professional may choose to broaden career opportunities include occupational therapy, physical therapy, and dietetics. Each of these professions requires the exercise science student to compete for entry slots into these academic programs. The exercise science curriculum usually provides an excellent base from which to compete. Two popular subdisciplines of exercise science that fall under the health rehabilitation category are athletic training and clinical exercise physiology.

Occupational Therapy

Occupational therapists help individuals recover or maintain working skills and daily function. They work with individuals who have physically, mentally, emotionally, or developmentally crippling conditions. In many cases, the occupational therapist teaches clients how to compensate for some temporary or permanent loss of function. They often help patients learn or regain the ability to perform functions of daily living, such as eating, dressing, and preparing meals.

Most occupational therapists work in hospitals, school systems, community health centers, adult daycare centers, and in long-term care facilities. Because medical advances are making it possible for more people to survive injury and illness, positions for occupational therapists are increasing along with the demand for rehabilitation and long-term services. This profession demands additional biologic and behavioral science course work. For more information contact the

Practical Application 5.3

HIGHLIGHTS OF A PERSONAL TRAINING INDUSTRY SURVEY[a]

Start-up business costs: minimal

Operational costs: moderate

Limitations of income: number of hours willing to work; effective business planning

Industry growth: high

College graduate: 42% (19% postgraduate degree)

Certified: 94% yes

Sex: 23% male, 78% female

Client occupations: professional (28%), homemaker (20%), owner/proprietor (13%), executive management (8%), middle management (5%), healthcare (5%), student (4%), clerical (4%), sales (3%), service (2%), other (6%)

Average age of clients: 41 years (52% of clients 35–44 years)

Sex of clients: 26% male, 74% female

Legal business plan: 49% sole proprietorship

Typical business policies: medical history (96%), informed consent (87%), lifestyle history (81%), physician release (72%), cancellation policy (69%), written contracts for services (55%), refund policy (20%), chronic tardiness policy (19%)

Marketing methods: predominantly referrals

Services offered: personal training, group training (2–5 clients), fitness assessment, dietary assessment, supplement sales, equipment sales, sports massage

Average session fee: $41

Payment method used: 66% collect in advance, 54% collect at session, 23% invoice

Highest revenue month: January (73%), February (68%), March (61%), October (52%), April (51%), August (69%), July (67%), December (51%), June (45%)

Primary Work Location: Multipurpose health club, clients' homes, training facility

Average Salary for 38.5 hr/week: $33,800

---

[a]Adapted from IDEA. Personal trainer business survey. IDEA Personal Trainer 1997;8:25–42.

American Occupational Therapy Association, 4720 Montgomery Ln., PO Box 31220, Bethesda, MD 20824-1220 (301-652-2682).

Physical Therapy

Physical therapists help clients improve mobility, reduce pain, and prevent or limit permanent disability. A wide variety of treatment plans for patients are designed after the professional conducts tests to measure the client's muscular fitness, range of motion, and function. The majority of physical therapists work in private offices and hospitals. Other employment settings include rehabilitation centers, home health agencies, long-term care facilities, and school systems. Owing to the growing demand for rehabilitation and long-term care services, the physical therapy profession has a bright future. All entry-level physical therapy academic programs are now at the master's degree level; therefore, exercise science students pursuing this profession must attend a graduate school. Extra science courses are also required. For more information contact the American Physical Therapy Association, 1111 North Fairfax St., Alexandria, VA 22314 (703-684-2782).

Athletic Training

Athletic trainers are sports medicine professionals who are involved in managing, recognizing, and preventing sports injuries. Athletic trainers work closely with coaches and physicians to best prepare athletes for practice and competition. Athletic training has a broad job market, with work opportunities in universities, colleges, secondary schools, professional sports, industrial health care programs, health clubs, and sports medicine centers. In addition to the exercise science curriculum, advanced courses in athletic injury prevention are required as well as approximately 800 hr of athletic training experience in a supervised setting. Refer to Chapter 14 for a comprehensive description of athletic training. For more information contact the National Athletic Training Association, 2952 Stemmons Fwy., Dallas, TX 75247 (800-879-6282 or 214-637-6282).

Clinical Exercise Physiology

Clinical exercise physiologists work with people who have a variety of chronic pathologic conditions, including cardiovascular, respiratory, and metabolic diseases, for which participation in physical activity has a known therapeutic or functional benefit. Clinical exercise physiologists keep appropriate records for the duration of treatment to determine the effectiveness of the treatment. Employment opportunities exist in hospitals, health centers, and cardiac rehabilitation centers. In addition to the exercise science curriculum, advanced courses in electrocardiography and pathophysiology are required. Certification is also becoming increasingly important to enter this job market. Refer to Chapter 11 for a comprehensive description of clinical exercise physiology. For more information contact the American Association of Cardiovascular and Pulmonary Rehabilitation (608-831-6989).

DIETETICS Dietitians develop and implement nutritional programs after assessing the nutritional needs of individuals in long-term care facilities, medical institutions, health departments, social service agencies, residential care facilities, school systems, or hospitals. They generally must coordinate their efforts with other healthcare practitioners who are treating the same clients. Dietitians also advise patients on a number of health-related conditions, including weight loss, diabetes control, high blood pressure control, and cholesterol reduction. They may educate special populations (e.g., the elderly and AIDS and cancer patients) about effective nutritional practices. Exercise science students pursuing this profession take additional courses in nutrition, chemistry, physiology, microbiology, and institution management. For more information, contact the American Dietetic Association, 216 West Jackson Blvd., Chicago, IL 60606 (800-877-1600).

Teaching and Higher Education

Two fields historically related to exercise science are health education and physical education. Degrees in these areas require students to pursue academic credentials in a teacher preparation program. Teacher certification must be attained by passing a national competency examination. This usually qualifies the individual for teaching assignments in grades K–12. Professionals in these fields may also be asked to perform some coaching assignments as part of their employment.

There are also a number of opportunities for exercise science professionals to teach at the community college level. Most of these opportunities require having a master's degree in the field. Individuals following this path primarily teach sports skills classes (e.g., tennis, volleyball, and badminton); lifetime physical activity classes (e.g., group exercise, jogging, and weight training); and introductory classes in health, nutrition, and exercise science. For more information about programs and job opportunities, contact the American Alliance of Health, Physical Education, Recreation and Dance, 1900 Association Dr., Reston, VA 22091 (800-321-0789).

Students who wish to pursue a research career must have an advanced degree in a particular area of exercise science. Individuals with doctoral training may choose from a number of disciplines, including exercise physiology, biomechanics, physical activity epidemiology, motor behavior, sports psychology, cardiac rehabilitation, environmental physiology, exercise biochemistry, neuroscience, occupational physiology, pediatric exercise physiology, psychology and behavior, therapeutic exercise, and exercise and aging. Advanced expertise in these areas usually leads to employment at universities, colleges, medical institutes, hospitals, and medical research centers. To learn more about graduate programs around the country that offer advanced education in the field of exercise science, contact the American College of Sports Medicine, PO Box 1440, Indianapolis, IN 46206 (317-637-9200; fax: 317-634-7817). For employment opportunities in higher education contact Human Kinetics, PO Box 5076, Champaign, IL 61825 (800-747-4457) or the Chronicle of Higher Education, 1235 Twenty-third St. NW, Washington, DC 20037 (202-466-1000).

Fitness Specialties

Fitness specialties include a multitude of nontraditional opportunities for the exercise science professional not covered in any of the above categories. Because the training of the exercise science professional is quite diverse, a number of specialty tracks are open for career direction. Some of these alternative tracks may entail additional education or training.

Considerations for exercise science professionals who wish to apply their abilities in related fields include chiropractic health, exercise equipment design, exercise science software development, fitness and nutrition center manager or owner, fitness product marketing and sales, fitness writing and publishing (newspapers, periodicals, and books), exercise science seminars and programs, military fitness, pharmaceutical sales, shoe company consultant, and sports nutrition. For more information on different vocations associated with the fitness industry, contact Fitness Management, 3923 West Sixth St., #407, Los Angeles, CA 90020 (213-385-3926) to obtain the *Fitness Management Source Guide.*

With all of the different career paths to choose from, the exercise science discipline is wide open for students who have the appropriate credentials. It is advisable for the exercise science professional to develop a career plan that includes interests and areas of expertise. Interview exercise science professionals in your area of interest, attend conferences, go to association meetings, and network with colleagues. By considering all of your career options early in your educational process, you will be more prepared for the challenging opportunities that await you.

SUMMARY POINTS

- As the world evolves from an industry-based economy toward an information-based society, exercise science professionals are developing more intercommunication and involvement with the other allied health professions.
- The exercise scientist plays a fundamental role in determining the appropriate sequencing and progression of interventions for improving and maintaining the adherence to and compliance with health and physical activity programs. In addition, the exercise science profession has become involved with enhancing the quality of life for seriously deconditioned and disabled populations.

- The four evolving career areas of growth in exercise science are health and fitness, health rehabilitation, teaching and higher education, and fitness specialties.
- Within the fitness industry, growing areas of career emphasis include elderly fitness programs, exercise programs for youth, and aquatic exercise programs.
- A growing career area for exercise science professionals is health rehabilitation. This catch-all category is for a specialization of exercise science professionals working with people who have special needs or are at higher health risks. The growth in health rehabilitation careers stems from a mission of the medical community to emphasize disease prevention and wellness through physical activity.
- Exercise science professionals choosing to follow a track of advanced education have numerous disciplines from which to select. Expertise in higher education areas usually leads to employment at universities, colleges, national medical institutes, hospitals, and medical research centers.

REVIEW QUESTIONS

1. Describe the expanding role of the exercise science professional.
2. Name and describe four evolving employment areas of growth in the field of exercise science.
3. Identify and describe the different career paths that may be pursued in the health and fitness domain.
4. Explain where the exercise science professional may work within the area of health rehabilitation.

References

1. U.S. Department of Health and Human Services. Healthy people 2000: national health promotion and disease prevention objectives. Washington, DC: GPO, 1991.
2. Curtis O, Penrose T. The field of exercise science. ACHPER Healthy Lifestyles J 1996;43:9–14.
3. Brock D, Guralnick J, Brody J. Demography and epidemiology of aging in the US. In: E Schneider, J Rowe, eds. Handbook of the biology of aging. San Diego, CA: Academic Press, 1990:3–23.

Suggested Readings

Fleck SJ, Kraemer WJ. Designing resistance training programs. 2nd ed. Champaign, IL: Human Kinetics, 1997.
Howley ET, Franks BD. Health fitness instructor's handbook. 3rd ed. Champaign, IL: Human Kinetics, 1997.
O'Brien TS. The personal trainer's handbook. Champaign, IL: Human Kinetics, 1997.
Wilson BRA, Glaros TE. Managing health promotion programs. Champaign, IL: Human Kinetics, 1996.

6

Management and Marketing Concerns

BRIAN C. LYONS AND KIRK L. WAKEFIELD

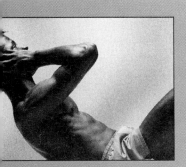

Objectives

1. Identify the role of management, including its major functions.
2. Explain the components of the program development cycle.
3. Explain the importance of leadership in the managerial process, both at the organizational and at the individual client levels.
4. Explain what risk management is.
5. Describe the basic components of a marketing strategy, including examples tailored for the exercise and fitness industry.
6. Describe the unique characteristics of sports marketing and how it differs from the marketing of other services.
7. Apply key marketing concepts to the management of sports, health, and fitness centers.

When one thinks of the field of exercise science, invariably the subdiscipline of exercise physiology, sports biomechanics, or motor behavior comes to mind. Perhaps thoughts of related course work in psychology, statistics, and the basic sciences also emerge. Rarely, however, does one ponder the importance of sound administration, **management,** and marketing skills to leisure, sports, and fitness programs and businesses. This is unfortunate because, although sports and exercise programs certainly rely on the expertise of the scientist, management facilitates the smooth achievement of the organizational mission, and marketing ensures that fiscal success is achieved. This chapter examines topics that are important to sound administrative practice in leisure, sports, and fitness programs.

SPORTS AND FITNESS MANAGEMENT

In today's marketplace success depends on the ability to manage. This section examines issues relevant for the aspiring sport manager.

The Managerial Role

Management can be considered the art and science of facilitating the effective and efficient achievement of organizational **goals.** It involves functions such as planning, organizing, leading, and controlling. Managers must be adept at generating human, fiscal, physical, and technological resources as well as judiciously using and allocating them (1).

The wording of this definition warrants deeper consideration. What is meant by *art, science, effective,* and *efficient?* The artistic dimension of the manager is being intuitive, flexible, creative, and innovative. The scientific aspect, in contrast, is being rational and determined. The term *effective* refers to behaviors and decisions that do, in fact, bring the organization closer to achieving its goals. *Efficiency* refers to the process of using minimal resources while being maximally effective. In other words, to be effective is "to do the right thing," and to be efficient is "to do the right thing right."

Human resources include exercise scientists, coaches, leisure leaders, administrative assistants, and many others. Fiscal resources involve money for salaries, equipment, and the maintenance of facilities. Physical resources can be natural or synthetic (e.g., hiking trails, pools, laboratories, classrooms, and gymnasia). Examples of technological resources are computer software, metabolic carts, cinematographic equipment, and fax machines.

An illustration of the managerial role should clarify these concepts. Managers operate under a general paradigm known as the **program development cycle** (Fig. 6.1). The program development cycle is an ongoing process that begins with an understanding of the purpose of the business or organization. Once the purpose is clearly defined, needs must be identified. Then goals and **objectives,** which are designed to address the needs, are developed. Planning, implementation, and **evaluation** of the program then occur.

> *Setting goals is not enough. Plans must engineer a path to goal achievement and devise means to keep the path clear.*

For example, a recent exercise science graduate is hired as the director of the newly opened Ironworks Body Shop, a commercial health club that caters to a middle-class, urban clientele. The new director will certainly need to address several issues immediately. What is the mission of the organization? How many other personnel will be needed to achieve the mission? What equipment is available and what equipment is needed? What are the actual and expected revenues and expenditures of the club? Can the revenue–cost relationship be improved? How? What other organizations offer similar services, i.e., who is the competition? What are the organization's strengths, weaknesses, opportunities, and threats? These are but a few of the questions that a manager must address.

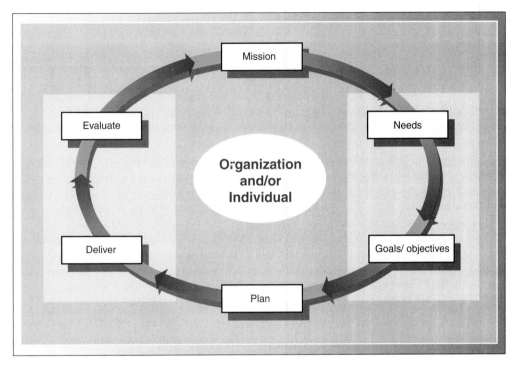

FIGURE 6.1 Program development cycle.

The mission, or purpose, of this organization is primarily to make a profit. Accomplishing this involves complex, innovative, creative, rational, and calculative decision making. Decisions that improve the clients' quality of life and, consequently, client satisfaction are generally effective. Wise and frugal decisions that result in improved client satisfaction and simultaneously use minimal organizational resources are not only effective but efficient.

The accomplishment of the mission requires a complement of professionals. One person acting alone cannot fulfill the mission. The director must decide, for example, if exercise physiologists, biomechanists, strength coaches, and administrative personnel are needed. Perhaps specialists are appropriate, but exercise leaders with a general exercise science background would suffice. Should the exercise leaders be certified, and should they be required to hold baccalaureate degrees? If hiring certified holders of college degrees is desirable, can the organization afford their salaries? Is the resistance training equipment safe, contemporary, technically sound, and attractive? What about the cardiovascular equipment? Is the facility adequate for the necessary programs? Who has the expertise to run the aquatic programs? Who should be in charge of **risk management?** In any organization, managers must prioritize their goals to fulfill the organization's mission effectively and efficiently. Often, the decisions involve costs and benefits, and it is the manager who strives to maintain the most auspicious benefit to cost ratio. Managers must be capable of seeing the "big picture," they must have vision, and they must think globally while acting locally.

The list of potential issues that leisure, sports, and fitness managers must address is well beyond the scope of this chapter. In fact, no text can provide all of the answers to the manager. Management involves a systematic approach designed to increase effectiveness and efficiency. The decision-making process is influenced by the philosophy, personality, and style of the manager, as well as the mission of the organization, available resources, competition, and clientele. In general, managers seek to satisfy wants and needs while simultaneously conserving resources. To accomplish this, managers must become proficient at planning, organizing, leading, and controlling. It is important to understand that these techniques can, to a significant extent, be learned.

There probably are no "natural born" managers; the growth and maturation of a manager comes only with time.

Organizational Program Development

Planning is necessary to realize organizational goals and objectives. An old managerial axiom proclaims that "Failing to plan is like planning to fail." It is logical that the formulation of organizational goals should be contingent on the mission of the organization, taking into account its strengths and weaknesses.

Thus the first task of a manger is to perform an organizational needs assessment. The assessment is designed to ascertain if the **leadership,** facilities, and programs are adequate and whether they can be improved. This assessment is most often informal and addresses the **organizational triad** (Fig. 6.2). All organizations are based on three foundational cornerstones: leadership, facilities and equipment, and programs. In the example of the Ironworks Body Shop, the director, personal trainers, marketing specialists, and janitorial personnel represent organizational leaders. The facilities and equipment can include weight rooms, aerobic studios, locker rooms, saunas, sand volleyball courts, and physiologic assessment rooms. The programs lie at the heart of this organization and could include exercise science workshops, stress management classes, a power-lifting club, and a martial arts class for children.

Once the assessment has been completed, goals and objectives are developed to focus the attention of the leaders and illuminate the direction of the organization. The goals and objectives address weaknesses and improve strengths, serving as a road map that facilitates the organization's effective and efficient journey to the desired destination, which is reflected in the achievement of the mission. Goals are broad, long-term general indicators of desired outcomes, whereas objectives tend to be short-term, more specific, and measurable.

Various types of goals are used to assist in the planning process. Common categories of goals include mission statements, **strategic goals, tactical goals,** and operational goals. Each of these types of goals reflects a different level of organizational management. For example, a **mission statement** is a written manifesto of the organization's purpose and reflects the organization's philosophy. Thus mission statements are most often generated by the organization's founders or the highest level of administrators. Strategic goals are generated by high-level managers and provide general direction for the organization. Tactical goals are generated by middle-level managers and provide guidance for achieving the strategic goals. Finally, operational goals, which are often re-

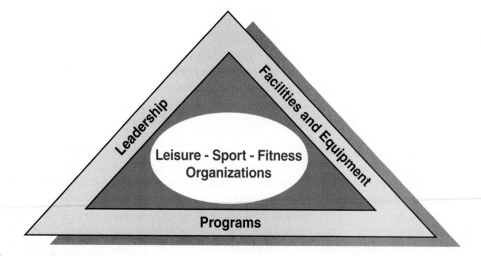

FIGURE 6.2 Organizational triad.

ferred to as objectives, are usually generated by supervisors and are designed to achieve the tactical goals. Operational goals are unique in that they are measurable and specific (1).

Refer to A Case in Point 6.1 for an example of how these various types of goals can work in a business. Notice that the goals are interrelated, hierarchical, and pyramidal; there is generally only one mission statement but many operational goals. The goals should be written and they should become increasingly more specific so it is possible to ascertain whether they have been achieved.

Organizational Planning

Although the development of goals helps focus an organization, goals alone cannot ensure that its mission will be accomplished. For each type of goal, there usually exists a corresponding plan. Thus strategic, tactical, and operational plans serve as blueprints for the achievement of goals. One of the most important aspects of plan formulation is the solicitation of input from all of the individuals who will have a role in affecting the realization of the goals.

Consider a simple example: A new, zealous director believes that revenues from memberships must be increased and decides that one way to accomplish this is to increase participation in all fitness-related programs. At first, this seems quite reasonable. However, the director, acting alone, creates and imposes a new goal stating that enrollment in the aerobic dance classes will increase 20%. He has not conferred with the supervisor of the aerobic dance instructors or spoken to the aerobic instructors. As it turns out, the aerobic dance classes are already extremely crowded, and new classes would be difficult to offer because the room is already being used for the children's karate classes and some yoga classes.

When the goal of increased aerobic dance participation is not achieved, who should be held responsible? Obviously, it is the director's responsibility, but an inept manager may attempt to shed responsibility and blame others. The situation is exacerbated if the aerobic dance instructors' salary increases are tied to goal achievement, i.e., if the aerobic instructors are denied salary increases because they did not meet a goal for which they had no input. Morale and performance will suffer greatly.

Planning can be a formidable and cumbersome process. The art of planning involves covering most of the concerns of the organization while, at the same time, requiring as little of the managerial team's time and effort as is reasonably possible. In other words, planning is essential, but managers cannot spend all of their time planning, which would also be counterproductive.

Delivery and Implementation

Eventually, the plans must be operationalized, or implemented, and the clients must be served. Acknowledging that the exercise science profession is a people profession, health and fitness clubs, cardiac rehabilitation programs, athletic programs, and personal fitness training all ostensibly involve the transformation of people. People are not simply biochemical machines but are whole beings with physiologic, psychological, and spiritual dimensions. The client is not interested in services but seeks a positive experience. An experience is stored in long-term memory; when positive, it is recalled repeatedly, and its recurrence is eagerly anticipated. When a person in a cardiac rehabilitation program is introduced to tai chi, the feeling of tranquility coupled with newfound vitality represents a positive experience. Ultimately then, most goals and their associated plans should be devised to provide positive experiences, not just services. Better equipment, clean and spacious facilities, and knowledgeable and courteous leaders all improve the clients' experience.

Evaluation

Once the goals have been formulated and the plans implemented, an evaluation should be undertaken to ascertain the efficacy of the programs. Have the goals been met? This explains why it is

Leadership Styles

It is generally agreed that three distinct leadership styles exist, although managers may employ various combinations of these styles. The autocratic leader is extremely task oriented and expects full compliance in carrying out orders or instructions. This is a militaristic type of leader. Little input is elicited before decisions are made. This individual lives by the my-way-or-the-highway philosophy. In contrast, the hands-off style, or **laissez-faire leadership** approach, is people oriented. This leader usually expects the group to come to a consensus rather than imposing his or her will on the group. Laissez-faire leaders serve the role of group facilitator, and input is elicited from those involved. The **democratic leadership** style falls somewhere in the middle. Generally, the democratic leader elicits input from those involved and then makes a decision (4).

The best leadership style probably depends on the situation. **Autocratic leadership** is expeditious and most appropriate when decisions need to be made quickly. If Ironworks Body Shop were to catch on fire and clients were in danger of being trapped, it would not be advisable to call a meeting to investigate possible options. Quick decisions would have to be made, and strict compliance with the orders would be expected.

Laissez-faire decision making promotes creativity and responsibility. Because the leader will not make the decision, the others involved must assert themselves and provide input. When deciding which type of resistance-training equipment should be purchased, input from all individuals affected should be sought, and a consensus should be reached. Unfortunately, the laissez-faire approach is slow.

The democratic style is reasonably expeditious and at the same time incorporates input from others. Most decisions in sports and fitness management should be reached via a democratic process.

If leadership involves influence, the power of the leader must be examined. **Leadership power** may be considered the degree to which the leader's techniques or behaviors are influential. Leaders with little power will have little influence, and those with much power will have greater influence. Power can be derived from several sources, and consequently there are several types of power (5).

Legitimate power is derived from the rank, or position, of the individual in charge. That is, by virtue of the fact that the person is the director, he or she has influence. This is the most tenuous type of power, and this power orientation is easily eroded by incompetence. Expert power results from having some knowledge or ability that is unique and needed. If a staff of exercise leaders includes only one person with knowledge of structural kinesiology, this individual will have the most influence when dealing with questions involving functional musculoskeletal anatomy as it relates to resistance training. Individuals gain referent power when others have positive feelings about them. A pleasant, humorous, helping personality often allows an individual to influence others. If the leader is well liked, he or she is likely to be influential. Finally, reward and coercive power is derived from the ability of the leader to provide praise and incentives and to dole out punishment. Leaders who influence promotions and make decisions concerning retention of employees have the ability to influence others. Obviously, a given leader can possess one or all of these types of power. The more power a leader has, the more influential he or she can be.

Leadership Theories

One of the earliest theories of leadership espouses that certain traits or characteristics are common among leaders. This approach has been referred to by several names, including the trait theory, great man theory, or universal behaviors theory of leadership (3,6). This theory states that great leaders have specific traits—such as honesty, intelligence, charisma, motivation, and vision. Research designed to test this viewpoint has revealed that certain characteristics are, in fact, somewhat common among effective leaders. These characteristics include intelligence, effective organizational skills, the ability to overcome situational inertia, the ability to engender and maintain organizational cohesiveness, and the ability to communicate (6–8). Although this viewpoint is appealing and the research seems to indicate that certain traits may be common among effective leaders, no particular characteristic or set of characteristics can adequately explain the variations among leaders. Trait theorists have failed to identify any specific characteristics that are essential to effective leadership, and this approach also fails to take into account the effect of numerous situational variables.

The contingency model of leadership looks at the leader's approach and the level of situational favorableness (9). Three factors serve to determine the degree of situational favorableness: the relationship between the leader and follower, the task structure, and the perceived or real power of the leader. In explaining the concept of situational favorableness, Lyons (2) states that "warm, trusting relationships, clearly defined tasks, and a leader in a position to reward and punish engender situational favorableness. In contrast, relationships characterized by mistrust and animosity, ambiguous objectives, and leaders with little authority clearly are not situations which are conducive to situational favorableness." The contingency model promotes the idea that, when situational favorableness is extraordinarily low or high, leader influence is optimized by using a task-oriented approach. When situational favorableness is moderate, an effective leader should employ a people-oriented approach to optimize influence. The contingency theory has been criticized for suggesting that leaders are either task oriented or people oriented, without taking into account that most effective leaders are simultaneously both (10). It has, nonetheless, elevated the importance of situational variables in the leadership equation.

The path–goal theory of leadership emphasizes the facilitative role of the leader. In this approach, the leader is seen as the individual who provides incentives for success while removing obstacles from the subordinate's path (11). The leader plays a facilitative role, whereby he or she works for the subordinate by supporting the staff member or client. Instead of the athletic director telling individual coaches what to do, he or she might ask what the individual coaches need and if there are problems. When problems arise, the athletic director would try to solve these problems, thereby removing obstacles that lie in the coaches' paths.

The life cycle theory of leadership, also referred to as the situational theory of leadership, was developed by Hersey and Blanchard (12), and it deals with subordinate maturity levels. Leadership, according to this approach, must evolve along with the evolution of the staff member or client. Subordinate maturity reflects the level of knowledge, skill, and ability accrued. Rookie baseball players, for example, have relatively low baseball knowledge, skill, and ability. Conversely, a 9-year, three-time league MVP in baseball has relatively high baseball knowledge, skill, and ability. Different approaches are warranted to lead the beginner and the expert.

According to the life cycle theory of leadership, managers manifest both relationship and task behaviors. Relationship behaviors include listening, supporting, and encouraging. Task behaviors include technical exercise instruction, use of computers, and advertising techniques. When dealing with a novice client, exercise and sports leaders should be task oriented, placing emphasis on explaining and demonstrating proper procedures and safe exercise techniques. As the client matures and develops skills and abilities, the leader should begin to emphasize relationship behavior and task development. The client still needs instruction regarding exercise technique but now also requires emotional support and guidance to adhere to the program and remain motivated. As the client develops even further, exercise technique is mastered, and adherence and motivation are the primary concerns of the leader, who must encourage and guide.

Finally, the client becomes a self-sufficient participant. When motivation is high and the technique has been mastered, the role of the exercise leader is minimized. Both task and relationship behaviors are attenuated. Thus when subordinates' knowledge, skill, and ability are low, the leader's behavior is task oriented and essentially autocratic; once subordinates' knowledge, skill, and ability have developed, the leader's behavior becomes more laissez-faire. The key point in this theory is that leaders must evolve as the clients or players evolve. No one approach or style will be effective under all circumstances.

Risk Management

An emerging concern of leisure, sports, and fitness managers is the concept of risk management (13). **Legal liability** refers to the responsibilities and duties that exist among people and that are enforceable by law. The manager of an organization that serves people has certain legal responsibilities; if those responsibilities are not met, legal action can be taken against the manager and/or the business. **Torts** are civil wrongdoings composed of three key elements: There must be a breach of legal duty, this breach of duty must be the proximate cause of an injury, and an actual injury must have occurred (13).

The type of tort that represents the greatest concern for leisure, sports, and fitness managers is **negligence.** Negligence exists when one acts or fails to act in a reasonable and prudent manner, and the result of this commission or omission is an injury (13). It is important to note that the injury can be physical, mental, and/or financial. Some examples of reasonable and prudent legal duties include a duty to warn of hidden dangers, a duty to provide proper instruction, a duty to maintain safe facilities, and a duty to employ competent leaders (see Practical Application 6.1).

If negligence has occurred, the injured party may sue for damages in civil court. Managers should be aware of what is referred to as the deep-pockets doctrine. When an injury occurs, it is not uncommon for the injured party's lawyers to sue all persons who are directly or even remotely associated with the incident. The purpose of suing everyone is to increase the chance that someone with the actual ability to pay damages will be found liable. In leisure, sports, and fitness liability cases, program sponsors, board members, independent contractors, administrators, supervisors, and leaders have been sued. Although being sued does not necessarily mean that one will ultimately be held liable, the mere process of defending oneself against such law suits is time-consuming, expensive, and personally and professionally taxing.

There are defenses against negligence claims. First the plaintiff does have to establish that an actual injury has occurred. If there is no injury, then there is no negligence. This defense is particularly important when the alleged injury is mental or financial in nature. Second, the injury

---

Practical Application 6.1

NEGLIGENCE

Every employee and participant must understand that safety is paramount. Safety is not simply the business of the manager, it is everyone's business. Facilities must be inspected regularly, and a written report of the results should be kept on file. Any unsafe situations must be handled expeditiously, and when appropriate action is taken it should be documented. Part of the organizational triad involves leadership. Managers must make every attempt to hire qualified persons, and managers must ensure that these persons continue to upgrade their knowledge, skills, and abilities. In other words, hiring someone who is certified in cardiopulmonary resuscitation (CPR) is fine, but if the certification expires, what good is it if someone has a cardiac event? Clients must be deemed healthy enough to participate in vigorous activities, pointing to the importance of administering a health status survey. If the client is not in the best of health but is still cleared to participate, all those who are likely to work with the client should be apprised of the client's condition. Clients must be provided with sufficient instruction regarding equipment and technique. Clients must be appropriately supervised at all times. Written emergency procedures should be well established and periodically practiced. Practice of such procedures should be documented. If an accident occurs, make sure a detailed accident report is filled out.

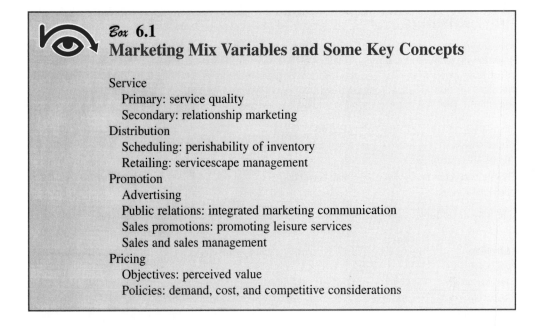

Box **6.1**
Marketing Mix Variables and Some Key Concepts

Service
  Primary: service quality
  Secondary: relationship marketing
Distribution
  Scheduling: perishability of inventory
  Retailing: servicescape management
Promotion
  Advertising
  Public relations: integrated marketing communication
  Sales promotions: promoting leisure services
  Sales and sales management
Pricing
  Objectives: perceived value
  Policies: demand, cost, and competitive considerations

do you expect management to do? Not all customer expectations are equally important. The service manager's job is to determine which are most critical to the target market and to manage them accordingly.

Expectations can be managed by informing and framing customers' expectations. Everyone who has been to a Disney theme park knows that the lines to the best rides can be long. But how does Disney manage your expectations? They post signs at turns along the serpentine waiting line that estimate how long the wait will be from that point. In fact, the wait typically takes less time than what was posted. Why? It is better for management to overestimate the time required and then provide the service under that time. In doing so, customer expectations and service goals have been set. When the service takes less time than expected, customers are satisfied. The worst waits are uninformed and boring waits (15). Consumers who are informed about the service process and are occupied while waiting (e.g., watching TV monitors of the game at concession stands) tend to underestimate waiting time.

Relationship marketing has been an important buzzword since about 1990, but the concept has been around since at least early biblical times. Relationship marketing focuses on making and keeping relationships with customers over the long term. People naturally want to conduct business with individuals they know and trust. Increasing employee–customer contact, providing consistently excellent service, handling complaints efficiently and effectively, and providing fair prices are all ways to enhance relationships. In short, the Golden Rule (treating others as you would like them to treat you if you were the customer) will lead to good customer relationships. A major motivating factor in relationship marketing is the fact that it costs more to get new customers than it does to keep current customers.

Distribution

Sports and fitness marketing is different from typical product marketing because of the **perishability of inventory** (16). The inventory of sports and fitness operators is time and space, which cannot be stored for future use. Whereas a retail outlet can store unsold merchandise to be available the next day, the inventory of sports operators perishes with each passing minute. That unsold box-seat or unfilled appointment time cannot be saved and resold later. As a result, managers must schedule and price service offerings in such a way as to maximize revenue.

▶▶ Sidelight 6.1

EVALUATING SERVICE QUALITY

Your university is providing a service (education) for which you pay a price (tuition, time, effort). How do you evaluate the service quality you are receiving? Service quality is evaluated on the basis of how well the service meets or exceeds customers' expectations. Students will likely enumerate a number of expectations they had when coming to the university and how well these expectations were met. The chart below gives some examples.

Expected	Received	Consequence
Small classes	Large freshmen classes	Dissatisfied
Professional instruction	Gifted professors	Satisfied
Boring basic courses	Boring basic courses	Neither dissatisfied nor satisfied
Personal advising	Group or impersonal advising	Dissatisfied

One way to understand this concept is to mark expectations on a scale like the one given here.

Attribute	Not at all what I expected				Just about what I expected			Much better than I expected		
Class size	1	2	3	4	5	6	7	8	9	10
Teacher quality	1	2	3	4	5	6	7	8	9	10
Social life	1	2	3	4	5	6	7	8	9	10
Dorm quality	1	2	3	4	5	6	7	8	9	10

The higher the mark on this 1 to 10 scale, the more satisfied you are likely to be.

The demand for service typically fluctuates on a weekly, monthly, and seasonal basis. People tend to recreate more on weekends than on weekdays. Paydays at the first and middle of the month tend to lead to increased business. People tend to be outdoors during the spring and summer. During high-demand periods, managers typically schedule events or programs priced at levels (i.e., full-price) that maximize attendance given a limited supply of time and space. During low-demand periods, prices are often reduced to maximize participation. For example, price discounts may be useful to attract customers to games or programs offered on Tuesdays or for games against poor opponents. High-quality services should be able to maintain prices (or even charge premiums) during prime time. Obviously, appropriate personnel must be scheduled to meet the expected demand at low and high periods.

For many sports and fitness venues, the customer essentially pays for admission to the facilities for a given amount of time. Customers are likely to base their willingness to commit themselves to spending time in a facility based on the quality of the **servicescape** (17). The servicescape is the ambience and design factors that make up the facility environment (18). Figure 6.3 shows an example of a customer survey that outlines the different aspects of the servicescape. Customers who perceive that the quality of the servicescape does not meet their expectations are unlikely to attend many games, join the club, or return frequently to the organization. Managers should periodically survey customers in a systematic fashion to determine their perceptions of the facility and its services. Without reliable customer input, managers tend to become accustomed to faults in the facility (e.g., cracking paint or broken machines or equipment) that may be motivating customers not to return.

Promotion

The promotion mix consists of four components: advertising, public relations, sales promotions, and sales and sales management. Organizations should strive for **integrated marketing communications** (IMC) in which all information presents a clear image with one voice (19). An objective of IMC is for customers to be able to consistently associate a positive image with the or-

Rate the facility on each of the items below

Poor   Excellent

Ambient Factors

Music selection	1	2	3	4	5	6	7	8	9	10
Music volume	1	2	3	4	5	6	7	8	9	10
Lighting	1	2	3	4	5	6	7	8	9	10
Temperature	1	2	3	4	5	6	7	8	9	10
Air quality	1	2	3	4	5	6	7	8	9	10
Food quality	1	2	3	4	5	6	7	8	9	10
Cleanliness	1	2	3	4	5	6	7	8	9	10
Staff appearance	1	2	3	4	5	6	7	8	9	10

Facility Design Factors

Location convenience	1	2	3	4	5	6	7	8	9	10
Parking access/exit	1	2	3	4	5	6	7	8	9	10
External appearance	1	2	3	4	5	6	7	8	9	10
Internal appearance	1	2	3	4	5	6	7	8	9	10
Layout accessibility	1	2	3	4	5	6	7	8	9	10
Seating comfort	1	2	3	4	5	6	7	8	9	10
Facility equipment	1	2	3	4	5	6	7	8	9	10
Directional signage	1	2	3	4	5	6	7	8	9	10
Overall Quality	1	2	3	4	5	6	7	8	9	10

FIGURE 6.3 Servicescapes.

ganization. For example, Nike maintains consistency with its trademark swoosh. Whenever you see a Nike ad, clothing, or shoes, you see the swoosh. All of Nike's communications are geared toward making its name and the swoosh mean quality.

Similarly, sports and fitness organizations need to integrate all of their communications to promote a clear, consistent image. Advertising messages should not conflict with sales promotion messages. For instance, an organization wanting to promote a high-quality service image to an upper-class clientele through their advertisements should not run frequent price discounts. Decisions regarding advertisements, sales promotions, personal selling, and public relations are not made independently. This is a particular risk for smaller firms in which managers can wear many different hats and consequently may not take the time to monitor and integrate all of their promotional activities. An organization should select an appropriate image and stick with it.

Customers patronize sporting events and fitness centers primarily for emotional rather than for functional reasons (19). Some customers may be motivated to exercise for their health, but many more are likely to be motivated by the consequences of being in shape, e.g., they will feel better about themselves and others will find them more attractive. Customers go to sporting events for the excitement and social interaction. The fact that these are more emotional, or psychosocial, motivations influences what kinds of sales promotions are likely to be effective in attracting customers.

A common misconception is that organizations must give price discounts to attract customers. This is often true for products for which there is little differentiation and which are bought with disposable income (e.g., groceries). However, products or services that are differentiated and bought from discretionary income can effectively attract customers with nonprice promotions that focus on delivering emotional benefits. For example, gift with purchase (or giveaways), extra programs, contests, celebrity appearances, and sweepstakes can all be used to generate excitement or interest without directly reducing revenue via price cuts. Unless the organization's objective is to be known as having the lowest prices around, price discounts should be carefully targeted for specific situations (e.g., grand openings or senior citizen groups).

Pricing

Perceived value can be defined as what one gives for what one gets (20). Consumers want to know that what they get is worth the money they pay for it. Consumers are likely to evaluate the value of a sporting event, fitness center, or health clinic based on employee service quality, servicescape quality, and any tangible product quality. In the sporting event setting, the employees include the players involved in providing the primary service and the service personnel supplying the secondary services. Conceptually, an organization should set prices that are in line with organizational goals and that produce value in the minds of consumers.

Having low prices does not necessarily mean high value to consumers. Consumers with ample income are willing to pay more for a Porsche than the sum total of its production costs. Think about some of the most popular restaurants in your area. Odds are that they do not necessarily have the lowest priced meals. Rather, they charge prices that reflect their customers' beliefs that they are getting their money's worth: excellent service, an interesting servicescape, and high-quality food. Unless the organization is pursuing an image as a low-cost provider, the ideal situation is to differentiate the organization on the basis of customer service, facility quality, and/or product quality, and price the product or service accordingly.

Many times, organizations set prices based on average cost considerations or customary pricing policies (e.g., 50% markup). Clearly, the organization's costs must be covered to remain in business. However, costs do not have to be directly covered on every service or product offered. For example, fitness center membership prices can be relatively low if profits from additional services purchased after gaining membership will provide indirect compensation. Similarly, tickets can be discounted to sell out an otherwise unfilled stadium when the team is playing against a weak opponent because selling one more ticket does not add any additional costs and additional revenue from concession sales might compensate for the opportunity cost of charging a lower ticket price than normal.

Consumers' perceived value of the organization's prices is strongly influenced by what the competition is charging. Remember, consumers will be dissatisfied when their expectations are not met. Consumers develop reference prices (or expectations) based on their shopping experiences. Consumers evaluate the prices offered by the organization by comparing the price to their reference price. If the price doesn't meet with what they expected, they will likely be dissatisfied and unlikely to buy. Thus organizations must frequently monitor competitors' prices and consumers' value perceptions.

SUMMARY POINTS

- Management is a dynamic process that involves creative, flexible, and logical decision making. Thus management is both an art and a science.
- Managers must understand the program development cycle to implement effective and efficient strategies that facilitate the pursuit of organizational and individual goals.
- Managers oversee diverse resources, including fiscal, physical, technological, and human resources. The management of human resources involves leadership, which is an important managerial function.
- Successful organizations have good leaders, facilities, and programs.
- Managers must understand that they have legal responsibilities and duties regarding their clients and players. Failure to meet these obligations can result in lawsuits.
- Sports and fitness marketing is more than just ballpark billboards and catchy advertising.
- Marketing strategies require a clear target market and a well-defined marketing mix.

- Marketers of sports and fitness operations must effectively design both the primary and secondary service offerings to meet the expectations of their customers.
- Enhancing customers' perceived value of the services provided by the sports or fitness operation is a key to success.

REVIEW QUESTIONS

1. What are some of the roles of the manager?
2. Explain the program development cycle.
3. What is leadership?
4. What are the differences among the autocratic, democratic, and laissez-faire leadership styles? Which is the best style?
5. What are the essential differences among the great man theory of leadership; the contingency model theory of leadership; the path–goal theory of leadership; and the life cycle theory of leadership?
6. What is risk management?
7. What is negligence?
8. Describe the search and experience qualities customers may associate with a fitness center or club. When do customers assess each of these qualities?
9. Why is sports marketing different from many other types of product and service marketing?
10. Outline a marketing strategy for a local sports team or fitness center, including explanations of each of the five components of a marketing strategy.
11. If you were managing a snow skiing resort, how would you price lodging and lift tickets according to demand fluctuations? When would be a good time to maintain or even increase prices? Cut prices?
12. Using Figure 6.3, rate a local fitness center or sporting event or stadium. What changes would you make to serve customers better?

References

1. Griffin RW. Management. 5th ed. Princeton, NJ: Houghton Mifflin, 1996.
2. Lyons BC. The death of leadership behavior in sport. J Miss Alliance Health Phys Educ Recreation Dance 1993;13:10–12.
3. Le Unes A, Nation J. Sport psychology. 2nd ed. Chicago: Nelson-Hall, 1996.
4. Horine L. Administration of physical education and sport programs. 3rd ed. Dubuque, IA: Brown & Benchmark, 1995.
5. Lord CG. Social psychology. New York: Harcourt Brace, 1997.
6. Iso-Ahola S, Hatfield B. Psychology of sports: a social psychological approach. Dubuque, IA: Brown, 1986.
7. Fiedler FE. Theory of leadership effectiveness. New York: McGraw-Hill, 1967.
8. Carron AV. Social psychology of sport. Ithaca, NY: Mouvement, 1980.
9. Bass BM. Stodgill's handbook of leadership. New York: Free Press, 1981.
10. Berry LM, Houston JP. Psychology at work: an introduction to industrial and organizational psychology. Dubuque, IA: Allyn & Bacon, 1993.
11. House R. A path-goal theory of leader effectiveness. Adm Sci Q 1971;16:321–380.
12. Hersey P, Blanchard KH. Management of organizational behavior. 6th ed. Englewood Cliffs, NJ: Prentice-Hall, 1993.
13. Davis KA. Sport management: successful private sector business strategies. Dubuque, IA: Brown & Benchmark, 1994.
14. Zeithaml VA, Parasuraman A, Berry LL. Delivering quality service: balancing customer perceptions and expectations. New York: Free Press, 1990.
15. Maister DH. The psychology of waiting lines. In: JA Czepiel, MR Solomon, CF Suprenant, eds. The service encounter: managing employee/customer interaction in service businesses. Lexington, MA: Lexington Books, 1985:113–123.
16. Lovelock CH. Services marketing. 3rd ed. Englewood Cliffs, NJ: Prentice-Hall, 1996.

17. Wakefield KL, Blodgett JG. The importance of servicescapes in leisure service settings. J Serv Marketing 1994;8:66–76.
18. Bitner MJ. Servicescapes: the impact of physical surroundings on customers and employees. J Marketing 1992;56:57–71.
19. Shimp TA. Advertising, promotion, and supplemental aspects of integrated marketing communications. 4th ed. Orlando, FL: Dryden, 1997.
20. Wakefield KL, Barnes JH. Retailing hedonic consumption: a model of sales promotion of a leisure service. J Retailing 1996;72:409–428.

Suggested Readings

Bass BM, Avolio BJ, eds. Improving organizational effectiveness through transformation leadership. London: Sage, 1993.
Camaione DN. Fitness management. Dubuque, IA: Brown & Benchmark, 1993.
Fisher RJ, Wakefield KL. Factors leading to group identification: a field study of winners and losers. Psychol Marketing 1998;15:23–40.
Galanes GJ, Brilhart JK. Communicating in groups: application and skills. 3rd ed. Dubuque, IA: Brown & Benchmark, 1997.
Marketing News. [Bimonthly trade journal that frequently has cutting-edge articles pertaining to sports and services marketing.]
Wakefield KL, Blodgett JG, Sloan HJ. Measurement and management of the sportscape. J Sport Manage 1996;10:15–31.
Wakefield KL. The pervasive effects of social influence on sporting event attendance. J Sport Soc Issues 1995;19:335–351.

7

Professional Issues

WALTER R. THOMPSON AND STANLEY P. BROWN

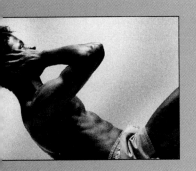

Objectives

1. Identify Flexner's six criteria that qualify an occupation as a profession.
2. Distinguish between a nonprofessional occupation and a professional occupation using the profession pyramid.
3. Explain role delineation and professional encroachment.
4. Explain the difference between certification and licensure.

- **Exercise Science as a Profession**
    What Is a Profession?
- **Certification or Licensure?**
- **Issues Regarding Encroachment**
- **Relationships with Other Allied Health Professions**
- **Role Delineation**
- **A Name for the Discipline**

Summary Points
Review Questions
References
Suggested Readings

This chapter addresses current issues important to the ongoing development of the field of exercise science. Issues such as the nature of a profession, certification, licensure, **encroachment,** and cooperation between healthcare professionals are discussed. The chapter also presents issues of nomenclature for exercise science in academic and employment settings. After reading this chapter, the student will have a better understanding of the complexity of these professional issues and will appreciate the encouraging future development of exercise science.

EXERCISE SCIENCE AS A PROFESSION

When discussing exercise science as a **profession,** it is important to note that the aim of this chapter is not to argue whether exercise science enjoys professional status equal to that held by the allied health professions (e.g., nursing, physical therapy, and occupational therapy) or the more established traditional professions (e.g., medicine and law). If one were to imagine a continuum on which were placed a number of different occupational groups, it would be clear that exercise science would fall somewhere after the established traditional professions but before nonprofessional groups, such as those that can be classified as crafts or blue-collar occupations.

As we consider current professional issues related to exercise science, the student should focus on particular subdisciplines rather than on exercise science as a whole. It is within these subdisciplines that the battles for professional status are currently being fought, some more successfully than others. At least one of the subdisciplines of exercise science (clinical exercise physiology) is in the process of forging a professional identity. In addition, another subdiscipline (athletic training) received recognition as a profession when, in 1990, the American Medical Association (AMA) formally recognized athletic training as an allied health profession. Whether exercise science in its entirety gains professional status any time soon remains speculative. For a discussion of the future development of the discipline of exercise science, the student is referred to Chapter 19.

What Is a Profession?

The term profession has its origin in the word *professor.* At institutions of higher learning, the professor is a teacher who holds the highest academic rank and is recognized as an expert in his or her field. In addition, a professional is someone who is characterized by and conforms to the technical and ethical standards of a profession. This idea was developed in the early part of the twentieth century by Flexner (1) who was writing specifically about social work as a profession. His ideas, however, are useful to consider here for exercise science. Flexner listed six criteria that an occupation must meet to qualify as a profession:

Intellectual pursuit and responsible actions.

Knowledge base derived from science and research.

Practice involves the use of practical skills—not solely academic skills.

Representative professional organization.

High level of communication with members in good standing.

Altruism.

According to Flexner's scheme not all occupations enjoy professional status. For example, a plumber, though possessing technical skills and useful expertise, is considered to be subordinate to the professionals who design the plumbing systems (i.e., the architect or engineer). Although plumbers may be employed to repair a problem in the system, they would not be asked to design the system. Rather than being viewed as professionals, plumbers and a host of other skilled technicians are considered craftsmen, often requiring a certain level of supervision. Their duties, unlike those of the professional, are not intellectually focused. In fact, their duties may be readily learned by most members of society with little or no formal education.

How does the craft of a plumber differ from the professional activities of an architect? The answer lies in the fact that, as a profession, architecture demonstrates all of Flexner's criteria for professional status. In a similar fashion, Purtilo and Cassel (2) mention five critical characteristics important for health professions: self-governed autonomy, social value, specialized knowledge, representative organization, and lifetime commitment. For a group to be classified as a health profession all five characteristics must be present.

Figure 7.1 illustrates how these characteristics are related to each other in a hierarchy. As you ascend to the top of the pyramid, the characteristic becomes less valued in terms of its importance to the professional status of the group. The base of the pyramid, self-governed autonomy, is critical to the claim of professional status. Self-governed autonomy refers to the freedom of a professional group to self-govern. Explicit in self-governed autonomy is the fact that professionals act independently and use sound judgment in their practice. Implicit in self-governed autonomy is the need for there to be control of the profession by people who are actually in the profession (see A Case in Point 7.1).

The claim to being a profession is also made in regard to the service provided to society, or the social value. Society benefits from the practice rendered by the professional. Physical therapy may serve as a good example here, because of its close association with exercise science and because physical therapy education requires course work in many of the exercise science subdisciplines. Also, both the discipline of exercise science and the profession of physical therapy have movement as their common knowledge base. Physical therapy is an allied health profession, whereas exercise science falls elsewhere on the profession/occupation continuum. Yet, both the discipline of exercise science and the profession of physical therapy have tremendous social value. A group's value to society increases when it is able to maintain a rigorous professional code of ethics that is enforced through its main professional organization. Has the American College of Sports Medicine (ACSM) taken on this role for exercise science (see Box 7.1)?

The third characteristic, specialized knowledge, relates to the fact that the professional has often endured long and intensive academic preparation. Ownership of a certain body of knowledge sets apart professionals from those in other occupations on the continuum. A body of knowledge is defined as the sum total of all the research and scholarship in a discipline. The body of knowledge in any discipline is dynamic and constantly changing as new scholarship expands it. Professionals essentially have intellectual ownership of this knowledge and use it in the prac-

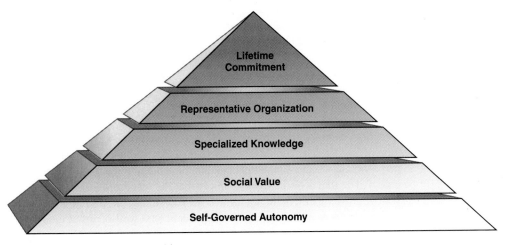

Figure 7.1 The profession pyramid.

A Case in Point 7.1

SELF-GOVERNED AUTONOMY—A GOAL IN THE PROFESSIONALIZATION OF EXERCISE PHYSIOLOGY

The complex issues surrounding the professionalization of particular subdisciplines of exercise science are evident in the recent attempts that are being made to advance exercise physiology to professional status. Questions of who rightly controls the future of this subdiscipline have led to the recent organization of the American Society of Exercise Physiologists (ASEP), a body of exercise physiologists that has as a major goal the professionalization of exercise physiology. Among the problems being addressed by ASEP members is the recognition that only exercise physiologists should govern the direction the field takes. A point of contention in this ongoing debate is whether the American College of Sports Medicine (ACSM)—an eclectic organization devoted to exercise science in its entirety and composed of at least 56 occupations (including exercise physiology)—has the right and ability to govern the development of exercise physiology as a profession (note the ACSM's recent and ongoing effort to develop a professional registry of clinical exercise physiologists). The debate continues and will not be settled here, but the argument is a key one any group desiring professional status must address. Autonomy, the ability of professionals to act independently in self-governance, is a key ingredient to gaining professional status.

Box 7.1
ACSM Code of Ethics

PRINCIPLES AND PURPOSES

Preamble: These principles are intended to aid Fellows and Members of the College individually and collectively to maintain a high level of ethical conduct. These are not laws but standards by which a Fellow or a Member may determine the propriety of his/her conduct, relationship with colleagues, with members of allied professions, with the public, and with all persons in which a professional relationship has been established. The principal purpose of the College is the generation and dissemination of knowledge concerning all aspects of persons engaged in exercise with full respect for the dignity of man.

Section 1: Members should strive continuously to improve knowledge and skill and make available to their colleagues and the public the benefits of their professional attainment.

Section 2: Members should maintain high professional and scientific standards and should not voluntarily associate professionally with anyone who violates this principle.

Section 3: The College should safeguard the public and itself against members who are deficient in ethical conduct or professional competence.

Section 4: The ideals of the College imply that the responsibilities of each Fellow or Member extend not only to the individual, but also to society with the purpose of improving both the health and well-being of the individual and the community.

Box 7.1
ACSM Code of Ethics (continued)

MAINTENANCE OF GOOD STANDING IN REGULATED PROFESSIONS
Any Fellow or Member required by law to be licensed, certified or otherwise
regulated by any governmental agency in order to practice his or her profession must remain in good standing before that agency as a condition of
continued membership in the College. Any expulsion, suspension, probation or other sanction imposed by such governmental agency on any
Fellow or Member may be grounds for disciplinary action by the College.

PUBLIC DISCLOSURE OF AFFILIATION
Other than for commercial venture, any Member or Fellow (FACSM) may
disclose his/her affiliation with the College in any context, oral or documented, provided it is currently accurate. In doing so, no Member or
Fellow may imply College endorsement of whatever is associated in context with the disclosure, unless expressly authorized by the College.
Disclosure of affiliation in connection with a commercial venture may be
made provided the disclosure is made in a professionally dignified manner, is not false, misleading or deceptive, and does not imply licensure or
the attainment of specialty or diploma status. Members and Fellows who
are ACSM Certified may disclose their certification status. Because membership and fellowship in the ACSM is granted to individuals, disclosure
of affiliation and/or use of the initials ACSM are not to be made as part
of a firm, partnership or corporate name.
Disclosure in violation of this article may be grounds for disciplinary action.

PUBLIC USE OF PROFESSIONAL EXPERTISE
Members and Fellows are encouraged to consult and share their professional
expertise beyond their workplace as opportunity provides, with or without compensation. In doing so, the professional expert is expected to
avoid misrepresentation and omission of relevant facts, involvements exceeding one's area of expertise, and conflicts of interest with or through
the ACSM when serving the ACSM in an appointed capacity.

DISCIPLINE
Any Fellow or Member of the College may be disciplined or expelled for
conduct which, in the opinion of the Board of Trustees, is derogatory to
the dignity of or inconsistent with the purposes of the College. The expulsion of a Fellow or Member may be ordered upon the affirmative vote
of two-thirds of the members of the Board of Trustees present at a regular
or a special meeting, and only after such Fellow Member has been informed of the charges preferred against him and has been given an opportunity to refute such charges before the Board of Trustees. Other disciplinary action such as reprimand, probation, or censure may be
recommended by the Committee on Ethics and Professional Conduct and
ordered following the affirmative vote of two-thirds of the members of
the Board of Trustees present at a regular or special meeting or by mail
ballot, provided a quorums take action.

tice of their profession as they provide a service to their clientele. As was explained in Chapter 1, the body of knowledge in the discipline of exercise science is movement. Regarding specialized knowledge, the road to professional status for any group takes on the following step-wise progression: identification of the specific body of knowledge; provision of a formal course of study ending in an academic degree; and an internship experience and a process of rigorous study to pass cognitive and practical examinations leading to certification or licensure that ultimately ensures competence, ends in professional employment, and protects the public from spurious practitioners. Although this process is certainly available for individuals interested in studying exercise science, the current lack of professional recognition is related to a perceived lack in one or more of the areas of the professional pyramid.

The remaining two characteristics are considered somewhat lower in terms of importance. A professional organization is essential to provide standards, regulations, structure and a means of communication (see Chapter 3). Also, professionals are often dedicated individuals who offer a lifetime of commitment to their community through the practice of their profession.

Certainly, different levels of competency occur within professions. Many professions are regulated by state law or national certification programs, many of which are voluntary. Such is the case with health and fitness professionals and, in most states, exercise science professionals working in a clinical setting.

CERTIFICATION OR LICENSURE?

In 1975, the ACSM published the first edition of *Guidelines for Graded Exercise Testing and Exercise Prescription* (3). It outlined detailed behavioral objectives (unobservable mental process) and specific learning objectives (behavior is described in observable terms) for physicians, **program directors,** and **exercise specialists.** Topics were arranged under the headings of functional anatomy, exercise physiology, behavioral psychology and group dynamics, emergency procedures, therapeutic exercise and exercise prescription, and exercise laboratory techniques. For the first time, an evolving profession (clinical exercise physiology) was given expectations from the academic community.

In that same year the ACSM introduced a national clinical certification for program directors and exercise specialists. This was followed in 1976 by certification for the exercise test technologist (now discontinued). In 1986, the ACSM first offered certifications for the health and fitness industry by introducing the **Exercise Leader, Health/Fitness Instructor,** and **Health/Fitness Director** certifications. The ACSM guidelines is now in its sixth edition (4).

The issue of certification and licensure has recently surfaced because of publications offered by the U.S. government and respected professional organizations. In 1991, the U.S. Department of Health and Human Services (DHHS) (5) published *Healthy People 2000: National Health Promotion and Disease Prevention Objectives,* which was followed by the American Heart Association's (AHA) (6) announcement that physical inactivity was (along with high blood cholesterol, hypertension, and smoking) a major risk factor in the development of heart disease.

In 1995, the Centers for Disease Control and Prevention (CDC) and the ACSM jointly published recommendations for physical activity and **public health** (7). In the same year, the President's Council on Physical Fitness and Sports announced a multimillion-dollar budget to promote youth sports and physical activity. After these developments, the U.S. surgeon general (8) announced an endorsement that all Americans would benefit from regular physical activity, and the U.S. Department of Agriculture (USDA) (9) included a statement about regular physical activity in its publication *Dietary Guidelines for American Adults.* By bringing exercise as a necessary component of disease prevention to the forefront of public awareness, these publications and statements solidified the exercise science professional's role in the future of public health.

It would appear, then, that exercise science professionals can only benefit from these certifications and from licensure. The licensing of professionals, however, is a state issue not a national issue, because only states can pass laws requiring licensure. Although many national organizations endorse state licensure, the licensing of a professional (and the requirements for licensure) must come from within the state. Certification, however, is a national issue that is governed only by the organization from which it is developed. Therefore, regulation of certified individuals comes from within the certifying agency.

In many instances, a certification program is used as a licensing examination. This is the case in Louisiana, which currently has the only license for clinical exercise physiologists. Louisiana uses as its licensing examination the ACSM Exercise Specialist certification. The following definitions are offered in the act:

> Clinical Exercise Physiologist: a person who, under the direction, approval, and supervision of a licensed physician, engages in the practice of exercise physiology.

> Exercise Physiology: the formulation, development, and implementation of exercise protocols and programs, administration of graded exercise tests, and providing education regarding such exercise programs and tests, in a cardiopulmonary rehabilitation program to individuals with deficiencies of the cardiovascular system, diabetes, lipid disorders, hypertension, cancer, chronic obstructive pulmonary disease, arthritis, renal disease, organ transplant, peripheral vascular disease, and obesity (10).

To qualify for a clinical exercise physiologist license in Louisiana, the candidate must *(a)* be at least 21 years of age; *(b)* be of good moral character; *(c)* be a citizen of the Unites States or possess a valid and current legal authority to reside and work in the United States; *(d)* have successfully completed a master's of science degree or master's of education degree in an exercise studies curriculum at an accredited school, which at the time of the applicant's graduation was approved by the ACSM or the Louisiana licensing board; *(e)* be certified as an Exercise Specialist by the ACSM, having taken and successfully passed the ACSM certifying examination as administered by ACSM or the Louisiana licensing board; and *(f)* have successfully completed an internship of 300 hr in exercise physiology under the supervision of a licensed exercise physiologist.

In this particular case, the state of Louisiana has adopted the ACSM Exercise Specialist certification as its own licensing examination, because there are no legal requirements for the state to prepare and provide its own licensing examination. Therefore, there is an alliance of sorts between a national certifying agency (which has no licensing authority) with a state that can issue a license. The ACSM Exercise Specialist certification program satisfies the Louisiana State Board of Medical Examiner's requirements for the licensed clinical exercise physiologist. Other professional organizations have similar relationships. The American Dietetic Association Registry Examination, for example, is often used as the qualification examination in states where the practice of dietetics is regulated by licensure.

The ACSM recognizes the importance of the clinical exercise physiologist and has recently added a study group within its committee structure to determine how the practice of clinical exercise physiology should be regulated from a national perspective (see Box 4.4). The process of developing and implementing a new healthcare credential began in the mid-1990s and took the rest of the decade to be completed; the first registry examination was given in June 2000.

Other states are currently using Louisiana as a model to design their own state license for clinical exercise physiologists. In addition, the North Carolina standards for programs of cardiopulmonary rehabilitation require that each program have a certified ACSM Exercise Specialist on staff. Some of the programs in that state are using consultants to fulfill this requirement. The North Carolina Cardiopulmonary Rehabilitation Association also awards $1500 per year to individuals seeking the Exercise Specialist certification.

In the 1990s, California, Florida, Utah, Kentucky, and Maryland attempted to enact legislation for licensing clinical exercise physiologists. All failed because, in each case, other professional groups effectively opposed the legislation.

ISSUES REGARDING ENCROACHMENT

The delineation of specific roles and the possible encroachment of professionals in other domains has long been an issue, particularly in healthcare. Any standard dictionary will provide a definition for *encroachment*. Although licensure often includes a rather narrow description of professional responsibilities, there is enough flexibility to allow licensed professionals to add additional tasks and responsibilities. It is this flexibility, however, that can create frustration for the exercise science professional.

The first definition for encroachment in Webster's dictionary is "to trespass or intrude (i.e., upon the rights, property, etc. of another individual). The second definition is "to advance beyond the proper, original, or customary limits."

For example, the Louisiana Clinical Exercise Physiologist Licensing Act provides that, under the supervision of a physician, the clinical exercise physiologist can administer a graded exercise test. The law (although this may not have been the intention) reads, "in a cardiopulmonary rehabilitation program." Does this mean that only the clinical exercise physiologist can administer a graded exercise test or can a health and fitness professional administer a test to that same person (with or without disease) outside of a cardiopulmonary rehabilitation program? Likewise, if a hospital or medical center does not offer a structured cardiopulmonary rehabilitation program, can a professional (e.g., physical therapist or registered nurse) other than a clinical exercise physiologist administer the same test? Unless previously governed by legislation, these questions can be answered only at the local site, taking into consideration all of the circumstances surrounding the actions in question.

RELATIONSHIPS WITH OTHER ALLIED HEALTH PROFESSIONS

The inclusion of physical inactivity as a major risk factor in the development of heart disease has increased awareness among Americans of the importance of regular exercise. It has also created a perplexing issue for healthcare professionals. In 1992, the AHA (6) published a position statement on the benefits of regular physical activity. In it, the expert panel wrote:

> Nurses, an integral part of the health care team, may assess physical activity habits, prescribe exercise, and monitor responses to exercise in healthy persons and cardiac patients. The services of physical and occupational therapists, and exercise scientists, and other health professionals may also be useful.

Clearly, this statement increased the awareness among the nursing profession and schools of nursing of the importance of exercise programs. The exercise scientist was recognized as an integral member of the healthcare delivery team with the necessary academic training and knowledge to prescribe exercise to cardiac patients. However, because smaller hospitals, medical centers, and for-profit hospitals often require cross training, nurses are now entering graduate programs in exercise science. In addition, many undergraduate exercise science majors seek a degree in, for example, nursing or physical therapy (see Practical Application 7.1).

Similar situations exist for other members of the healthcare delivery team. For the comprehensive development of programs for cardiac rehabilitation, pulmonary rehabilitation, and rehabilitation for metabolic disorders, the student of exercise science should refer to the American Association of Cardiovascular and Pulmonary Rehabilitation (AACVPR) (11,12). This professional organization has clearly outlined the distribution of responsibilities for all members of the

Practical Application 7.1

CROSS TRAINING AND ENCROACHMENT

Cross training and encroachment are important and weighty matters that students should grasp along with other professional issues. Students should be aware that the person who is qualified to do several things often has the advantage in the job market. In the case of the healthcare job market, the exercise science student has definite contributions to make in the team approach to healthcare. This is evident in that more and more of the other allied health professions are encroaching or cross training and entering the job market in cardiopulmonary rehabilitation, often taking jobs that were once largely held by individuals trained in exercise science. On the one hand, this speaks well for the position exercise now enjoys as a preventive and rehabilitative tool. On the other hand, many of these positions are not going to exercise science trained individuals but to people who may have little academic preparation in the concepts taught in courses such as exercise prescription, cardiopulmonary rehabilitation, and exercise physiology. The academic content most often used in cardiopulmonary exercise therapy today was developed within exercise physiology, and is most competently applied by the exercise physiologist. In addition, cardiopulmonary rehabilitation as a healthcare process largely developed as a consequence of the emergence of clinical exercise physiology as a subdiscipline of exercise science, which emerged out of physical education. Yet job classifications involving professionals who deliver exercise treatment within cardiopulmonary rehabilitation are being blurred as other allied health practitioners assume these roles. Cross training occurs when a person with an exercise science degree seeks training in another field of study (e.g., nursing or physical therapy). It also may occur in the opposite direction, when physical therapists or nurses, for instance, become students in exercise science programs. Although there is nothing wrong with this development, indeed it is a major advancement for the job prospects of exercise personnel, the student of exercise science probably needs to play catch up in terms of his or her ability to compete for jobs. Unfortunately, this may mean additional training in another clinical area if a clinical position is desired.

healthcare delivery team. For example, program direction and coordination of cardiac rehabilitation programs are provided by a professional with a "Bachelor's degree in an allied health field, such as exercise physiology" (12) as a minimal requirement. Preferred qualifications include an advanced degree in a relevant allied health field of study. Minimal certification includes the ACSM Exercise Specialist certification, and other acceptable certifications include the advanced cardiopulmonary speciality of the American Physical Therapy Association or the American Nursing Credentialing Center.

The student of exercise science should be aware of the concept of **role delineation.** Role delineation describes the services the healthcare professional is expected to deliver to the patient. Often, however, the roles of professionals working as part of the healthcare delivery team are not well defined. The local situation may dictate a set of circumstances that either increase or decrease the scope of practice, and careful analysis of job skills and performance expectations is necessary.

ROLE DELINEATION

In the evolution of the exercise sciences, it has become critical to fully evaluate the roles and expectations of professionals who work in the related subdisciplines. The student of exercise science has many options upon graduation from a baccalaureate degree program (see Chapter 5 for a discussion of employment opportunities). Although advantageous for the student, it has created a somewhat perplexing issue for prospective employers. Most academic programs have taken the typical, historical approach to undergraduate education (the **educational pyramid**). This model suggests that the undergraduate should be exposed to great breadth with little depth of knowledge; depth comes with graduate education. The pyramid model allows for exposure to a large body of knowledge, but the undergraduate student is exposed to little depth of knowledge. Prospective employers then must determine how much continuing education to provide after employment and who provides the service.

The issue of role delineation has been avoided by national groups who have attempted to develop clinical guidelines or consensus statements. For example, the Agency for Health Care Policy and Research (AHCPR) contracted with the AACVPR to develop clinical practice guidelines for cardiac rehabilitation (13). The members of this group included some of the most respected professionals in cardiac rehabilitation. The result provided a focus for future cardiac rehabilitation programs and will, perhaps, enlighten third-party insurance carriers to provide this service to their clients. However, the guidelines failed to adequately define the specific responsibilities of the multidisciplinary team. A National Institutes of Health (NIH) consensus statement did much the same (7). Although these two government publications were well received, they fell short of defining specific responsibilities of this new healthcare team.

As managed care and preferred providers of healthcare become more commonplace, third-party payers (i.e., insurance carriers) will be seeking professionals for the delivery of services who are both productive and cost-effective. State law may dictate some of the responsibilities for medical decisions and treatment. In the evolving role of the exercise physiologist on the healthcare delivery team, it will be critical for job descriptions to accurately reflect the education and experiences of this position. A comprehensive role delineation study for exercise physiology and other exercise science subdisciplines interested in the clinical arena (for instance, clinical biomechanics) has not yet been accomplished by any national organization.

A NAME FOR THE DISCIPLINE

For two decades, specialization within the recognized subdisciplines of exercise science has been hotly debated (14). Although the debate over the proper designation for the discipline has recently begun to subside, no conclusion by any national professional organization has been offered. For example, in a published debate, Higgins et al. (15) favored alternative names for what appear to be similar academic programs. Higgins suggested "movement science" as the most descriptive name for the discipline that houses these collective subdisciplines, whereas Kretchmer suggested "exercise and sport science." Newell favored "kinesiology" as the correct title, and Katch chose to defend "exercise science."

In addition, many individuals working within the established subdisciplines of exercise science have their own mini-debates, favoring some titles for the subdisciplines over others. Exercise physiology, biomechanics, ergonomics, motor integration, exercise biochemistry, and sensorimotor biofeedback are some examples suggested for the names of various subdisciplines and for the academic departments that house them (see Box 7.2). Part two of this text provides the student with a succinct description of the most widely recognized subdisciplines of exercise science.

At this time two of the most accepted titles for the academic discipline that studies human movement are *exercise science* and *kinesiology.* We have chosen exercise science as the proper name for the discipline, because of the name's breath and all inclusiveness. In Higgins et al. (15), the most persuasive argument was made for *exercise science* being the proper designation for the discipline, which is made up of several subdisciplines, including biochemistry of exercise, exercise physiology, motor integration, ergonomics, sensorimotor biofeedback, and biomechanics. The debate is significant simply because it is important for people in and out of the field to grasp, with one title, the essence of a discipline. However, the debate is likely to continue.

Lost in many more contemporary arguments, however, is the term *sports medicine,* the designation of the leading exercise science umbrella organization. Although this term once had a comprehensive connotation, it now is used more narrowly to identify professionals working within athletic training and physicians who practice in sports medicine. Athletic training as a subdiscipline of exercise science emerged as an important element within the ranks of coaching. When athletic trainers became accepted as an integral part of the sports medicine team by physicians who cared for athletes, an alignment was necessary. Therefore, athletic trainers adopted the title of sports medicine professionals. Sports medicine is considered in this text to be an important knowledge base, although functioning under the umbrella of exercise science (see section V).

SUMMARY POINTS

- A profession manifests these five characteristics: autonomy, social value, specialized knowledge, representative organization, and lifetime commitment.
- As the professions interested in wellness, fitness, health, and movement studies evolve, certification and licensure will become more important.
- Professional responsibilities include certification, licensure, and adherence to a code of conduct.
- The multidisciplinary team approach to medical care and health services delivery is now the acceptable strategy for patient care.

Box **7.2**
Some Academic Department Titles

Movement Science
Exercise and Sport Science
Kinesiology
Exercise Science
Sports Medicine
Sports Science
Bioscience
Human Biodynamics
Movement and Sports Science
Exercise Technology
Kinesiology and Health
Human Performance

Exercise physiology is an important subdiscipline within the discipline of exercise science. As a major field of scientific inquiry, exercise physiology has made many significant contributions to both basic and applied physiology. These contributions have advanced our knowledge of sports performance and the relationship between exercise and health. Largely owing to the considerable expansion of the field of exercise physiology since the 1970s, exercise has become inculcated into the culture of Western society. During this time, the number of exercise-related research studies supported by national granting agencies skyrocketed. This has had a vast influence on our nation's healthcare policy and on the lifestyles of many people. The result of these developments is that people of all ages and backgrounds enjoy exercise on a regular basis. This chapter presents a definition and description of exercise physiology, introduces concepts of bioenergetics as the basis for movement, presents important organ systems supporting metabolic processes, and includes important advances made in this field.

DEFINITION, DESCRIPTION, AND SCOPE

Taking its content from the parent disciplines of biochemistry and biology, exercise physiology is the study of the function of the body under the stress of acute and chronic physical activity. Exercise physiology is equally concerned with: how the body responds to the intense demands placed on it by physical activity and the changes that occur in the body as individuals regularly participate in exercise training.

Physical activity takes many forms. Activities as diverse as a slow stroll, a fast paced run, a dock worker's heavy physical labor during an 8-hr workday, an Olympic weight lifter's 200-kg snatch, an elite bodybuilder's grueling 3-hr workout, and a marathoner's 26.2-mile run are but a few examples of the activities to which the principles of exercise physiology can be applied.

Most of the physical activities we engage in are not related to sports performance but are normal everyday activities of life. The diverse forms of physical activities in which we are all involved require our bodies to make major physiologic adjustments. These processes are complicated. The role of the exercise physiologist is to examine specific physiologic responses in an attempt to delineate the adjustments made with acute exercise. In this way, scientists have a better understanding of the chronic adaptations that occur with exercise training.

With this definition as a base, we can now more fully describe exercise physiology by surveying its scope. Figure 8.1 identifies the content areas typical of exercise physiology undergraduate courses. Within each of these units, students learn the basics of the physiologic systems involved, exercise responses and adaptations within these systems, and more specialized topics or applications related to exercise. The arrows are meant to represent the general order of influence from one system to the next.

At the outset of our survey of exercise physiology, two important questions should be asked: What are the boundaries that delineate exercise physiology as a subdiscipline of exercise science? Who benefits from the scientific inquiries made within these boundaries?

Acute Responses and Chronic Adaptations

To describe exercise physiology we need to first identify its boundaries. We can begin this process by examining the terms *acute* and *chronic*. Acute refers to performing a single bout of exercise. This may take a few seconds (as in putting the shot or running a 40-yard dash) or many hours (as in an ultramarathon run). Within the realm of acute exercise responses, one of the purposes of the science of exercise physiology is to investigate how the body makes internal adjustments in the face of the massive disruptions in **homeostasis** that occur with acute exercise.

The study of acute exercise responses has taken a giant leap forward in recent years with the advent of important technological advances. This, in turn, has greatly expanded the knowledge base of exercise physiology to include such areas as molecular biology and genetics. These

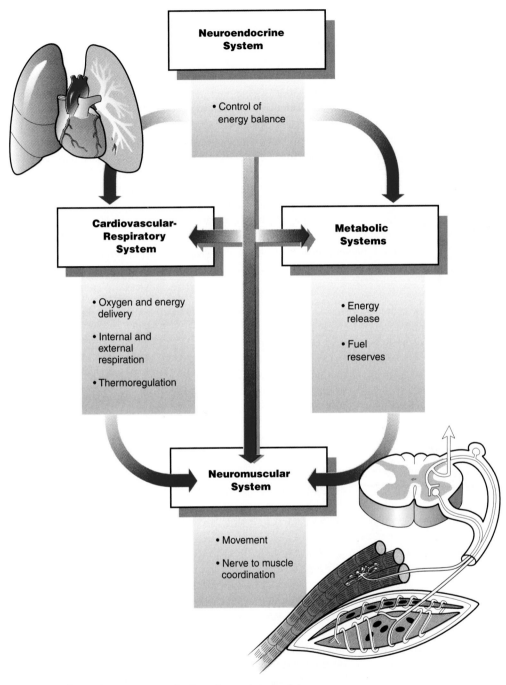

FIGURE 8.1 General content organization of exercise physiology courses.

technological advances have led to a better understanding of the physiology of sports performance and of how to better enhance the health of the average individual through appropriate exercise recommendations. These advances have helped chart a bright course for the continued development of exercise physiology. Box 8.1 lists just a few of the hundreds of important
exercise-related research questions scientists have attempted to answer regarding acute physiologic responses.

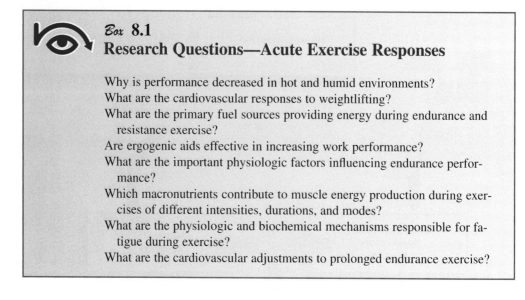

Box 8.1
Research Questions—Acute Exercise Responses

Why is performance decreased in hot and humid environments?

What are the cardiovascular responses to weightlifting?

What are the primary fuel sources providing energy during endurance and resistance exercise?

Are ergogenic aids effective in increasing work performance?

What are the important physiologic factors influencing endurance performance?

Which macronutrients contribute to muscle energy production during exercises of different intensities, durations, and modes?

What are the physiologic and biochemical mechanisms responsible for fatigue during exercise?

What are the cardiovascular adjustments to prolonged endurance exercise?

The study of acute responses is only about one half of what interests the exercise physiologist. Also of great concern is the way the body adapts to being chronically exposed to exercise stress. The term *chronic* refers to a certain length of time over which changes take place in different physiologic systems during an exercise training program. These changes generally can be interpreted as an improvement in the body's function, both at rest and during submaximal and maximal exercise. Box 8.2 presents some important questions related to chronic adaptations (bodily changes) after exercise training.

Box 8.2
Research Questions—Chronic Exercise Adaptations

Can muscle fibers be converted from one type to another by specific training practices?

Is cross-training harmful or helpful in sports performance?

Is the muscle fiber type distribution different in athletes of different specialties?

Does weight training increase maximum oxygen consumption?

What are the causes of the gender difference in maximum oxygen consumption?

Is the increase in maximum oxygen consumption after endurance training limited by central (heart and lung) or peripheral (muscular) adaptations?

What are the physical changes produced by fitness training?

How has the heart of a weightlifter adapted compared to the heart of an endurance athlete?

What are the physiologic consequences of overtraining?

What combinations of training duration and frequency are best for improving cardiorespiratory fitness?

What combinations of training duration and frequency are best for weight control?

What physiologic factors best predict success in endurance activities?

Using the framework of acute responses and chronic adaptations, the exercise physiologist applies the knowledge gained from the basic sciences to problems in exercise physiology, thereby gaining insights into how the body functions during exercise. This can then be used as a basis for developing the best training practices to enhance athletic performance and health, two areas of special interest to the exercise physiologist. Later in this chapter, I examine research involving several of these questions.

The Activity Continuum

Acute responses and chronic adaptations are not the only boundaries established for the study of exercise physiology. Exercise physiologists are interested in studying all forms of physical activity, including everyday life activities, sports activities, and exercise activities. The differences in the acute responses and chronic adaptations among physical activities are often astounding. I'll begin this section by briefly examining some of these differences.

It is possible to place all exercises, athletic activities, and general physical activities on a continuum. This activity continuum is useful for classifying exercise in two important ways: the metabolic and hemodynamic responses produced by a given activity. In terms of metabolic responses, the physical activity continuum ranges from activities that are largely **anaerobic** to those that are largely **aerobic** (Fig. 8.2). The second way we can classify exercise and activity is from a physiologic standpoint by examining the hemodynamic responses produced by the activity (Fig. 8.3). The terms *metabolic, aerobic, anaerobic,* and *hemodynamic* are explained later in this chapter.

Metabolic Response

Figure 8.2 illustrates physical activities as energetic events. Furthermore, the activities are placed in a time frame that depicts the duration of the maximal effort during the event. The descriptors *power, speed,* and *endurance* communicate how intensely the activity is performed. Track and field events are good examples of the use of these descriptors and their time frames.

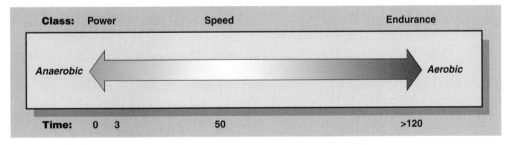

FIGURE 8.2 Physical activity continuum of metabolic responses.

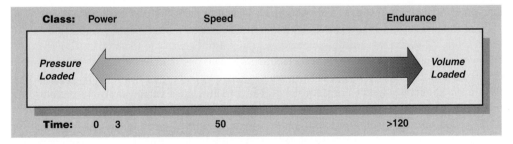

FIGURE 8.3 Physical activity continuum of hemodynamic responses.

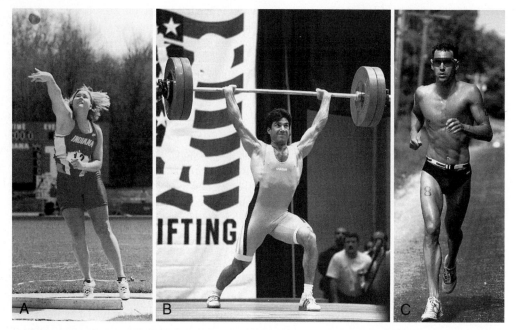

FIGURE 8.4 **A,** Indiana University athlete Allison Morgan competing at the 1997 NCAA men's and women's outdoor track championship. Courtesy of Paul Riley, Indiana University Photographic Services. **B,** Tony Gerasia performing a clean and jerk at the 1997 Senior National Championship (135-kg class). Courtesy of East Coast Gold Weightlifting Team. **C,** Endurance runner. Courtesy of Steve Handwerker, SLH Communications.

For instance, the shot-put takes only 2 to 3 sec to perform. In that time frame, the athlete extends maximal effort to get across the ring to displace the shot with as much force as he or she can produce.

What makes this a power event and not a speed event? The answer lies in the time frame required to perform the event and, ultimately, the definition of the term *power*. Power is the application of a force relative to time. If the force is applied in a short time frame, more power is generated. When it takes more time to apply the force, power output drops off accordingly.

Across the continuum of physical activities, there are a number of examples of power events. Events in which maximal efforts are produced over a short time frame include the shot-put and Olympic weightlifting (Fig. 8.4). Some running events may also be included in this category. For instance, the 40-yard dash and simply running up the stairs qualify as power activities. In contrast, speed events require a longer time period. Because of this, the power generated during the event is much lower. Examples of speed events are sprints (100 to 200 m) and longer runs such as the 400-m run. Weightlifting performed as an exercise involving many repetitions also qualifies as a speed event, because the time frame is longer (many seconds) than in power lifting. Endurance events are much longer than power and speed events and, therefore, are placed at the other end of the continuum. The 1500-m run and runs of longer duration are put in this category (Fig. 8.4).

Figure 8.2 shows that metabolic responses range from anaerobic to aerobic. Activities are, however, not mutually exclusive in a metabolic sense; no one activity relies solely on a single energy system. In addition, use of the physical activity continuum to illustrate types of activities from a metabolic standpoint does not mean that activities are limited purely by the muscle's **metabolic capacity.** For instance, although success in Olympic weightlifting requires a well-developed anaerobic system, muscle strength, power, and lifting technique are as important for success. In the next section, I briefly survey several **metabolic pathways** and explore how they produce energy for muscular activity.

The exercise physiologist, therefore, is interested in a wide range of activities that produce different acute metabolic and hemodynamic responses. Again, it is important to consider the time frame. Some of these activities are of long duration but are not particularly intense and thus are largely aerobic, whereas others are of short duration but extremely intense and thus are largely anaerobic.

In terms of metabolic responses, activities may fall at either end of the continuum or at some point in the range from aerobic to anaerobic **metabolism.** For instance, weightlifting, as one form of **resistance exercise** is understood to be primarily anaerobic, whereas jogging and walking, two forms of **endurance exercise,** are primarily aerobic. Exercises, activities, and sports events can also fall at different points on the activity continuum. For example, is soccer play aerobic or anaerobic? What about basketball? What about a maximal-effort mile run? One can readily see that some activities fall into a gray zone, with the energy output depending on both anaerobic and aerobic sources. Generally, the shorter the activity, the greater the contribution of anaerobic energy production. The longer the activity, the greater the contribution of aerobic energy production. The type of training program one adopts to improve performance in an activity or sport event depends heavily on where the activity falls on the continuum in terms of the acute metabolic response.

SPECIFICITY   An important concept that relates to both the type of exercise training employed and the physical activity continuum is specificity. Specificity is one of several basic training principles that must be heeded if a physical training program is to produce optimal results. The specificity principle states that to maximize benefits, training should be carefully matched to an athlete's specific performance needs or an individual's goals. This concept is important because the kinds of physiologic adaptations one achieves from training are related to the specific responses produced by acute exercise. That is, the physiologic adaptations that arise out of an exercise training program are highly specific to the nature of the training activity (1).

Specificity is simple to comprehend when one understands that the quickest way to achieve success in athletic pursuits is to practice the activity itself or to perform ancillary activities that closely simulate the athletic event.

This is a concept that is simple to understand, but often violated. For instance, there is a common misconception that weight training will produce aerobic or cardiovascular benefits. The reasons why this is false are physiologic and biochemical in nature and relate to the fact that specific kinds of adaptations (i.e., the aerobic benefits that supposedly are produced by weight training) follow only if there is a demand made on the bioenergetic processes and the physiologic system thought to be adapting. Cardiovascular benefits do not result from weight training because weightlifting does not sufficiently engage aerobic bioenergetic pathways. Bioenergetic processes are briefly explained later in this chapter.

Hemodynamic Response

The second way we can classify exercise and activity on the activity continuum is from a physiologic standpoint (Fig. 8.3). The degree to which an activity promotes blood movement and affects blood pressure are important considerations when attempting to understand acute responses. As shown in Figure 8.3, this classification scheme relies on the hemodynamic response produced by a given activity. *Hemodynamic* refers to the circulation of blood and may also encompass the forces restricting or promoting its circulation.

Exercises that promote a great deal of blood movement involve endurance activities. These are also associated with moderate elevations in blood pressure. These exercises are classified under the volume load heading, which refers to the fact that the heart is loaded, or stressed, during

FOCUS ON SCIENCE

The meaning of the term *energy* is difficult to grasp, yet the concept of energy is vital for a sound understanding of how the body functions during muscular activity. In fact, although movement can be understood in physiologic terms, the most rudimentary understanding of movement can be reduced to the study of the biochemical processes that release bound or **potential energy** and convert it to **free energy,** which is involved at any moment in all biologic processes, including muscular activity. It is in this context that energy is best understood as the ability to perform work (or exercise).

The concepts of *work* and *energy* are directly related. As work increases, so does the transfer of energy. Table 8.1 lists some forms of energy important in biologic processes. The conversion of energy from one form to another takes place according to the laws of thermodynamics that govern the transformation of energy. The first law states that the many different forms of energy are interchangeable, i.e., energy can be converted from one form to another. As energy is transformed from one form to another, it is said to be conserved, so that no energy is lost. This principle can be illustrated in the body by briefly exploring where we get energy for movement and how free energy release in the muscles leads to muscular contraction.

Energy for Movement

It is important to understand that our body's bioenergetic systems are part of the thermal processes that govern life on the entire planet. The sun is the ultimate source of energy for life on earth. The massive amount of thermonuclear energy on the sun is released during fusion reactions. These reactions release energy to the surroundings. Some of this energy radiates to the earth, where it drives the reactions of photosynthesis, the process that makes **carbohydrates** in plant life.

In this way, the energy from one reaction, characterized as energy releasing, is transformed to another form via energy-absorbing reactions. The energy-releasing and energy-absorbing reactions are then said to be coupled, or linked. In the example of photosynthesis, radiant energy from fusion reactions on the sun is transformed to chemical energy in the form of carbohydrates.

Why is this important in the study of exercise physiology? The same coupling of energy-releasing and energy-conserving reactions takes place in our bodies, and movement—brought on by muscle contraction—is the ultimate outcome.

Energy for movement comes from the food we eat (animal and plant sources), which provides energy-rich nutrients in the form of carbohydrates, **fats,** and proteins. In this section, I focus on how energy is derived from the breakdown of carbohydrates and fat, the two main energy nutrients used during exercise. In the digestive processes, these three energy nutrients are broken down to their constituent building-block molecules. These molecules enter the body from the digestive tract and are processed by the liver for storage and use in the body. These building-block molecules (Fig. 8.5) are rich in potential energy that is available to be converted to free energy for future muscular work. The energy bound in the building-block molecules, however, cannot be directly used for muscular activity. It must first be converted to another chemical, which

Table 8.1	ENERGY FORMS AND BIOLOGIC PROCESSES

Energy Form	Biologic Processes
Mechanical	Skeletal muscle contraction; heart muscle contraction
Chemical	Muscle contraction; metabolism; digestion
Electrical	Nervous conduction; thinking
Thermal	Maintenance of body temperature
Solar	Vitamin D production

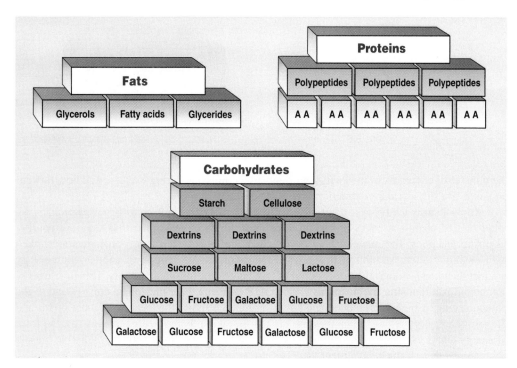

FIGURE 8.5 Energy nutrient building blocks.

can then become the direct source of energy for muscular activity. For a closer look at the amount of energy reserve we possess see Box 8.3.

The sum of the chemical processes that convert energy from indirect sources (the energy nutrients) to the source that can be used directly to do muscular activity is metabolism. Metabolism refers to all of the chemical reactions that take place in the body. It is the sum of all catabolic and anabolic processes. Catabolism is the process of breaking down the large energy nutrient molecules to their smaller constituent building blocks. In this process, a transfer of energy takes place. In this section I will briefly review the catabolic reactions that are important in

Box **8.3**
How Much Energy Do We Have?

Potentially, one half of our body weight functions as an energy reserve. The energy nutrients—fats, proteins, and carbohydrates—contain approximately 9, 4, and 4 kcal/g, respectively. The total amount of available energy reserve in the body of the average reference man (65 kg body weight and 13% body fat) equals about 78,150 kcal, exclusive of protein reserve. This calculates to be 76,050 kcal for 8.45 kg of fat and 2,100 kcal for 0.525 kg of carbohydrates. If this person were to endure a forced starvation regimen, the energy reserve would be gone in < 50 days. This assumes the man is resting quietly the entire time. If only minimal activity is performed, the survival period would be reduced to < 12 days. In addition, notice that very little carbohydrate is actually stored, making it essential that it's replenished on a regular basis.

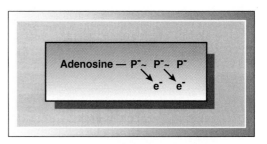

FIGURE 8.6 ATP energy.

the transfer of energy from the energy nutrients to the muscles during exercise and how this energy is active in muscular contraction.

Anabolism is the process whereby smaller molecules are built up to larger molecules. An input of free energy is necessary to produce these kinds of reactions; thus they are energy-requiring reactions. For movement to occur, catabolic (energy-releasing) processes are linked with anabolic (energy-trapping) processes for the purpose of producing another high-energy product that then becomes the direct donor of free energy for muscular activity. This high-energy compound is **adenosine triphosphate** (ATP). ATP contains three phosphate units bound to the core molecule by high-energy chemical bonds. Figure 8.6 shows the location of these bonds and the resultant energy release when they are broken. Breaking them releases free energy, the form of energy that is available to the cell for powering all kinds of cellular activity, including muscle contractions that produce movement.

ATP is an energy-rich compound that provides cells with a means of storing and conserving energy. As we will see, the subsequent breakdown of ATP releases its bound energy, converting it to free energy, which is then used for all of the energy-requiring processes. How ATP is created in the cell to power muscular activity is one of the major topics in the study of biochemistry, one of the parent disciplines of exercise physiology. The processes that produce ATP can proceed by anaerobic means or by aerobic production. These biochemical processes are controlled by mechanisms inside the cell that regulate energy storage and by important organ systems. All of this activity is precisely integrated for the most efficient production of ATP for a given sports activity or exercise.

Anaerobic Production of ATP

Some of the bioenergetic processes in our muscles can produce ATP by means that do not require oxygen, which is to say that ATP can be produced anaerobically. The anaerobic production of ATP is an important means of powering movement. It gives us a greatly expanded repertoire of activities. Table 8.2 provides a list of activities that are powered by the anaerobic production of ATP. These are divided into power and speed activities. Without the anaerobic production of ATP, activities such as sprints, high jumps, and heavy weightlifting would not be possible. What

Table 8.2	Examples of Anaerobic Activities		
Activity	**Power**	**Speed**	**Duration, sec**
Weight training, Olympic style	X		<5
Track and field throwing events	X		<10
Pole vault	X		~10
100-m sprint	X		
200-m sprint		X	>20
Weight training, body building		X	>30
400-m run		X	>45

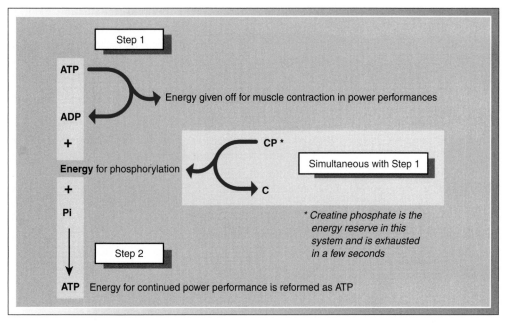

FIGURE 8.7 The phosphagen system.

makes power and speed activities possible is the rapid production of ATP in the cell by means of anaerobic metabolic pathways.

PHOSPHAGEN SYSTEM   Figure 8.7 shows the first and simplest anaerobic pathway, the **phosphagen system,** so named because it uses two important high-energy phosphate compounds that are stored in muscles. Upon its breakdown, ATP releases energy that causes muscle fibers to shorten (contract). Every cell in the body contains a quantity of ATP and other high-energy phosphates. These quantities are small; and because the high-energy phosphates cannot be supplied from other areas of the body, ATP must be continuously remade in muscle and every other cell. The energy charge of the cell, therefore, is directly related to ATP concentration. From an energy standpoint, when ATP concentrations are low, the energy charge is low, and vice versa. A central role of metabolism is to guarantee that the cell is properly charged by the conversion of bound energy from the energy nutrients to adenosine diphosphate. This produces ATP by the chemical process called **phosphorylation.**

The phosphagen system is important for anaerobic activities such as sprinting and weightlifting. Because anaerobic activities are highly intense, they require a rapid resupply of ATP for the rate of activity (e.g., running speed) to be sustained. Aerobic activities are much less intense; therefore, ATP production can proceed slowly through the coordinated integration of both cellular and organ system interactions. Because of the very nature of highly intense activity, ATP must be produced rapidly.

To understand these differences more fully, it is important to introduce the concept of **metabolic power** versus metabolic capacity. Simply stated, metabolic pathways are relatively more powerful if they have the ability to rapidly supply ATP during highly intense activity. Power, then, relates to how quickly the system can produce ATP. Capacity, however, refers to the ability to make large quantities of ATP. Power and capacity are inversely related. That is, metabolic pathways that are the most powerful also have the least capacity, and vice versa. The anaerobic pathways, therefore, are far more powerful but have a limited capacity for ATP production. They produce relatively little ATP, but the amount they do produce is produced rapidly.

The most intense activities can be sustained for only a few seconds. Try running 200 m at the same velocity that you run 40 m, and you will quickly learn that during the longer run your velocity reduces considerably. This is true even for the elite athlete. Why is that? The answer to that question involves biochemical concepts and concerns another important high-energy phosphate found in muscle in even greater quantities than ATP. This compound is **creatine phosphate,** and because its concentration in muscle is three times that of ATP, it serves an important cellular function, that of an energy reservoir.

ATP is referred to as the energy currency of the cell, because the free energy released from its breakdown powers cellular functions, including muscular activity. But because the concentration of ATP is low in muscle, it is possible to deplete it rapidly in highly intense exercise. The depletion rate of ATP during intense activity would be much greater if it were not for creatine phosphate serving as an energy reservoir. You can see from the reactions of the phosphagen system how this simple system works to sustain ATP concentrations during short, but intense power activities. The breakdown of creatine phosphate serves to sustain ATP levels in the muscle until the reservoir (creatine phosphate) is depleted. When the reservoir is depleted, ATP concentration decreases precipitously and so does the power output of the activity. In essence, the runner in a 200-m run cannot complete that run at 40-m sprint velocities because of rapidly declining ATP concentrations. The cell, in effect, is running out of energy. In fact, we will see that without the presence of the next anaerobic metabolic pathway, a 200-m run could not be completed with much intensity of effort at all, and neither could other anaerobic activities.

LACTIC ACID SYSTEM   The 200-m sprint and longer distance sprints can be completed in an intense fashion because our muscles have the capability to break down glucose to produce ATP in intense activity. The breakdown of glucose is termed **glycolysis** (Fig. 8.8). During intense activity lasting longer than 10 sec, exercising muscles rely more and more on glycolysis to pick up where the phosphagen system left off. This has important implications, because without glucose breakdown in intense activity we would have to severely curtail our running velocity before we finished our 200-m run. In effect, our range of anaerobic activities would be limited to activities that could be completed with high intensity of effort before our reservoir of creatine phosphate ran out, which is only a few seconds. Thus we would not be able to engage in the speed activi-

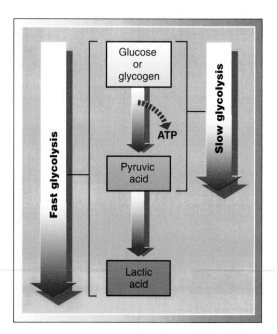

FIGURE 8.8 The lactic acid system.

ties (intense activities that are more enduring than the power activities, but of much shorter duration than the endurance activities). Fortunately, the glycolytic pathway provides an adequate backup.

According to the concept of power versus capacity, glycolysis, although capable of rapidly supplying ATP, is less powerful than the phosphagen system. One reason is that glycolysis is a far more complicated metabolic pathway. It involves the use of 11 enzymes (10 if glycolysis is slow; see Box 8.4), whereas the phosphagen system needs only 2 to produce ATP. But remember that when power is low, capacity is high. This means that the capacity of fast glycolysis to produce ATP is much greater than the phosphagen system. The reason is that there is a lot more energy reserve stored as glucose, so much so that its storage quantity is not a limiting factor for intense activity. This means that glycolysis will be limited or forced to cease during intense activity before glucose is depleted in the cell. Recall that the reason ATP production via creatine phosphate breakdown stopped was that creatine phosphate exists in limited quantities in muscle. These facts make glycolysis an ideal backup to the phosphagen system for producing ATP anaerobically. Furthermore, as stated earlier, our range of anaerobic activities is greatly increased. Now, let's turn to the question of what limits glycolysis.

The cell's capacity for glycolysis is crucial beyond the initial 10 to 15 sec of intense activity and up to approximately 90 sec. However, there is a limit to the ability of glycolysis to sustain ATP production in intense activity. This limitation is brought about by the end product of fast glycolysis: **lactic acid.** When glucose is metabolized in muscle during intense activity, lactic acid, formed in the last of 11 reactions, gradually increases in concentration in the muscle and spills over into the blood circulating through the muscle. Because this is an acid buildup, the pH of the cell significantly decreases to the point at which muscle contraction begins to be compromised for at least two reasons. First, the buildup of the acid in the muscle cell causes any further chemical breakdown of glucose to be hampered by decreasing the activity of the enzymes responsible for glucose breakdown. Second, as the watery medium of the muscle cell (the sarcoplasm) becomes more acidic, the ability of the muscle to continue to contract forcibly is reduced (3). The net result of this is that exercise intensity (e.g., running speed) must be reduced.

Lactic acid is a fatiguing substance; and in this respect, its buildup is detrimental. The ability of the cell to form lactic acid early in intense activity, however, is actually what provides the cell with the capability to continue to make ATP rapidly. Therefore, lactic acid can be seen as both necessary initially and detrimental later in intense activity. Beyond its use inside the cell,

---

Box 8.4
Glycolysis

Although glycolysis is introduced at this point as the second of the anaerobic pathways, it also functions with the aerobic system. This means that there are two forms of glycolysis. During endurance activity, slow (aerobic) glycolysis ends in a substance called pyruvate, because oxygen tensions are adequate in the muscle. In this instance glycolysis is said to be slow, a term that does not relate to the speed of ATP development, but rather to the fact that glycolysis is at that point linked to the aerobic production of ATP via pyruvate. During intense activity, the energy demand of the working muscles exceeds the oxygen supply, or its rate of use. As a result, a product called lactic acid is formed, and glycolysis is said to proceed fast. The descriptor *fast* is a term that relates to the ability of glycolysis to continue under conditions in which lactic acid is formed in the cell in great quantities.

Box 8.5
The Importance of Glucose in Prolonged Exercise

Glucose is stored in the liver and muscles as glycogen (animal starch). Liver glycogen is capable of being broken down into individual glucose molecules to keep the concentration of blood glucose adequate (an important function of the liver). The glucose that is used to fuel either intense (anaerobic) or slow (aerobic) activity, however, comes primarily from stores inside the muscles. When these stores are depleted, as can happen in prolonged, marathon-length activities, fatigue occurs. At this point the muscles start to take up the circulating blood glucose, which can lead to a condition known as hypoglycemia, low blood glucose levels. Hypoglycemia is associated with severe symptoms that make it nearly impossible to maintain the exercise bout. Marathoners often complain of "hitting the wall" at about the 20-mile mark. This is in large measure caused by running out of muscle and liver glycogen. Any exercise training and dietary regimen that enhances glycogen stores in the liver and muscle will increase one's capacity for prolonged exercise.

---

however, lactic acid serves as an important source of energy by other tissues in the body that can absorb it from the general circulation.

Aerobic Production of ATP

When we engage in exercise at an intensity level that can be maintained continuously for long periods of time, ATP is produced in muscles through **cellular respiration,** a process that uses oxygen. In terms of power versus capacity, the aerobic production of ATP has by far the least power. That is, it is not capable of providing ATP rapidly. In turn, the capacity of this system far exceeds the anaerobic systems. Glycolysis releases only approximately 5% of the energy in the glucose molecule. When the exercise intensity is lower, the rest of this energy is liberated by cellular processes that are located in specialized cell structures called **mitochondria.** Glucose breakdown continues in the mitochondria during activity that can be extended for long periods of time. Glucose metabolism, however, may become hindered during prolonged exercise (see Box 8.5)

The processes of cellular respiration are complex, involving the integration of cellular aerobic metabolism with several organ systems designed to coordinate fuel (energy nutrient) and oxygen delivery to the working muscles. Cellular respiration involves five separate metabolic pathways in the breakdown of the two main energy nutrients used during **steady-state** (endurance) exercise: triglycerides (fat) and glucose. We have already considered glycolysis, which breaks down glucose. The breakdown of triglycerides is termed **lipolysis.** In this process, fatty acids are released from the triglyceride molecule. This takes place primarily in adipose (fat) tissue where the fatty acids are released to the blood and transported to muscle cells, where they are metabolized. The breakdown of fatty acids is termed **beta-oxidation.** In this process acetylcoenzyme A (acetyl-CoA) is formed. The other pathways involved in the aerobic production of ATP are the **Krebs cycle** and the **electron-transport chain.**

Beta oxidation and slow glycolysis are coordinated in that both funnel their end products to the respiratory mechanisms inside the mitochondria. Slow glycolysis ends in the formation of pyruvate, whereas beta-oxidation ends in the formation of acetyl-CoA. Pyruvate is placed into the mitochondria where it is converted to acetyl-CoA. Therefore, acetyl-CoA is referred to as the *common degradation product,* because it is derived from both carbohydrate and fat catabolism.

In the aerobic production of ATP during endurance types of activities, both of these energy nutrients are metabolized simultaneously with common end products entering cellular respiration.

As noted earlier the aerobic production of ATP is quite complicated, because the reactions involve many separate metabolic pathways, each with many enzyme steps that are located in different parts of the cell and the body. For instance, fatty acids are mobilized from fat cells during lipolysis and are catalyzed via beta-oxidation in muscle during exercise. Muscle stores of triglycerides are also used. Recall that both anaerobic pathways were located in the sarcoplasm of the muscle fiber and had relatively few steps. This allowed ATP to be produced rapidly for quick muscular activity. Thus power was increased at the expense of capacity. In the aerobic system this is turned around, with the advantage toward capacity. In fact, once fat is being used as a fuel substrate, the energy source is almost unlimited. This great increase in capacity, however, comes at the expense of decreases in power.

In many ways the Krebs cycle can be considered the beginning of the aerobic system, because it is the point of entry for all metabolic intermediate compounds that serve as fuel substrate to be completely broken down in cellular respiration. Starting in the Krebs cycle, these compounds are further broken down to form additional energy-rich carrier molecules: nicotinamide adenine dinucleotide (NADH) and flavin adenine dinucleotide (FADH). These high-energy carrier molecules funnel hydrogen ions to the inner mitochondrial wall, where the electron-transport chain makes large quantities of ATP molecules in a process called oxidative phosphorylation.

The Krebs cycle is also significant because it is the process whereby carbon dioxide is produced. The aerobic system is aptly named, because a regular supply of oxygen is needed in the mitochondria to serve as a final repository for the hydrogen atoms that are stripped off of the energy nutrients during metabolism. With enough oxygen, NADH, and FADH present, oxygen serves as the final acceptor of hydrogen atoms as these atoms are passed along a series of intermediate acceptors. Throughout this process, ATP is generated, and metabolic water is produced. This process, therefore, uses the oxygen we breathe in and delivers to the working muscles. In this process, oxygen is said to be consumed. In the next section, I examine the physiologic systems that deliver oxygen to the muscles, where it is extracted from blood and used in aerobic metabolism. Figure 8.9 illustrates the interrelationships between the different metabolic pathways during cellular respiration. The ATP supplied to the muscles provides the energy for contraction to occur. Sidelight 8.1 provides some detail as to how this ATP energy is used in the engines (the muscles) that allow movement to occur.

The Cardiorespiratory System

To meet the demand contracting muscles have for oxygen during endurance exercise, major organ systems must provide an adequate supply of oxygen. The organ systems responsible for delivery of oxygen into blood (pulmonary system) and blood to the working muscles (cardiovascular system) are controlled to precisely match the increased metabolic demand for oxygen. These systems work as a coupled unit to maintain oxygen and carbon dioxide homeostasis in the body (Fig. 8.10). The function of the pulmonary system is to provide a means of gas exchange between the external environment (the atmosphere) and the internal environment (the various tissues of the body). Part of this function is the process of **external respiration,** whereby oxygen diffuses from the air into the lungs and then into the blood circulating through the lungs. The function of the cardiovascular system is to deliver adequate amounts of oxygen and nutrients to the body and remove heat and waste products.

The integration of the pulmonary and cardiovascular systems in the delivery, extraction, and use of oxygen can be depicted by an equation that expresses the relationship between three important variables: **oxygen consumption, cardiac output,** and the amount of oxygen extracted from the blood as it bathes the working muscles. The blood delivered depends on the cardiac output (the volume of blood circulated per minute). The amount of oxygen extracted depends in

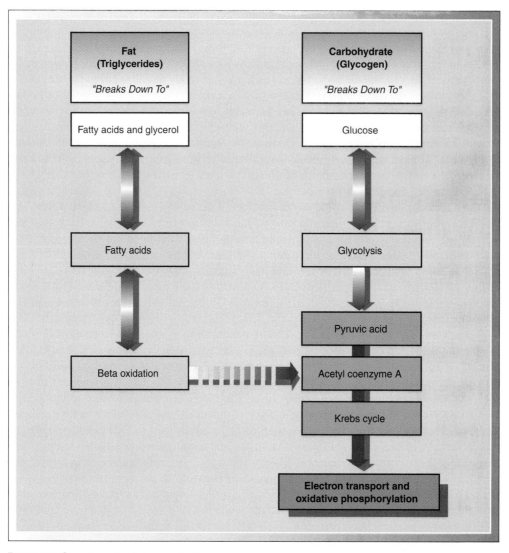

FIGURE 8.9 Overview of cellular respiration.

large part by the ability of the muscles to absorb and use oxygen. Let's now review how these variables are linked to aerobic metabolic processes in the cell.

Oxygen consumption = Amount of blood delivered × Amount of oxygen taken out of the blood by the working muscles

With endurance exercise, there is an immediate need to meet the increased demand for oxygen with an adequate supply. To do this, there is an integrated response from the cardiovascular and pulmonary systems. Three things happen immediately. First, the **heart rate** and the strength of cardiac contractions increase so that the cardiac output closely matches any level of oxygen consumption. The increased strength of cardiac contractions produces a greater cardiac **stroke volume.** Cardiac output is the product of heart rate and stroke volume. These factors result in an increase in the delivery of blood to the working muscles and constitute the central factor (pertaining to the heart itself) for the increase in oxygen consumption that occurs with exercise. The increased delivery of blood is accomplished not only by an increase in blood flow (cardiac

MUSCLES AS MOLECULAR MOTORS

We have already seen that energy for muscular contraction comes from the breakdown of ATP. This occurs in muscles, where the two proteins responsible for shortening the muscle fiber are located. These proteins make up the contractile mechanism of the muscle fiber, and the theory that best explains how muscles contract or shorten is called the *sliding filament theory*. Actin (the thin filament) and myosin (the thick filament) are arrayed in muscle fibers as bundles known as myofibrils. Within the myofibril, the thin filaments are secured in repeating units called sarcomeres. The sarcomere is the smallest contractile unit of muscle. When muscles shorten, thousands of sarcomeres, which are arranged end-to-end along the entire length of the fiber, contract. The thick filaments lie in a parallel position in between the thin filaments and in close proximity. The sliding filament process is part of a greater sequence of events referred to as excitation-contraction coupling, which explains the manner in which skeletal muscles are stimulated by the nervous system to contract.

A nervous transmission arriving at the junction between a nerve and a muscle causes the muscle to reach an electrical condition called the threshold. When this happens, the membrane of the muscle fiber and the interior of the fiber are electrically stimulated. This causes calcium to be released to the interior of the muscle and mix with the contractile elements. Calcium is important for contraction to occur, because it uncovers a spot on the actin filament that was previously covered in the resting state, preventing contraction. This spot is referred to as an active site, because it is the place on the actin filament that binds the ATP molecule. Once the site is uncovered in the excitation process, short projections from the myosin filament called cross bridges attach to the site. These cross bridges are globular portions of the myosin filament that are in a constant state of oscillation. That is, they cyclically vibrate to and fro, attaching, rotating, and reattaching to the active site positions. These cross bridges are the molecular motors of the muscle fiber that are responsible for producing tension. At any given time only about 50% of the cross bridges are in contact with the actin filament. Once in contact, tension is developed by a tilting action of the cross bridge, which has the effect of pulling actin over the myosin filament. The pulling of actin shortens the sarcomeres and thus the entire fiber. When fresh ATP is added to the active site, detachment of the cross bridge occurs. ATP breakdown with the release of free energy re-cocks the myosin cross bridge, and the attachment and tilting action begins again. This continues for as long as calcium is present. Once the nervous stimulation stops, calcium is removed, and the muscle relaxes.

output) but also by the massive redistribution of blood away from areas that do not participate in producing movement (e.g., the gastrointestinal tract, bone, and skin) and toward the working muscles. The increase in cardiac output, heart rate, and oxygen consumption during endurance activities is proportional to exercise intensity. For instance, both cardiac output and oxygen consumption increase in a step-by-step fashion as walking or running rate increases. However, during weightlifting, a resistance exercise that is largely anaerobic, oxygen consumption is much lower for a given level of heart rate.

Second, as exercise intensity increases, more oxygen is extracted from the blood as the blood passes through the **capillaries** of the working muscles. This can be measured as a larger difference between the oxygen content of the arteries feeding the muscles and oxygen content of the veins leaving the muscles. This greater difference in the oxygen content of arteries versus veins constitutes the peripheral factor (away from the heart) for the increase in oxygen consumption that occurs with exercise.

Third, the increase in oxygen consumption with exercise results from an increase in pulmonary ventilation. Pulmonary ventilation is the bulk flow of air into and out of the lungs. Upon the initiation of exercise, both the rate and depth of breathing increase, which results in an increase in pulmonary ventilation. As the exercise intensity during endurance activity increases, more air is passed in and out of the lungs. The increased rate at which the lungs are ventilated allows more oxygen to be delivered to the working muscles. Exercise physiol-

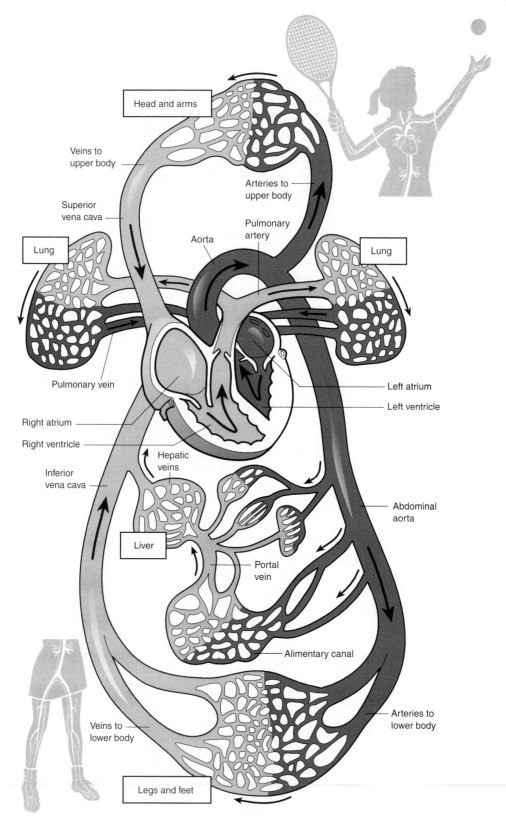

FIGURE 8.10 Cardiorespiratory system.

***Box* 8.6**
Important Measurements in Exercise Physiology

Oxygen consumption is an important variable measured in exercise physiology research. Oxygen consumption (Vo_2) is the rate at which oxygen is used during aerobic ATP production. The maximum rate at which oxygen can be consumed (Vo_2max) is recognized as the single best indicator of one's cardiorespiratory fitness level. A high Vo_2max indicates a more optimal functioning of the cardiovascular, pulmonary, and muscular systems during endurance exercise. One's oxygen consumption level during exercise is also a key indicator of how hard the exercise session is. The intensity at which we perform endurance exercise is usually expressed using qualitative descriptors of the level of oxygen consumption, such as low, moderate, heavy, and maximum. A range of values is typically given to these descriptors in terms of a percentage of Vo_2max. For instance, low-intensity endurance exercise is anything less than about 50% Vo_2max, whereas moderate ranges from 50% to 75% Vo_2max, heavy is anything greater than 80% Vo_2max, and maximal is 100% Vo_2max.

Another important measurement exercise physiologists make is carbon dioxide (CO_2) production. Recall that carbon dioxide was produced in the Krebs cycle. When both the production of carbon dioxide (Vco_2) and consumption of oxygen (Vo_2max) are measured, the exercise physiologist can calculate the respiratory exchange ratio (R). This measure is useful for describing the energy nutrients being used to fuel endurance exercise. It then becomes possible to know how the exercise is being fueled, whether by fat or carbohydrate, or the relative percentages of both.

ogists are interested in these kinds of variables because they help quantify exercise responses (see Box 8.6).

Thermoregulation

All mammals are **homeothermic.** This means that we must maintain our internal body temperatures within narrow limits for survival, regardless of the state of the external environment. This is often quite challenging when we're faced with extremes of temperatures. As stated earlier, one of the functions of the cardiovascular system is to remove heat from the body. This function is especially important during aerobic exercise, because of the large amount of heat produced and subsequently trapped in the body.

Part of the energy liberated during aerobic exercise is used to perform useful work; however, this portion of the energy expenditure is relatively small (only 20 to 30%). This means that the remaining part of the energy produced is stored as heat and must be eliminated to maintain our **core temperature** within reasonable levels. If this is not done adequately the result may be some form of **heat illness** or possibly even death.

When aerobic exercise is performed in environmental conditions that are favorable (low to moderate air temperature and relative humidity) the body's ability to thermoregulate is sufficient to keep core temperature increases to a minimum. In this case, the increase in core temperature is linked to the intensity of exercise in terms of the relative percentage of maximum oxygen consumption. For instance, exercise at 50% of one's maximum oxygen consumption means a core temperature increase of only 1°C. This represents a successful thermoregulatory effort. Practical Application 8.1 describes what would happen during exercise if there were no system to regulate core temperature.

If, however, environmental conditions are at the extremes of temperature, relative humidity, or both, thermoregulation is much harder to accomplish. The result of exercising in environmental extremes is an increase in core temperature, with a reduction in work output. The reduced work output is a direct result of the extra burden placed on the cardiovascular system, which not only must supply oxygen to the working muscles to sustain the work output but now has the even more important role of delivering heat to the superficial regions of the body to dissipate the heat. In Figure 8.11 one can readily see that the ability to deliver blood to the working muscles is reduced in the heat. This has the direct effect of reducing maximum oxygen consumption and reducing exercise performance. In this case, two areas of the body are competing for the same cardiac output: the muscles, to sustain the exercise intensity, and the skin, to dissipate the heat being carried by the blood. As the skin region receives more of the cardiac output, there is of necessity, a reduction in endurance performance.

Evaporation

The ability to adequately dissipate the extra heat produced during aerobic exercise depends on the evaporative transfer of heat to the environment as water is vaporized from the respiratory passages and from the surface of the skin. Evaporation of water (sweat) off the skin is especially important because it represents the major way heat is removed from the body during exercise, except in hot, humid environments. Anything that retards this process hinders exercise performance and carries a certain amount of risk to the exerciser.

Evaporation is aided when the vapor pressure gradient from the skin surface to the air is large. This occurs when the relative humidity of the air is low. In this condition sweat easily evaporates to air that is relatively more dry than the skin. With the transfer of water off the skin, heat is also transferred to the surroundings, thus the body is cooled. Exercising in conditions of low relative humidity is, therefore, desirable. This problem is independent of environmental temperatures, because deaths have occurred in high humidity conditions even when temperatures have been moderate (4).

Practical Application 8.1

HEAT PRODUCTION AND LOSS DURING EXERCISE

The following is a hypothetical situation that proves a serious point. For an average jogging session it is possible for a runner (70 kg body mass) to consume 120 L of oxygen for a 1-hr run (2 L of oxygen/min for 60 min). On the average, 1 L of oxygen equals the liberation of 5 kcal of energy (120 L × 5 kcal/L = 600 kcal). This represents an extra 600 kcal of body heat to be eliminated by the thermoregulatory system. The specific heat of body tissue is 0.83 kcal/kg/°C, giving this individual a value of 58.1 kcal/°C (0.83 kcal/kg/°C × 70 kg). This means that for every 58.1 kcal produced, the 70-kg runner's body temperature would raise 1°C, for a total increase for this exercise session of 10.3°C (600 kcal ÷ 58.1 kcal/°C); that is, if that the runner did not have a functioning thermoregulatory system. On the other hand, without a thermoregulatory system, this athlete would not likely have made it to the point of engaging in exercise in the first place, given that at rest there is a 0.5° to 0.6°C increase in body temperature for each hour of life. Without the ability to dissipate this heat, death would quickly follow.

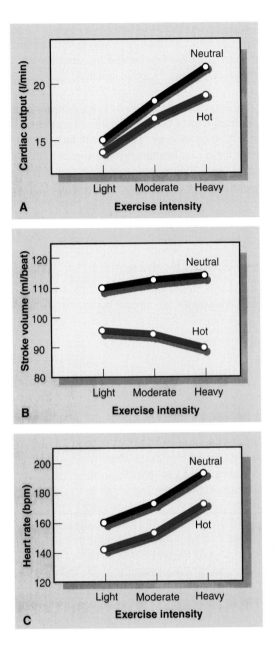

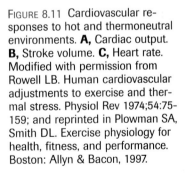

FIGURE 8.11 Cardiovascular responses to hot and thermoneutral environments. **A,** Cardiac output. **B,** Stroke volume. **C,** Heart rate. Modified with permission from Rowell LB. Human cardiovascular adjustments to exercise and thermal stress. Physiol Rev 1974;54:75-159; and reprinted in Plowman SA, Smith DL. Exercise physiology for health, fitness, and performance. Boston: Allyn & Bacon, 1997.

Inappropriate clothing greatly retards the evaporation of sweat from the skin. Different types of clothing are more effective in setting up a microenvironment around the skin than others, resulting in evaporation being retarded even when the outside environmental conditions are favorable. Certain types of athletic wear are specifically designed to provide a vapor barrier that completely stops the evaporative cooling process (see Practical Application 8.2).

Water Intake

One of the most important things that one can do when exercising in a hot environment is to drink plenty of water. The importance of this cannot be stressed too much. Studies have shown that water replacement is effective in keeping to a minimum the increase in core temperature that occurs with exercise. One study in particular demonstrated that when subjects maintained a water balance (water intake that matched water loss) core body temperature increases were minimal (5).

On the other hand, subjects who were allowed to drink water ad libitum (whenever they wanted) and those who were not allowed to drink water experienced a significantly greater body core temperature. This study underscores the fact that the thirst response lags behind the need for water during exercise. Physiologic conditions were improved when subjects maintained their water balance.

In conclusion, I highlighted in this section the important link between several physiologic systems and the energy processes that occur in muscles during various forms of exercise. Let's now turn our attention to two advances made in exercise physiology. The first, the link between muscle fiber types and sports performance, although not recent, continues to be a fruitful area of investigation. The second, overtraining, is currently being heavily researched and promises to shed light on an important concern for athletes and nonathletes alike.

ADVANCES IN EXERCISE PHYSIOLOGY
Muscle Fiber Types: A Determinant of Sports Performance

Not all athletes are alike. We know this intuitively. But what about muscles, are all muscles alike? The answer to this question is not readily apparent. It is an important concern because it has much

---

Practical Application 8.2

THE USE AND MISUSE OF VAPOR BARRIER CLOTHING

Different types of exercise training apparel are on the market today that effectively create a microenvironment around the body when worn. This so-called vapor barrier clothing is designed to prevent evaporation and conserve body heat by creating a condition of 100% humidity in the space between the suit and the skin. These suits are commonly worn by athletes and adults who want to cause weight loss or prevent rapid cooling. To be an effective vapor barrier, the suits typically are made of a vinyl material. If used to aid in weight loss efforts it should be realized that, though effective, the weight loss is temporary, lasting until natural rehydration occurs. In addition, the weight loss is reflective of a significant reduction in plasma volume, which accompanies an increase in the demand on the heart, even in the resting state. Because most people wear these clothes while exercising, the added stress on the heart is compounded. Although the average young athlete may have enough cardiac reserve to overcome the extra demands, older individuals often do not. Herein lies the danger in wearing vapor barrier clothing. Such clothing should not be worn in the summertime for any reason, especially by older adults. This practice places the individual at an increased risk for heat exhaustion or stroke. In the winter, however, it can be an effective means of remaining warm during exercise bouts in very low temperatures, as long as one realizes that exercise will naturally heat the body. Certainly in subfreezing temperatures these suits may serve a valid purpose. Such clothing is useful for athletes (baseball pitchers and football quarterbacks, for example) in cooler weather as a means to prevent muscular cooling and stiffening during inactive periods.

to do with success in sports performance and with our innate athletic potential. Since the mid-1970s, there has been a tremendous amount of research investigating muscle fiber types and sports performance. Not all muscle fibers are alike. With the advent of the percutaneous needle biopsy technique to sample human skeletal muscle fibers before, during, and after exercise, exercise physiology research has been able to establish a link between muscle fiber types and sports performance. Let's briefly review this research and see how exercise physiology has advanced our understanding of how muscle fiber makeup may lead to differences in athletic potential.

Although it may be apparent that not all muscles are alike, it is not apparent that muscles are composed of fibers with strikingly different characteristics. There are different types of muscles in the body. Some are skeletal, as in the biceps brachii (muscle of the upper arm responsible for flexing the elbow), and some are smooth, as in those that line the arteries. The heart (cardiac) muscle is a third type. In addition, the major skeletal muscles are also obviously different, having different shapes, sizes, and functions. The deltoid (shoulder muscle), for instance, is not at all like the gastrocnemius (muscle of the lower leg). Within each skeletal muscle there are at least three general types of fibers that have been characterized in humans (6,7). This knowledge has led to a more complete understanding of the physiology of athletic performance.

The main muscle fibers that have been characterized are slow oxidative, fast oxidative glycolytic, and fast glycolytic. These fibers have characteristically different mechanical, metabolic, and morphologic makeups. The descriptors *slow* and *fast* are used to relate how quickly these fibers reach their peak tension (Fig. 8.12). For instance, fast glycolytic fibers reach peak tension in about 50 msec, whereas slow oxidative fibers take up to 110 msec. This contraction speed is supported by metabolic properties appropriate for each. Fast glycolytic fibers have a much higher capacity to breakdown glucose to lactic acid, whereas the slow oxidative fiber has a much higher capacity to use oxygen in the aerobic breakdown of energy nutrients. Fast oxidative glycolytic muscle is also referred to as intermediate, because it has a slightly greater oxidative capacity and slightly lower glycolytic capacity than the fast glycolytic fiber (the true anaerobic fiber). The metabolic and contractile properties of these fibers can influence exercise performance. In fact, being born with a preponderance of one fiber type may set a genetic limit for particular kinds of athletic endeavors.

Research has shown that fiber type makeup is characteristic for particular events (Fig. 8.13) (8). This strongly suggests that athletic prowess is linked to muscle fiber type. Athletes who compete in long distance events have predominantly slow oxidative fibers. The calf muscle of these athletes has been shown to contain 90% slow oxidative fibers. Just the opposite has been shown for sprint athletes and other athletes who engage in power performances, such as weightlifters. For these athletes the percentage of slow oxidative fibers in the calf muscle may be as low as 25 to 45%.

Can individuals be counseled into sports activity based on the fiber type distribution of their muscles? It would appear that if muscle fiber type were the only factor that dictated athletic success the answer would be yes. Unfortunately, predicting athletic success is not that simple. Many other factors, such as cardiovascular function, body size, and other important physiologic and biomechanical factors play important roles (see A Case in Point 8.2). What we do know is that fiber type distribution is important. Therefore, this research has advanced our understanding of the physiology of sports performance.

Overtraining: Is More Really Better?

Athletes often want more of a physiologic return for their training time. To do this they often fall prey to the old adage that "More is better." But is this really the case? There is a fine line between optimal training and overtraining for both the athlete and nonathlete. When that line is crossed, decrements in performance capacity will occur along with myriad other problems, some medical and physiologic and others psychological (see Box 8.7).

The problem of overtraining has been the focus of a substantial amount of research aimed at increasing our understanding of the physiologic, pathophysiologic, nutritional, immunologic,

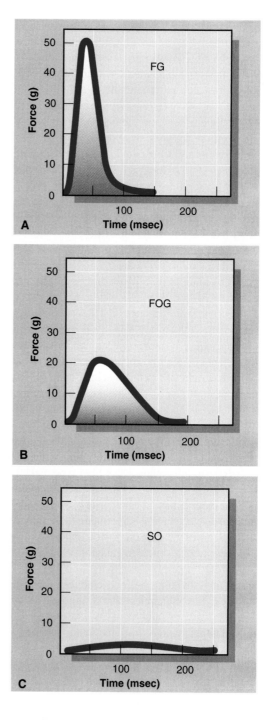

FIGURE 8.12 Muscle performance characteristics. **A,** Fast glycolytic fibers. **B,** Fast oxidative glycolytic fibers. **C,** Slow oxidative fibers. Modified with permission from Edington DW, Edgerton VR. The biology of physical activity. Boston: Houghton Mifflin, 1986.

and psychological consequences of overtraining in endurance and strength and power athletes (9,10). This research promises to have application for people who exercise a great deal but are not considered athletes. This increase in research activity was amply illustrated by an international conference devoted solely to overtraining that was held the week before the Centennial Olympic Games in Atlanta in the summer of 1996.

The overtrained condition is more than just an acute problem that can be alleviated with short-term rest. It is also more than a slight decrease in competition-level performance capability. Rather the problem is chronic and cannot be easily remedied. As more research is accom-

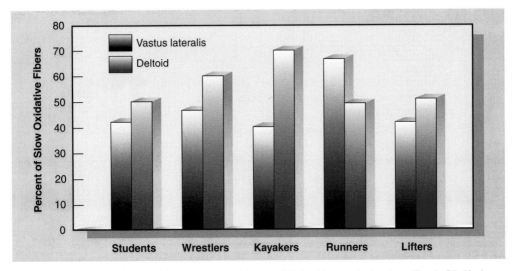

FIGURE 8.13 Muscle fiber type by athletic specialty. Modified with permission from Tesch PA, Karlsson J. Muscle fiber types and size in trained and untrained muscles of elite athletes. J Appl Physiol 1985;59:1716–1720; and reprinted in Plowman SA, Smith DL. Exercise physiology for health, fitness, and performance. Boston: Allyn & Bacon, 1997.

plished in this important area, strategies and guidelines are likely to be developed to help avoid and overcome this malady.

In conclusion, this chapter has considered only a small part of the total content of exercise physiology. The focus was on information related to the basic foundations of this subdiscipline of exercise science. There is much more to be learned than what was introduced here. Chapters 9 and 11 present other information with a physiologic knowledge base that is important to the

A Case in Point 8.2

PREDICTING SUCCESS IN ENDURANCE RUNNING[a]

In 1972 Frank Shorter was a world-class marathon runner, even though by objective standards his success may have seemed less than likely. The reason is that compared to other elite marathoners, he had a modest maximum oxygen consumption of approximately 65 mL/kg/min. Although much higher than the average person, this value did not seem to ensure much success against the competitors, whose values were in the high 70s and low 80s. Shorter, however, went on to win the Gold Medal at the 1972 Munich Olympic Games. How was this possible?

Success in endurance events is multifactorial from a physiologic standpoint. In fact, four factors seem to be needed for success: high Vo_2max value, high lactate threshold, high economy of effort (low Vo_2 value for the same rate of work), and high percentage of slow-twitch muscle fibers. Shorter's unusually high lactate threshold allowed him to run at more than 90% of his Vo_2max and still have blood lactate levels that were not different from resting levels. This means that compared to his competitors—who had higher aerobic capacities but lower lactate thresholds—he could run at a greater velocity without significant blood lactate buildup and thus win the race.

[a]Daniels JT. A physiologist's view of running economy. Med Sci Sports Exer 1985;17:332–338; Daniels JT, Yarbrough RA, Foster C. Changes in max Vo_2 and running performance with training. Eur J Appl Physiol 1978;39:249–254.

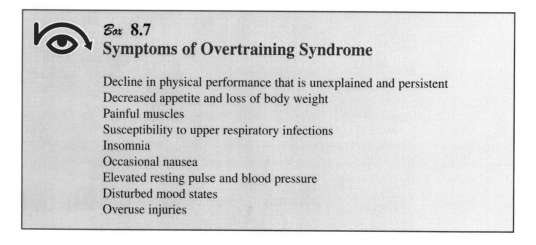

Box **8.7**
Symptoms of Overtraining Syndrome

Decline in physical performance that is unexplained and persistent
Decreased appetite and loss of body weight
Painful muscles
Susceptibility to upper respiratory infections
Insomnia
Occasional nausea
Elevated resting pulse and blood pressure
Disturbed mood states
Overuse injuries

fitness and health. Those chapters will round out the discussion of the important physiologic areas of exercise science.

SUMMARY POINTS

- Exercise physiology is the science of how the body functions during exercise and sports activity and how it changes during chronic exercise training.
- The activity continuum allows us to visualize acute exercise as power, speed, or endurance events in terms of metabolic and hemodynamic responses.
- Energy is released from the energy nutrients during cellular mechanisms and, in turn, captured again in the form of ATP.
- The breakdown of ATP powers muscular contraction.
- ATP is made in the muscles by processes that are linked to important physiologic systems (neural, endocrine, cardiovascular, and pulmonary).
- The specific way ATP is made is dictated by the kind of activity in which one is engaging.
- During intense activity, ATP is made primarily by creatine phosphate and glucose breakdown.
- For long-duration exercise, ATP is produced by cellular respiration.
- Aerobic metabolism is integrated to systems that supply oxygen—the pulmonary and cardiovascular systems.
- Thermoregulation is an important function for maintaining near-normal core temperatures as we exercise.
- Exercise in the heat and humidity results in increased cardiovascular stress and reduced exercise performance.

REVIEW QUESTIONS

1. Define exercise physiology.
2. List five activities each that can be classified as power, speed, and endurance activities.
3. Using the activities listed in question 2, identify the predominate metabolic pathway.
4. Explain the differences between acute and chronic exercise.
5. Describe how the body uses energy to produce movement. What is the relationship between muscle contraction and energy production?
6. Explain how the cardiorespiratory system is coordinated with energy production.
7. Explain the importance of thermoregulation during exercise.

References

1. Bouchard C, Godbout P, Mondor JC, et al. Specificity of maximal aerobic power. Eur J Appl Physiol 1979;40:85–93.
2. Falkel JE, Fleck SJ, Murray TF. Comparison of central hemodynamics between powerlifters and bodybuilders during resistance exercise. J Appl Sport Sc Res 1992;6:24–35.
3. Bertocci LA, Gollnick PD. pH effect on mitochondria and individual enzyme function. Med Sci Sports Exer 1985;17:244.
4. O'Donnell T, Clowes G. The circulatory abnormalities of heat stroke. N Engl J Med 1972;287:734–737.
5. Fox E, Bowers R, Foss M. The physiological basis for exercise and sport. Madison, WI: Brown & Benchmark, 1993.
6. Colliander EB, Dudley GA, Tesch PA. Skeletal muscle fiber composition and performance during repeated bouts of maximal, concentric contractions. Eur J Appl Physiol 1988;58:81–86.
7. Costill DL, Fink WJ, Pollock ML. Muscle fiber composition and enzyme activities of elite distance runners. Med Sci Sports Exer 1976;8:96–100.
8. Jansson E, Sjokin B, Tesch P. Changes in muscle fiber type distribution in men after physical training. Acta Physiol Scand 1978;104:235–237.
9. Hooper SL, Mackinnon LT, Howard A, et al. Markers for monitoring overtraining and recover. Med Sci Sports Exer 1995;27:106–112.
10. Lehmann M. Overtraining in endurance athletes: a brief review. Med Sci Sports Exer 1993;25:854–862.

Suggested Readings

McArdle WD, Katch FI, Katch VL. Exercise physiology: energy, nutrition, and human performance, Baltimore, MD: Williams & Wilkins, 1996.
Powers SK, Howley ET. Exercise physiology: theory and applications to fitness and performance. Madison, WI: Brown & Benchmark, 1997.
Wilmore JH, Costill DL. Physiology of sport and exercise. Champaign, IL: Human Kinetics, 1994.

9

Sports Nutrition

STELLA L. VOLPE

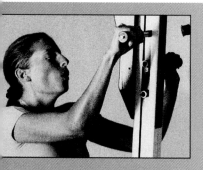

Objectives

1. Describe what is required to become a sports nutritionist.
2. Distinguish between carbohydrate, fat, and protein needs of athletes.
3. Identify the vitamins and mineral needs of athletes.
4. Explain the hydration needs and regimen of athletes and why hydration is important.
5. Classify improper weight loss regimens and explain why these are dangerous and not helpful to athletic performance.
6. Classify and describe the popular ergogenic aids and discuss their efficacy.
7. Classify and describe various body composition assessment techniques.
8. Describe the use of stable isotopes of minerals in sports nutrition research.

Sports nutrition, in addition to being a subspecialty of the multidisciplinary field of nutrition, has developed since the 1980s as an important subdiscipline of exercise science. Although sports nutrition is one of the newest of the exercise science subdisciplines, there is currently a great amount of research being conducted in this field, pointing to the importance of nutrition in optimal sports performance and the general interests this field has come to have. In the arena of high-level collegiate and professional sports, it is important for athletes to maintain the competitive edge that proper nutrition gives them. This competitiveness, however, sometimes leads athletes to disregard sound nutritional practices in lieu of the latest supplement that purports to enhance performance. Today, with a plethora of "health food" choices at our disposal, competitive athletes, as well as the general public, may put themselves at risk by following what usually proves to be spurious nutritional advice. This chapter takes the guess work out by covering important facets of sports nutrition, including the role of sports nutritionists; the carbohydrate, fat, and protein needs of athletes; the mineral and vitamin needs of athletes; hydration; weight loss and athletic performance; and the use of **ergogenic aids** to increase exercise performance.

> *Nutrition is a science consisting of a number of subspecialties, including clinical nutrition, nutritional biochemistry, community nutrition, nutrition in the food service arena, nutritional management, and nutrition counseling.*

DEFINITION, DESCRIPTION, AND SCOPE

Sports nutrition is concerned with applying nutritional principles to sports and deals mainly with the following aspects: *(a)* how nutrition affects exercise performance at all levels, novice to elite athlete; *(b)* how nutrition affects physical performance (e.g., for individuals who have jobs that require a great deal of physical exertion); and *(c)* the effects (including dangers) of ergogenic aids on nutrition and physical performance. What we take into our bodies has a vast influence on our overall health and well-being. This is true for people in all walks of life, making knowledge about nutrition among the general public a high priority within public health. As our society has become more and more prosperous, leading to an increased interest in leisure time activities and sports, our understanding of the role of proper nutrition for exercise, general physical activity, and sports has increased. This trend, however, has also resulted in an increase in the exploitation of the public in the area of nutritional supplementation. Fads, misconceptions, and lack of knowledge help proliferate **quackery,** which is the promotion of nutritional products without regard to the facts.

Nutritional quackery is the propagation of questionable scientific information as important evidence for the effectiveness of a particular product. This problem is especially acute in athletics, where the pursuit of superior performance leads individuals to consume a wide variety of nutritional supplements. One has only to read about the latest record-breaking performance in the sports pages to learn about the newest hot nutritional ergogenic aid.

> *Faddism in the context of sports nutrition is an exaggerated belief in the effects of nutrition on maintaining health and enhancing performance, whereas quackery is usually applied to people or advertisers who may be sincere but are misguided in their beliefs about the efficacy of a sports nutrition product.*

To properly define sports nutrition, we should begin with a good working definition of *nutrition,* which is "the science that interprets the relationship of food to the functioning of the living organism" (1). Because nutrition is a multidisciplinary science, this interpretation is viewed in a broader sense by the American Dietetic Association (ADtA; see Chapter 3), which views nutrition as being affected by many factors, including psychological, sociologic, and economic aspects. Because food consumption and athletic performance are often intricately intertwined with psychological state, the athlete's psychological status often affects nutritional status. The focus of this chapter, however, is on the biochemical and physiologic functions of food and how they may affect athletic or physical performance. Figure 9.1 describes a typical undergraduate sports nutrition course. Notice that the figure is not all-inclusive but gives only a basic idea of what a sports nutrition course might include; the main focus centers on the hard science content.

Sports nutrition is a field that is virtually skyrocketing, largely because ours is a sports-conscious culture and a media-driven society. Although sports nutrition is everywhere seen in the popular culture, not everything the general public sees and hears should be interpreted as being sound advice. But what of legitimate sports nutrition? Typically, sports nutritionists work with athletes at the high school, collegiate, Olympic, and/or professional level. Sports nutritionists also work with individuals who exercise and/or have jobs that are physically demanding. Sports nutritionists may be individuals who research the effect of nutritional interventions on exercise performance or registered dietitians who counsel athletes to ensure optimal performance through sound nutrition. Within these two main areas are a number of subareas in which qualified individuals can specialize. For example, a researcher may focus on mineral metabolism to see

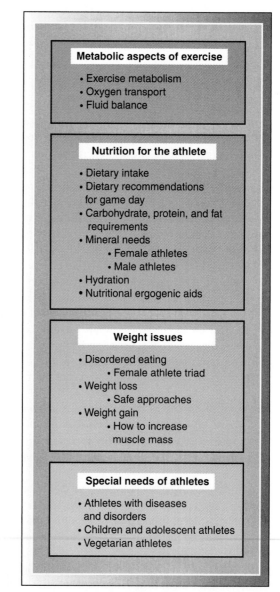

FIGURE 9.1 General content organization of a sports nutrition course.

HOW TO BECOME A SPORTS NUTRITIONIST

The first step to becoming a sports nutritionist is to receive a bachelor's degree in nutrition and/or nutrition and dietetics from a program accredited by the American Dietetic Association (ADtA). Academic prerequisites for these programs include inorganic and organic chemistry, biology, and biochemistry. Programs that offer a specialized degree in sports nutrition typically require additional courses to the ADtA-recommended curriculum. Students in a general nutrition or dietetics program that does not have a sports nutrition specialty may take exercise science classes to gain a better understanding of exercise nutrition. As an alternative, students in such a program may pursue a double major (in exercise science and in nutrition), which accomplishes the same goal.

During their senior year, sports nutrition students apply to specific dietetic internships to prepare them to take the registered dietitian (RD) board examination. These internships generally last 10 to 12 months. The status of registered dietitian demonstrates that the individual has undergone rigorous and proper training in nutrition, has passed the board examination for registered dietitians, and is qualified to teach and counsel on nutrition in a variety of areas. In addition, after gaining registered dietitian status, individuals are required to maintain their credentials by obtaining an established number of credits every 5 years (e.g., by attending conferences pertinent to their speciality).

After earning the necessary credentials to practice dietetics, professionals interested in sports nutrition may decide to pursue a master's degree in exercise physiology or science. This additional academic preparation allows dietitians to validly market themselves as sports nutritionists. Furthermore, it is always a good idea to gain practical experience by working in a clinical (hospital) setting before starting a sports nutrition career. The knowledge gained from clinical experience offers a great advantage to the novice sports nutritionist.

whether mineral supplementation improves oxygen transport and use in the body and how it may contribute to bone strength, thereby reducing exercise injuries. In addition, there has been a plethora of nutritional ergogenic aids developed over the last few years. For example, much research has examined compounds containing creatine, which is thought to enhance power and speed performances. The role of sports nutrition in this day of fast-moving sports and activity pursuits by a large segment of the population is indeed great. Sidelight 9.1 gives some valuable advice for exercise science students interested in sports nutrition as a career. The following section looks at **macronutrients** and exercise performance, an important topic in the science of sports nutrition.

FOCUS ON SCIENCE

"There is a common belief that there are sport-specific diets. The truth is that there are only people-specific diets. The first nutritional requirement for athletes and their sports fans is a well-balanced diet that contains a wide range of foods and covers daily energy expenditure" (2). This statement is an excellent one because, although athletes may require more carbohydrates and protein than their sedentary counterparts, athletes' diets should still be healthy and contain a wide variety of nutrients for improving performance and health. Athletes will often forget about their health, so to speak, and will do anything to win. Consuming a wide variety of foods will improve athletic performance and overall long-term health; both should be emphasized to athletes. This section discusses the macronutrients—carbohydrates, fats, and protein—and **micronutrients**—minerals and vitamins. The importance of water consumption is also discussed.

Before discussing the specific macronutrients, it is imperative to teach athletes that they need to consume enough total energy to match their energy expenditure. If the athlete does not do this, a detriment in both mental and physical performance may result (see Practical Application 9.1).

Practical Application 9.1

EATING BREAKFAST: A HOT TOPIC?

Many athletes have their own agenda and are concerned only about performance and not long-term health; however, the job of the qualified sports nutritionist is to focus the athletes' attention on both performance and overall health. Athletes are often looking for a magic bullet to place them first among their competitors.

When an athlete records his or her diet, the diet typically is lacking in many major foods. The first thing a nutritionist may notice is that the athlete does not eat breakfast. This may sound like a boring topic, because we have all been told many times, "Eat your breakfast!" Well, this simple phrase has really proven to be true. Athletes who consume breakfast prepare their bodies and minds for the rest of the day (including practices). Athletes who fuel their bodies in the morning tend to have good concentration and don't crash and burn when practice rolls around. Eating breakfast helps athletes avoid overeating after practice. For example, many athletes skip breakfast and eat a small lunch, which leads to overconsumption of foods from about 7:00 to 9:00 P.M. These individuals generally not only eat more calories than needed but also eat nutrient-poor foods. All of this can lead to fatigue and poor performance. Because of overeating in the evening, these athletes are not hungry in the morning.

Note that breakfast need not be right at 8:00 A.M. every morning. For example, if an athlete gets hungry at 10:00 A.M., he or she can eat breakfast then. And if an athlete has early morning practice (e.g., at 7:00 A.M.), eating at 8:00 may not be realistic. So the athlete must plan accordingly. If early morning practices are the norm, then a small breakfast—say some water, a banana, and a breakfast powder mixed with skim milk—may be a good start. After practice, the athlete can eat a fuller breakfast of fruit plus cereal and skim milk, pancakes, or French toast. Furthermore, typical breakfast foods are not the only foods that can be consumed in the morning. If an athlete likes peanut butter and jelly with milk for breakfast, that is just fine. It provides the protein, fat, and carbohydrates needed to start the day.

With all this said, many athletes with an inadequate overall dietary intake will be quick to look to supplements because they are supposed to lead to better performance. When consulting athletes, sports nutritionists must first examine their clients' dietary intake to assess what they are actually consuming. A lot of women athletes, for example, do not consume enough protein; conversely, a lot of male athletes consume too much protein. Balance is the key. Thus consuming a varied diet and the proper amount of calories and fluids will lead to peak performance. Eating breakfast still is the best advice, even in this day of high-tech nutritional supplements.

Carbohydrates: Fuel for the Body

Carbohydrates are foods needed to maintain **glycogen stores** in the body. Glycogen is used for energy and is the storage form of carbohydrates found in the liver and muscles. Carbohydrate foods need to be eaten so there is enough **blood glucose** available, not only for exercise but also

| *Table 9.1* | GOOD FOOD SOURCES OF CARBOHYDRATES[a] |

Food	Serving Size	Carbohydrates, g
Applesauce, sweetened	½ cup	125
Barley	1 cup	135
Pancakes, whole wheat	4 (1 inch)	52
Pasta, cooked, enriched	1 cup	40
Potato, baked with skin	1 medium	51
Pretzels, hard, salted	2 ounces	44
Grape-Nuts cereal	1 cup	93
Bread, whole wheat	2 slices	24
Milk, skim	1 cup	12
Hummus, fresh	½ cup	6
Ice cream, chocolate	1½ cups	56
Rice pudding	1 cup	66

[a]Reprinted with permission from Wardlaw GM. Perspectives in nutrition. 4th ed. Boston: McGraw-Hill, 1999.

for the brain and entire central nervous system. The central nervous system uses glucose as its primary fuel source. Table 9.1 lists foods that are good sources of carbohydrates.

Dietary Carbohydrate

Why are carbohydrates so important in exercise? Carbohydrates, in the form of glucose, provide fuel (energy from adenosine triphosphate; see Chapter 8) for your muscles. Low-carbohydrate diets such as the Zone Diet or Protein Power are not appropriate and can even be harmful to a person's health. In the 1970s, for instance, high-protein, low-carbohydrate diets became popular. The public was shocked, however, when some people died from heart failure while on these diets. What is often viewed by the public as benign may often be quite dangerous, requiring proper counseling by a knowledgeable professional. For example, nutritionists are often called on to counsel athletes with conditions such as diabetes mellitus, a disease of carbohydrate metabolism. Athletes who have type 1 or 2 diabetes have special needs; therefore, a qualified registered dietitian should be consulted to help these individuals.

> *Diabetes mellitus is a disease in which insulin—a hormone made by the islets of Langerhans and used to help deposit glucose into cells for energy—is not made in sufficient quantities by the body. When a person's body is not synthesizing enough insulin, he or she requires insulin injections and has insulin-dependent, or type 1, diabetes mellitus. When there is enough insulin, but the insulin receptors are not working properly, he or she has non-insulin-dependent, or type 2, diabetes mellitus.*

At rest, carbohydrates supply about 40% of the energy our bodies need. When a person engages in low-intensity exercise, the percentage of fat is more important; however, as exercise intensity begins to increase, carbohydrate use increases to about 50% or more. At higher intensities, more than 70% of a person's maximum consumption of oxygen, carbohydrates become the primary fuel for the body. In essence, then, your body is always using carbohydrates; however, the greater the intensity of the exercise, the greater the use of carbohydrates.

Every gram of carbohydrates provides the body with 4 **kilocalories (kcal)** of energy. For example, 400 g of carbohydrates provides 1600 kilocalories (400 g carbohydrate × 4 kcal/g of carbohydrate = 1600 kcal).

Athletes should consume a mixed meal (carbohydrates, protein, and fat) a few hours before competition or practice. This meal should be followed by about 200 kcal of carbohydrates every hour during an endurance event. The carbohydrates can be in a liquid (e.g., a sports drink), if that is preferred. Athletes should consume high-carbohydrate foods 15 min to 2 hr after an event so they can properly replenish their glycogen stores.

It is typically recommended that 60 to 65% of an athlete's total calorie intake should consist of carbohydrates. Thus if 2000 kcal of food are consumed per day, then 1200 to 1300 kcal (60 to 65%) should be from carbohydrates, which is equal to 300 to 325 g of carbohydrates per day. Many researchers prefer that athletes consume 7 to 10 g of carbohydrates for every kilogram of body weight per day (see Box 9.1) (3,4). Note that most of the carbohydrates consumed should be complex carbohydrates (e.g., grains, pasta, whole grain breads, potatoes, rice, or bagels). Complex carbohydrates provide a more sustained release of glucose (simple form of carbohydrates) over time and provide more nutrients than do simple carbohydrates (e.g., pastries, cakes, and candy).

There are a number of ways to increase the amount of carbohydrates in the diet. First, snacks and meals should be based around nutritious carbohydrate foods like whole grains and breads, fruits, legumes (e.g., kidney beans, pinto beans, lentils), pasta, and rice. These types of foods should cover about half of the diner's plate (5).

Carbohydrates are necessary to maintain energy levels in both athletes and nonathletes alike. Without carbohydrates, a person will feel tired and light headed, because the brain relies on blood glucose for energy. In addition, without enough stored carbohydrates in the form of glycogen, athletes will feel listless and lethargic. But can athletes eat too much carbohydrates? After all, if some is good, isn't more better? Well, the answers are yes to the first question and no to the second question. First, there are a number of athletes who believe that eating as much carbohydrates as possible is the best thing for their performance. They also believe that they should not consume any fat, so, essentially, their diet consists of carbohydrates, protein, and very little fat. This is not a good dietary practice. As was discussed earlier, a balance of carbohydrates, protein, and fat is needed for optimal performance and overall health. For some athletes, a typical day's diet is as follows: four plain bagels and orange juice for breakfast; a turkey sandwich with mustard, pasta, juice, and soft drink for lunch; and baked chicken breast, rice, bread, milk, and water for dinner. This diet may seem fine at first glance, but it is lacking in many things, including fruits, vegetables, water and other liquids, and fat.

Athletes tend to overconsume carbohydrates with the thought that it will be better for their performance. Although carbohydrates should make up the major portion of an athlete's diet, it should not be more than 65% of the total. When too many carbohydrates are consumed, the athlete misses out on many key nutrients required for optimal performance and health and may become fatigued and sluggish. Thus it is important that athletes are educated by qualified sports nutritionists on eating well and eating balanced.

Carbohydrate Ingestion and Exercise Performance

Since the 1980s, one of the most rewarding areas of research in sports nutrition has been the role of carbohydrate ingestion before and during exercise. Carbohydrate loading, also called glyco-

---

Box 9.1
Calculating an Athlete's Daily Carbohydrate Needs

First convert the athlete's weight from pounds to kilograms: If the athlete weighs 150 lb, then 150 lb ÷ 2.2 lb/kg = 68.2 kg. Assume a daily requirement of 7 to 10 g of carbohydrates per kilogram body weight: 7 g/kg × 68.2 kg = 477 g and 10 g/kg × 68.2 kg = 682 g. Thus this athlete should consume between 477 and 682 g of carbohydrates per day.

Table 9.2   METHODS OF CARBOHYDRATE LOADING FOR ENDURANCE EVENTS

Days Before the Event	Classic Method[a]		Modified Method[b]	
	DIET	EXERCISE	DIET	EXERCISE
0	High CHO meal before event	Event lasts 60–90 min	High CHO meal before event	Event lasts 60–90 min
−1	Continue previous day's plan	Rest	Continue previous day's plan	Rest
−2	Continue previous day's plan	Rest	Continue previous day's plan	Continue previous day's plan
−3	> 10–12 g CHO/kg/day	Rest	8–10 g CHO/kg/day	20 min at 75% $\dot{V}O_2$max
−4	Continue previous day's plan	Continue previous day's plan	Continue previous day's plan	Continue previous day's plan
−5	Continue previous day's plan	Continue previous day's plan	Continue previous day's plan	40 min at 75% $\dot{V}O_2$max
−6	> 2 g CHO/kg/day	90–120 min at 65–85% $\dot{V}O_2$max	Continue previous day's plan	Continue previous day's plan
−7	50% CHO mixed diet	Exercise to exhaustion	4.5 g CHO/kg/day	90 min at 75% $\dot{V}O_2$max

[a]Introduced in Bergstrom J, Hermansen L, Hultman E, Saltin B. Diet, muscle glycogen and physical performance. Acta Physiol Scand 1967;7:140–150.
[b]Introduced in Sherman WM. Carbohydrates, muscle glycogen, and muscle glycogen supercompensation. In: MH Williams, ed. Ergogenic aids in sport. Champaign, IL: Human Kinetics, 1983:3–26.
CHO, carbohydrates

gen supercompensation, is a practice followed by many serious and amateur road runners who compete in endurance events lasting 60 to 90 min. The goal is to temporarily modify one's diet by eating more complex carbohydrates than normal to obtain additional stored glycogen, sometimes four times the usual level. The higher than normal glycogen content in the muscles and liver helps delay fatigue during long-duration exercise. Performance is enhanced, because the extra glycogen allows the athlete to maintain race pace for a longer time. Both the classic and the modified versions of glycogen loading are presented in Table 9.2. The modified method represents the better approach, because it does not require an exercise bout to exhaustion designed to deplete glycogen at the start (on day −7) of the 8-day regimen. Nor does it require the athlete to eat extremely low (on day −6) or high (on days −3 to −1) amounts of carbohydrates, which some people are not able to tolerate. It does cause glycogen supercompensation, increasing glycogen stores to values that are consistent with good performance. It is important to emphasize that if the endurance athlete is already consuming 60 to 65% of his or her daily caloric intake as dietary carbohydrate, he or she is already receiving enough to ensure adequate liver and muscle glycogen stores.

Carbohydrate ingestion during exercise is also very important when the exercise duration is long term. As glycogen levels decrease in the muscles, the athlete starts to rely on glucose delivered by the blood and supplied from the liver stores of glycogen. When liver glycogen decreases during prolonged exercise, the athlete may experience hypoglycemia. This condition occurs when blood glucose levels become seriously low, which affects the central nervous system. At that point, the athlete needs another source of glucose, and the only source available is exogenous (outside the body). Glucose ingestion during exercise of long enough duration to cause liver and muscle glycogen depletion has been shown to be an important technique for delaying fatigue. One typical study showed that when glucose was ingested during a 15-min break in exercise (between two 45-min continuous exercise sessions) a superior cycle sprint performance

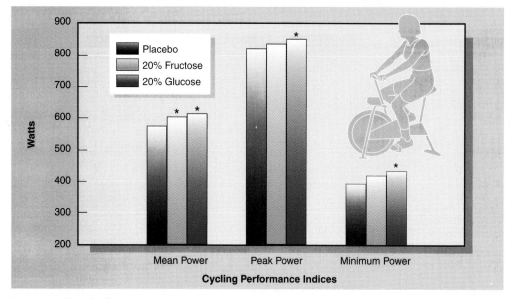

FIGURE 9.2 Results from a 40-sec cycle sprint test conducted after 90 min of cycling. Each subject consumed a fructose or glucose solution during a 15-min break in the exercise session. Although fructose improved performance, glucose gave more consistent results. Adapted from Sugiura K, Kobayashi K. Effect of carbohydrate ingestion on sprint performance following continuous and intermittent exercise. Med Sci Sports Exer 1998;30:1624–1630.

(40-sec sprint test) was achieved (Fig. 9.2). If an athlete does not consume glucose during a long-distance event, protein breakdown becomes a source of energy. Protein breakdown means that muscle is being broken down for energy, which is not a desirable situation.

⚷ Symptoms of hypoglycemia may include acute fatigue, light-headedness, nausea, and marked irritability. The symptoms may be severe, as in the case of an individual with diabetes, who may experience delirium, coma, and possibly death.

Fats: You Do Need Them

A diet that is more than 65% carbohydrates may rob the athlete of other important nutrients, including fats and proteins, which are essential for optimal athletic performance and maintaining good health. Fat, like carbohydrates, is a macronutrient required by the body and needed for energy. Fats provide 9 kcal/g, which is twice as much as carbohydrates provide and the reason why many people think they should not have any fat in their diet. Fat is extremely important for the body and is involved in such processes as hormone production and proper nervous system function. Fat is required to maintain a number of important bodily functions. Between 20 and 30% of your total calories should be from fat. Going below 20% can have negative effects. An athlete who consumes 2000 kcal per day needs to consume 400 to 600 kcal of this as fat, which is equal to 45 to 67 g of fat per day.

There are different types of fat in foods: saturated, monounsaturated, and polyunsaturated (see Box 9.2). Fats are composed mainly of chains of carbon atoms connected by chemical bonds. In addition, hydrogen atoms are linked to each carbon atom on the fat. A fat is considered saturated if all of the spaces on the carbon atoms are filled with hydrogen atoms. In non-scientific terms, a saturated fat will be solid at room temperature. Some examples of saturated fats are listed in Table 9.3. Because saturated fats tend to increase blood cholesterol levels, they should make up only about 7% of the total daily caloric intake.

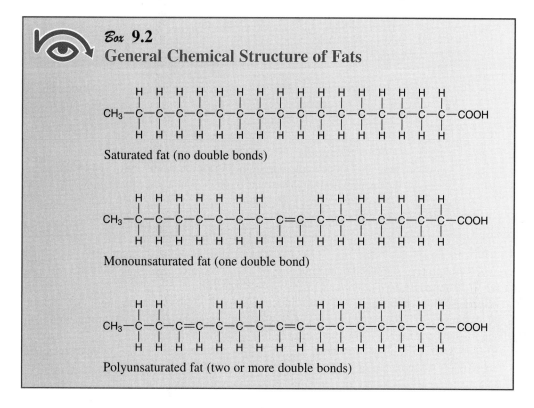

Box **9.2**
General Chemical Structure of Fats

Saturated fat (no double bonds)

Monounsaturated fat (one double bond)

Polyunsaturated fat (two or more double bonds)

Food manufacturers use a process called hydrogenation to change a fat from one form to another; information about hydrogenation will appear on the food label. For example, when a label on a box of processed food reads "hydrogenated soybean oil," hydrogen atoms were added to soybean oil (a polyunsaturated fat) to make it behave more like a saturated fat, which gives the product a more butter-like flavor and increases its shelf life. Hydrogenated fats may increase blood cholesterol levels more than saturated fats, but this is still under debate (see Box 9.3).

Monounsaturated fats should make up about 13% of the total daily caloric intake. Some studies found that monounsaturated fats have no effect on blood cholesterol levels, but others found that they may decrease total cholesterol and increase the good cholesterol (**high-density lipoprotein;** HDL) in the blood. Finally, polyunsaturated fats should make up about 10% of the total daily caloric intake. Although polyunsaturated fats can lower total cholesterol, they can also lower HDL. The effects of fat consumption on blood cholesterol levels help determine the risk of heart disease later in life. The type of fat consumed does not necessarily affect athletic per-

Table 9.3   EXAMPLES OF SATURATED, MONOUNSATURATED, AND POLYUNSATURATED FATS[a]

Saturated Fats	Monounsaturated Fats	Polyunsaturated Fats
Butter	Olive oil	Soybean oil
Fat from meats (e.g., lard)	Canola oil	Safflower oil
Coconut oil	Peanut oil	Sunflower oil
Palm oil	Walnut oil	Corn oil
Palm kernel oil	Avocados	Margarine

[a]Reprinted with permission from Wardlaw GM. Perspectives in nutrition. 4th ed. Boston: McGraw-Hill, 1999.

Box 9.3
Hydrogenation

The term *hydrogenation,* meaning to add hydrogen to fats, is a term seen on the labels of many prepared foods. Food manufacturers hydrogenate oils to make the oil taste more like butter and to increase the shelf life of the product. In addition, hydrogenating oils is less expensive than using butter. The process of hydrogenation makes a polyunsaturated fat more like a saturated fat. In the chemical process of hydrogenation, the configuration of the original fat changes somewhat. This change in configuration may make hydrogenated fats more unhealthy than saturated fats; however, this is still being debated by scientists.

---

formance, but athletes should be concerned about being healthy throughout their life, not just during the competitive years.

Some scientists have suggested that athletes may benefit from increasing their consumption of fat, because each gram of fat provides 9 kcal, but research results have been **equivocal.** Although a recent reported noted that a diet higher in fat content did not significantly increase blood lipid levels in endurance athletes, the study was conducted for only 3 months, which is probably not long enough to assess the long-term effects of a high-fat diet (6). Therefore, because a high-fat diet does not seem to improve athletic performance and probably leads to negative health consequences (i.e., coronary heart disease), it does not seem prudent to increase fat intake above 30% of the total daily calories consumed.

Protein: More Than Just Muscle

Proteins, macronutrients required for a number of physiologic functions, consist of amino acids, which are linked in specific ways to make up a particular protein. There are 20 **essential amino acids** and **nonessential amino acids** (Table 9.4). The protein needs of the average healthy person are about 0.8 g/kg of body mass per day; however, the protein needs of athletes have been under much debate. Athletes appear to require more protein in their diets than do sedentary individuals because they suffer tissue damage caused by exercise, have increased energy needs during exercise, and must recover and repair damaged tissue after exercise (5). However, because

Table 9.4   **THE AMINO ACIDS**[a]

Essential	Nonessential
Histidine	Alanine
Isoleucine	Arginine
Leucine	Asparagine
Lysine	Aspartic acid
Methionine	Cysteine
Phenylalanine	Glutamic acid
Threonine	Glutamine
Tryptophan	Glycine
Valine	Proline
Serine	Tyrosine

[a]Reprinted with permission from Wardlaw GM. Perspectives in nutrition. 4th ed. Boston: McGraw-Hill, 1999.

Table 9.5	GOOD FOOD SOURCES OF PROTEINS[a]	

Food	Serving Size	Protein, g
Tuna, light meat, canned in water	3 ounces	25
Barley	1 cup	23
Navy beans	1/2 cup	10
Pasta, enriched, cooked	1 cup	6
Almonds, toasted, unblanched	1/2 cup	14
American cheese, processed	2 ounces	13
Grape-Nuts cereal	1 cup	13
Milk, skim	1 cup	8
Tofu, fresh, firm	1 ounce	4
Hummus, fresh	1/2 cup	6
Egg, hard boiled	1 large	6
Peanut butter, any style	2 tablespoons	8

[a]Reprinted with permission from Wardlaw GM. Perspectives in nutrition. 4th ed. Boston: McGraw-Hill, 1999.

most people in the United States consume more than the **Recommended Dietary Allowance** (RDA; recently replaced by the **Dietary Reference Intake,** DRI) for protein, athletes already may be consuming what they need. Nonetheless, researchers state that endurance athletes may require from 1.0 to 1.4 g/kg/day of protein and that strength-training athletes (e.g., body builders) may require 1.1 to 1.7 g/kg/day of protein (7). Table 9.5 lists some foods high in protein. Caution must be taken not to increase protein to above what is needed, because too much protein in the diet leads to increased urinary calcium excretion (8). This means that bone density will be lost, which may cause early osteoporosis.

Many athletes who are trying to keep their weight low may be consuming too little protein. It is important that athletes are made aware that nutrition plays a major role in optimal athletic performance. If an eating disorder is suspected, the athlete should be counseled by someone who is trained in the area of the disorder (usually a registered dietitian, physician, and psychologist are required) (see Sidelight 9.2).

Protein supplement powders have become extremely popular since the 1990s. Many athletes, especially athletes who require increased muscle tissue and strength for their sports (e.g., body builders, football players, basketball players), believe it is necessary to obtain their dietary protein from these powders. Protein supplementation is not necessary for increased muscle mass and increased dietary protein. Athletes can consume more protein from the food they eat (such as those listed in Table 9.5), which will be more than adequate to meet their protein needs. Protein obtained from foods not only provides the necessary dietary protein intake but also is less expensive and contains other nutrients that can help athletes maximize their performance and health. Furthermore, athletes who believe they must increase their protein intake can make their own inexpensive protein shakes with skim or soy milk, instant breakfast powder, yogurt, powdered milk, and fruit. But remember, there is no need to consume more protein than is necessary to maintain nitrogen balance. In addition to eating more healthily, athletes should increase or decrease the time spent training or alter their workouts to optimize gains in muscle tissue and strength.

Minerals and Vitamins: Do Athletes Need More?

Minerals are micronutrients that are used in many metabolic reactions in the body. It is important to note that minerals do not provide energy—as do carbohydrates, fats, and proteins. Minerals are involved as **cofactors** in metabolic reactions that increase energy in the body, but

THE ATHLETE TRIAD: A NEW PERSPECTIVE

In the early 1990s, the American College of Sports Medicine (ACSM) coined the term *female athlete triad*. This term formally linked eating disorders and menstrual irregularities with the development of osteoporosis. Women who have eating disorders can develop osteoporosis at a young age. The ACSM's triad, however, is not just for females. Male athletes, too, are at risk for developing osteoporosis. Let's take a closer look at each leg of the triad stool.

EATING DISORDERS

Eating disorders include more than anorexia nervosa (severe calorie restriction) and bulimia nervosa (binge eating—eating larger than normal quantities of food—followed by purging via self-induced vomiting, abuse of laxatives, and/or overexercising). Eating disorders are better understood as existing on a continuum. Some individuals do not eat quite enough throughout the day or eat a limited variety of foods each day, thereby not providing their bodies with the appropriate amount of calories or nutrients needed for optimal health and athletic performance. Other individuals may overeat but still not consume the proper variety of foods necessary for optimal health and performance. Eating disorders are characterized by obsessive thinking about food, i.e., affected individuals base their day around food, even if their total consumption is minimal.

Any pattern of eating disorder can lead to depressed immune function, increased emotional stress and depression, and decreased overall health. In addition, overall athletic performance will be drastically affected. Even though the athlete may not seem to be fatigued, his or her performance will not be optimal. Eating disorders, then, can lead to the next legs of the triad stool: hormone disorders (amenorrhea or decreased testosterone levels) and osteoporosis.

HORMONAL DISORDERS

Several research studies have stated that too little fat in the diet can lead to menstrual irregularities in women (especially amenorrhea, which means "absence of menses"). Many athletes have a preconceived notion that fat is bad for them. On the contrary, everyone needs some fat in the diet for many metabolic processes in the body. Athletes, and all individuals in general, should consume between 20 and 30% of their total daily calories from fat. So, if a person consumes 2500 kcal/day, 500 to 750 kcal/day should come from fat (55 to 83 g of fat per day). The type of fat consumed should come from sources such as olive oil, canola oil, avocados, walnuts, almonds,

minerals do not provide the energy directly. Athletes may need more of some minerals than do sedentary individuals, but research results are equivocal.

The **major minerals** include calcium, phosphorus, potassium, sulfur, sodium, chloride, and magnesium. The **trace minerals** include iron, zinc, copper, selenium, iodide, fluoride, chromium, manganese, molybdenum, boron, and vanadium. This chapter describes the general needs of minerals for athletes and does not discuss each mineral in detail.

Minerals are a part of many metabolic reactions in the body. Some functions of minerals include working in combination with enzymes in the body, becoming part of the organizational matrix of cells, speeding up reactions in the body, and being part of the **antioxidant** system of the body. Minerals also act directly in many of the reactions involved in energy metabolism, such as glucose, lipid, and protein metabolism.

There is an abundant amount of research in the area of mineral needs for people who are physically active. In general, researchers have stated that athletes do not appear to need more minerals than nonathletes. However, athletes (or nonathletes) who do not consume enough minerals from foods should take a multivitamin and mineral supplement, not exceeding the dietary requirements. For female athletes, the minerals that are often a concern are calcium, zinc, and iron. It is important that female athletes obtain the proper amount of all minerals but they should be especially concerned about these three minerals, because low intake could result in reduced bone mineral density and anemia. Male athletes who are in sports in which losing weight is common should also be aware of appropriate mineral intake. Taking more minerals will not help athletic performance. In fact, taking too much minerals may be harmful to performance and over-

corn oil, and soybean oil with limited amounts of butter, meat fats, palm kernel oil, and hydrogenated fats.

Fat, however, is not the only cause of hormonal imbalances. Athletes who do not eat a varied, balanced diet with enough calories (i.e., relative to the amount of energy they expend) will experience a decrease in their estrogen (women) or testosterone (men) level. These hormones are vital to a number of metabolic processes in the body.

Decreased estrogen or testosterone can also be caused by overtraining. Overtraining increases the rate of injury, which means the athlete will spend more time on the bench than on the field. Furthermore, overexercise can lead to a depressed immune response and a greater likelihood of upper respiratory tract infections, which also put the athlete out of commission.

OSTEOPOROSIS

Osteoporosis, the third leg of the triad, is defined as "porous bones," leading to an increased risk of fracture. These fractures can be major (hip or vertebral crush fractures) or minor (stress fractures often seen in the foot or wrist). Any of these fractures can be a result of an eating disorder and/or overtraining. Estrogen and testosterone are vital for maintaining normal bone mineral density; thus a reduction in these hormones leads to decreased bone mineral density and an increased risk of fractures. There have been reports of young women in their teens and 20s who have bone mineral densities similar to women 70 years of age and older. Remember that men who have decreased testosterone levels are also at risk for low bone mineral densities. The good news is that if affected athletes begin to eat healthily and decrease their training, bone mineral density will increase, although it may not be back to normal.

Note that many athletes drink a lot of soft drinks (diet or regular), which replace milk in their diets. A study of athletes has shown that an increased consumption of soft drinks was significantly linked to an increased risk for fractures and osteoporosis. So athletes need to drink skim milk or soy milk for their bones and should stay away from the soda pop.

For both men and women, unhealthy or imbalanced eating and overtraining can lead to hormonal irregularities. These irregularities can result in a greater risk of osteoporosis and impaired athletic performance and health, even at a young age.

Modified with permission from Volpe SL, Levine RE. Sports Nutr Newslett 1999;3:174.

---

all health, because minerals can compete with each other in the body. For example, high doses of iron affects the body's copper and zinc status. In addition, there are no ergogenic benefits of taking more minerals. Consumption of real foods is the best way to obtain minerals, and they are in their best **absorptive** form in foods, as well.

Vitamins are also micronutrients required by the body. Like minerals, vitamins do not provide energy but are involved in energy-producing reactions. Athletes may have higher vitamin requirements than nonathletes, but there is no consensus among researchers and practitioners. It is important that athletes get what their bodies require; however, as with minerals, taking more vitamins than required can be harmful. Thus athletes must be guided by qualified sports nutritionists to ensure consumption of the proper balance of all nutrients, including vitamins and minerals, for optimal performance and health.

The water-soluble vitamins include vitamin B_6, vitamin B_{12}, folate, thiamin, riboflavin, niacin, pantothenic acid, biotin, vitamin C, and choline. The fat-soluble vitamins include vitamins A, D, E, and K. Again, overconsumption of vitamins can be harmful, but this is especially true of the fat-soluble vitamins, because they are stored in the body in higher amounts than are the water-soluble vitamins.

Hydration: Drink Before You Are Thirsty!

It was once thought that athletes should not consume water during practices so that they would toughen up. Thankfully, this practice has long since been abolished, and athletes are now encouraged to drink all day: before, during, and after they practice or workout. It is imperative that athletes drink before they are thirsty. By the time athletes become thirsty, their body cells require water and they are **hypohydrated**—they have probably already lost about 2% of their body weight (9). Obviously, the thirsty athlete should drink water and/or a sports drink, but it is better that he or she remains well hydrated all the time. Being hydrated actually helps athletic performance tremendously; conversely, being hypohydrated can result in impaired muscular endurance, impaired aerobic exercise performance, and decreased mental functioning (5).

Many people (athletes and nonathletes alike) are chronically hypohydrated. Athletes, however, sweat more than sedentary people; therefore, getting more fluids into their bodies is especially important. Drinking water is an excellent way to hydrate the body. However, sports drinks that contain between 6 and 8% carbohydrates have been shown to be absorbed at least as quickly as water during exercise (10). If exercising for more than 1 hr, a sports drink for hydration and carbohydrate replenishment is needed. If exercising for less than 1 hr, water should be sufficient. But if drinking a sports drink or diluted 100% fruit juice will make the athlete drink more, then that's fine. Beware, however, of colas and alcohol, because they are poor and possibly dangerous choices for rehydrating. They can result in underhydration, and alcohol also results in decreased coordination, among other things.

> *An ideal fluid-replacement beverage has the following qualities: good taste, does not cause gastrointestinal discomfort if taken in large volumes, promotes rapid fluid absorption and maintenance of extracellular volume, and provides energy.*

If hypohydration is suspected, follow these two suggestions. First, be aware of the color and frequency of urination. Athletes who have dark-colored urine and do not frequently urinate are underhydrated. Urine should be light colored and well-hydrated athletes should urinate frequently throughout the day. Second, athletes can weigh themselves before and after their workouts. For each pound lost, athletes should drink about 2 cups of water or other fluid (11).

During long-distance events, athletes may need between 500 and 1000 mL of fluid per hour (about 8 ounces every 15 min). However, it is good to drink enough fluids to match sweat loss; therefore, long-distance athletes may need more fluid. Athletes should drink 500 to 1000 mL of fluid up to 15 minutes before practice or competition, and they should drink the same amount or more afterward. Also athletes should take in about 1 qt water for every 1000 kcal used (11). The more energy expended in workouts, the more fluids will be needed before, during, and after workouts. Noticeable differences in exercise performance will be observed if the athlete stays well hydrated. Furthermore, the athlete will be healthier and will decrease his or her chances of suffering from hypohydration-related injuries, which can be serious.

There have been cases of **hyponatremia** in athletes who consumed only water during long-distance events (usually marathons and triathlons), because water will not replace **electrolytes** (like sodium and potassium) in the body (see A Case in Point 9.1). Thus during long-distance events (longer than 1 hr), water *and* sports drinks should be consumed. Sports drinks provide glucose, which means the muscles will use the glucose in the blood (provided by the drink), sparing the muscle glycogen stores and preventing fatigue.

Weight Loss and Athletic Performance

There are a number of different sports that require athletes to maintain a certain body weight, whether for aesthetics or for performance reasons. These sports include wrestling, body building, rowing, ice skating and ice dancing, gymnastics, and ballet. Athletes in these sports often use inappropriate methods of weight loss, such as starvation, hypohydration, saunas, excessive spitting, excessive exercising (including in the heat with a lot of clothing on), laxatives, and **diuretics** (12). These methods of weight loss are not only ineffective (the athlete is losing water weight) but extremely dangerous.

A Case in Point 9.1

WATER INTOXICATION

Athletes who compete in long-distance events, such as marathons, ultramarathons, triathlons, and cycling, require more than just water to rehydrate. These athletes are competing for a number of hours continuously and thus need both fuel and fluids for optimal performance. If these endurance athletes consume too much water—especially in the form of a hypotonic fluid (low levels of electrolytes, especially sodium)—during these events, they could suffer from hyponatremia (lower than normal levels of sodium in the blood) as

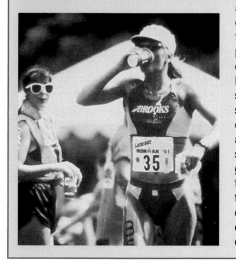

a result of too much water being driven into the cells. Normal levels of sodium in the blood range from 135 to 145 mEq/L. Because sodium is important in so many reactions in the body and can enhance glucose and fluid absorption, if levels become too low, athletes can suffer from seizures, respiratory arrest, very low blood pressure, coma, and even death. An easy way for endurance athletes to maintain optimal fluids, fuels, and normal blood levels of sodium is to consume sports drinks that contain the proper amounts of glucose and sodium. Thus hydration is important for all sports, but fueling the body is also important in long-distance events. This should be accomplished by consuming sports drinks and other carbohydrates that the athlete is able to digest easily.

Starvation is not something that is healthy for anyone, nor does it necessarily mean to not eat at all. Starvation can also mean that the body is being starved of necessary nutrients. So athletes who consume too few calories can starve their bodies of precious fuels needed for optimal performance and long-term health. In addition, when a person undergoes starvation, the first thing to go is not fat but protein (muscle).

In the fall of 1997, three collegiate wrestlers at three different universities died as a result of inappropriate weight loss practices. This was probably because the electrolytes in their bodies were imbalanced. The imbalance in electrolytes leads to heart **dysrhythmias,** which can result in death. Although death is the worst-case scenario for inappropriate weight loss practices, other negative consequences can result, including impaired athletic performance, decreased mental functioning, decreased lean muscle mass, slowed metabolic rate, and hypohydration.

If weight loss is something that an athlete strives to do, he or she should seek the counseling of a registered dietitian who specializes in sports nutrition and/or weight loss. Weight loss can be achieved safely and in a slower manner well before the beginning of the competitive season. In addition, if the athlete cannot lose all of the desired weight then he or she should consider competing at a more natural weight. The NCAA has recently revised their rules on weight loss for collegiate wrestlers to minimize any negative consequences and eliminate inappropriate weight loss practices (12). *Taking it to the Mat: The Wrestler's Guide to Optimal Performance* (13) is a guidebook written to address safe and healthy weight loss practices for wrestlers and other athletes. It is important that athletes (and nonathletes) know that proper weight loss can be achieved, but that it takes time to lose weight properly. A weight loss of no more than 1 to 2 lb per week is ideal and minimizes loss of muscle tissue and water. This means the athlete will be able to maintain weight loss over time and be able to perform better than if inappropriate methods of weight loss were used.

Ergogenic Aids: Do They Really Work?

Athletes are always striving to achieve optimal performance and rapid recovery. Because of this, erogenic aids are a popular area of discussion in the sports nutrition arena. In this section, some of the more popular nutritional ergogenic aids are discussed to allow you to become familiar with what is being used and/or touted as the "best" performance enhancers. The ergogenic aids discussed in this section are classified either as nutritional (e.g., boron) or physiologic (e.g., creatine), but the list is not exhaustive. Pharmacologic and psychological ergogenic aids are not included in this chapter. The ones discussed here are considered within the "spirit" of competition. That is, if these substances produce an ergogenic effect, the athlete is to be congratulated for incorporating sound nutritional practices into his or her training routine. Note that some ergogenic aids are illegal and are outside the "spirit" of competition. Athletes using them are sanctioned, if caught. They include such illegal substances as cocaine and growth hormone.

⚬—ₘ *Ergogenic aids may be classified as nutritional (discussed in this section), pharmacologic (e.g., anabolic steroids), physiologic (e.g., blood doping), and psychological (e.g., drugs that stimulate the central nervous system).*

Creatine Monohydrate

One of the most popular ergogenic aids of the 1990s was creatine monohydrate. Creatine is used as part of the creatine phosphate system (see Chapter 8), which helps regenerate adenosine triphosphate (ATP) during exercise of high intensity and short duration. The creatine phosphate system is used for short bursts of energy (e.g., sprinting and weightlifting) that last 1 to 10 sec. Creatine phosphate also acts as an intracellular buffer to maintain a proper pH in the body.

Creatine is derived from the diet; the best sources are meat and fish (or "muscle" foods). Creatine is also synthesized in the body from the amino acids arginine, glycine, and methionine. It is probable that vegetarians do not consume enough creatine in their diets and may have lower creatine stores in the body, but this has not been definitively shown. Furthermore, some recent studies have shown that caffeine ingestion may inhibit the resynthesis of phosphocreatine, which would reduce the ergogenic effects of creatine.

So, why do some athletes take creatine as a supplement? It has been shown that creatine supplementation can result in improved athletic performance in the higher-intensity sports that have short bursts of exercise (e.g., football, weightlifting, and sprinting) and may increase muscle mass. For instance, creatine supplementation was shown to improve cycle sprint performance measured as 6 sec of stationary cycle sprinting over the first 5 sets of a 12-set protocol; each set was separated by a 30-sec rest period (Fig. 9.3). In this study, subjects not only improved exercise performance after taking creatine for 28 days but also made positive changes in the amount of lean tissue they were carrying and in several measures of strength. Note, however, that the increase in muscle mass with creatine supplementation could be the result of water retention, although other researchers have reported increases in fat-free mass. Creatine does not act as an ergogenic aid in long-distance events, which makes sense, because creatine phosphate is used for high-intensity short bouts of exercise. In addition, it has not yet been shown that creatine will increase peak power output.

Although a number of research studies have shown positive results from creatine supplementation for activities that are of short duration with repetitive bursts of high-intensity exercise, caution must be taken. First of all, the long-term effects of high doses of creatine have not been fully determined, although some long-term studies are now under way. High doses could lead to adverse effects on the heart, liver, and possibly kidneys; but to date, no scientific data have shown

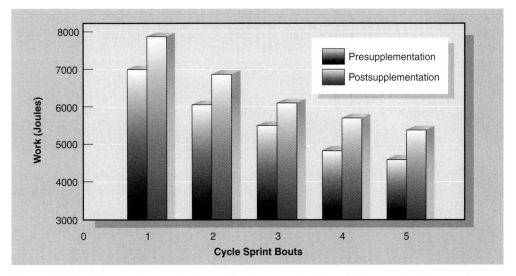

FIGURE 9.3 Creatine supplementation for 28 days improved cycle sprinting over the first 5 sprint bouts of a 12-bout session. *Light bars,* significantly greater work output after supplementation. Adapted from Kreider RB, Ferreira M, Wilson M, et al. Effects of creatine supplementation on body composition, strength, and sprint performance. Med Sci Sports Exer 1998;30:73–82.

a negative effect of creatine supplementation on these organs. It has been shown that the body's own production of creatine decreases with creatine supplementation, but it appears that production returns when creatine supplementation is discontinued. Nonetheless, repeated bouts of creatine supplementation could eventually be detrimental to the body's ability to produce creatine. More research is needed in this area.

The amount of creatine taken during the "loading phase" is generally 5 g of creatine monohydrate four to six times per day for a week or several weeks, although some people are now using lower dosages. The 5 g of creatine is equal to 1.1 kg of uncooked meat, which is almost 2.5 lb of meat, and that is only one dose! Thus, during the loading phase, athletes consume the equivalent of 10 lb or more of raw meat per day! Needless to say, our bodies are not equipped to handle that amount of creatine. Although some individuals argue that an athlete would not consume that much meat and that the amount of creatine consumed during the loading phase does not have the same effect as that much meat, there is presently no long-term research to assess this.

In addition, some trainers have stated that gastrointestinal upset, nausea, and muscle cramping are common complaints of athletes who have supplemented with creatine, but these are only anecdotal reports that have not yet been supported by scientific data. Athletes can increase creatine in their diets by increasing the number of servings of lean meat and fish they eat. In addition, altering training results in improved athletic performance.

It is interesting that creatine supplementation is finding its way into medical treatment, because of its propensity to help maintain lean body mass. In this way creatine supplementation may be of use in the treatment of diseases like cancer and AIDS, which are associated with muscle wasting.

Caffeine

Caffeine is in a number of products, including coffee, colas, some medications, and chocolate. Caffeine has been well studied as an ergogenic aid, and it seems to work by increasing free fatty acids in the blood to be used for energy, thereby sparing muscle glycogen (14). Caffeine has been classified as a restricted drug by the International Olympic Committee (IOC). The IOC has designated 12 μg/L of caffeine in the urine as the tolerable limit. Because 12 μg/L (six to eight cups of coffee) is actually quite a high amount, the IOC does not keep athletes from using caffeine as an ergogenic aid. Ingestion of about 2 cups of coffee has been shown to improve endurance performance (14). Because plasma concentrations of caffeine peak 45 to 60 min after caffeine ingestion, an athlete who uses caffeine needs to consume it about 1 hr before the athletic event to receive any ergogenic benefit. It is important to note that caffeine use can result in negative side effects such as high blood pressure, very rapid heart rate, nervousness, gastrointestinal upset, and hypohydration (owing to its diuretic effect). These side effects are probably the result of high doses of caffeine (more than 2 cups). Nonetheless, in individuals who are caffeine naive (do not consume caffeine regularly), smaller doses could result in some of these negative side effects. Although some research shows that caffeine has beneficial effects in aerobic (endurance) sports, the risk:benefit ratio of its use and side effects must be considered before recommending that an athlete use it as an ergogenic aid. Furthermore, the mechanisms of how caffeine may enhance endurance exercise have not been definitively validated (15).

L-Carnitine

L-Carnitine is a protein that is required to bring fatty acids into the mitochondria of the cell. Recall that the mitochondria are the powerhouses of the cells and that with aerobic exercise training the mitochondria within cells increase in size and increase in number, which is a physiologic

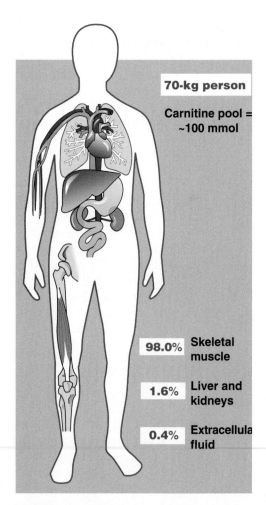

FIGURE 9.4 Carnitine distribution in the body.

Table 9.6   **DRI FOR CHOLINE**[a]

Age Group	Daily Requirement, mg
Infants	
0–6 months	125
7–12 months	150
Children	
1–3 years	200
4–8 years	250
Males	
9–13 years	375
14–70+ years	550
Females	
9–13 years	375
14–18 years	400
19–70+ years	425
Pregnancy	450
Lactation	550

[a]Reprinted with permission from Yates AA, Schlicker SA, Suitor CW. Dietary reference intakes: the new basis for recommendations for calcium and related nutrients, B vitamins, and choline. J Am Diet Assoc 1998;98:699–706.

effect of training. Fatty acids are brought into the mitochondria of the cell where they are metabolized (the process of beta-oxidation).

For most individuals, more than 50% of the daily need of carnitine is provided by the diet (meat, fish, poultry, and some dairy). The rest of one's carnitine needs are synthesized from the amino acids methionine and lysine. In a 150-lb person, the carnitine pool equals about 100 mmol, 98% of which is in skeletal muscle (Fig. 9.4).

Because of carnitine's role in fat oxidation, many people think that it may help them lose weight, but carnitine supplements do not result in weight loss. Athletes, on the other hand, think that carnitine supplementation will increase fatty acid oxidation, thereby leading to improvement in endurance performance. However, numerous research studies have been conducted on carnitine, and there were no reported effects on fuel use at rest or during exercise. Furthermore, D-carnitine can be toxic and lead to depleted L-carnitine stores, resulting in a carnitine deficiency. Therefore, supplementation with carnitine does not appear to be warranted because it is not an effective ergogenic aid.

Choline

Choline is considered an **amine** and is found as part of **phospholipids** in animal and plant foods. It can be synthesized from the amino acid methionine. Before 1998 there were no dietary requirements for choline. The present choline requirements range from 125 mg/day for infants to 550 mg/day for adult men (Table 9.6). Because it is a precursor of acetylcholine and lecithin, choline may affect nerve transmission, thereby increasing strength and facilitating body fat loss (16). Some researchers reported a decline in blood choline levels after long-distance running and swimming, but others reported no fall in blood choline levels after short or long bouts of cycling (17,18). Some reports noted that choline supplementation improved long-distance running and swimming times but did not improve strength or facilitate loss of body fat (16,18). It is still best to obtain choline from foods, not supplements. More long-term studies are needed to ascertain if choline supplementation above recommended requirements will result in negative health effects.

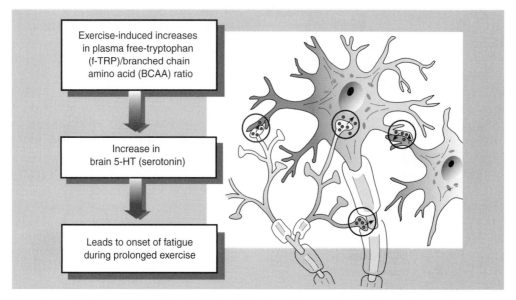

FIGURE 9.5 Hypothesis of onset of fatigue in relationship to BCAAs. Modified from Newsholme EA, Actworth IN, Blomstrand E. Amino acids, brain neurotransmitters and a functional link between muscle and brain that is important in sustained exercise. In: G Benzi, ed. Advances in myochemistry. London: Libbey Eurotext, 1989.

Branched-Chain Amino Acids

The branched-chain amino acids (BCAAs) are leucine, isoleucine, and valine. Unlike other amino acids, BCAAs are **transaminated** only on the muscle. The use of BCAAs may reduce the onset of fatigue during endurance exercise (Fig. 9.5) (19). It is hypothesized that if there is an increase in the ratio of plasma (blood)-free tryptophan to BCAA, there will be an increase in **serotonin** (5-HT) levels, leading to fatigue during prolonged exercise (19).

Serotonin is synthesized in the brain by the amino acid tryptophan. With prolonged exercise, tryptophan increases in the blood. More tryptophan in the blood means that more will go into the brain and be synthesized to serotonin, which makes people feel tired. Some human and animal studies do support this theory; however, the underlying mechanism behind it has yet to be determined.

How is all this connected to BCAAs? Well, the increase in tryptophan going into the brain means that less BCAA will cross the blood–brain barrier, and thus there will be more conversion of tryptophan to serotonin. That is why the ratio of free tryptophan to BCAA is important. Although this theory may seem logical, there is no definitive evidence that supplementation with BCAA will improve endurance performance; thus supplementation with BCAA is not warranted as an ergogenic aid. Nonetheless, some researchers have shown that supplementation with BCAA can increase blood BCAA levels, which could possibly be used as an energy source during exercise. Furthermore, some researchers have shown an improvement in cognitive performance with BCAA supplementation.

Dihydroxyacetone and Pyruvate

Dihydroxyacetone and pyruvate are three-carbon intermediates from glycolysis (the process that breaks down glucose). They have been studied to assess their effects on increasing muscle glycogen, which would help endurance athletes. Studies have shown that a combination of dihydroxyacetone and pyruvate may enhance muscular endurance and decrease perceived exertion (how difficult the exercise feels to the athlete) (20). Despite these positive results, more studies of longer duration with larger study groups are needed.

Many individuals are taking these substances to promote fat loss. However, the dosages used in studies are much greater than those recommended by the companies making these products. Once again, more well-controlled studies using manufacturer-recommended doses are needed.

Glutamine

Glutamine is an amino acid that, like the other amino acids, has a number of functions in the body. There may be an increased need for glutamine for individuals who exercise, because glutamine reserves in the muscle may become depleted (21). Some athletes may suffer from overtraining syndrome (OTS), meaning that they may have low levels of glutamine in their blood for a long period of time (months or years), which can lead to increased risk of disease and infection, because glutamine plays a major role in the immune system. Glutamine has been shown to induce glycogen resynthesis (22). More studies in this area are needed before definitive conclusions can be made. Note that individuals who do suffer from OTS may benefit from supplementation, if they indeed have low blood levels of glutamine. Athletes without OTS may benefit from increased protein in their diets to avoid competition of glutamine with other amino acids in their bodies.

Glycerol

Glycerol is another nutritional ergogenic aid that has become popular in the last several years. It is used by athletes to hyperhydrate, because it attracts water and is quickly absorbed in the body (16). Glycerol may enhance endurance performance better than water alone because of its hyperhydration effects, but some researchers have found no effects of glycerol on enhancing athletic performance (23). In addition, nausea, vomiting, and bloating are some of its side effects. The IOC has banned the infusible glycerol product but not the oral glycerol supplement.

Medium-Chain Triglycerides

Medium-chain triglyceride (MCT) oil has been available for years in the clinical setting, because it is used for patients who are unable to properly absorb fat from their diets. Because MCTs do not need to follow the same absorption pathway as long-chain triglycerides, they are absorbed more rapidly (almost as fast as glucose), which is good for individuals who cannot properly absorb fat. Recently, MCT oil has become popular in the athletic arena. Most studies have found no ergogenic benefit of using MCT. One study that used high doses of MCT did find an improvement in performance, but researchers also noted gastrointestinal upset, which adversely affected athletic function (24,25). MCT oil is expensive; and supplementation for its use as an ergogenic aid does not seem prudent, because most researchers have shown no improvement in athletic performance with its use.

Coenzyme-Q

Coenzyme-Q (ubiquinone) is required for ATP production in the mitochondria. A number of studies have been conducted on coenzyme-Q's effectiveness as an ergogenic aid, with equivocal results. Some studies have shown improvements in time to exhaustion and increased fat utilization in endurance exercise, but other studies have shown no improvement in exercise performance and no changes in fuel use (e.g., fat, carbohydrate, or protein). More research is required to assess coenzyme-Q's effectiveness with different types of exercise and over longer periods of time.

Ginseng

Ginseng is an herb that has been purported to improve energy; it has recently become popular because some professional athletes promote its alleged benefits. Mixed results have been reported in the literature about ginseng's ergogenic effects. Some researchers noted that there is no strong evidence that ginseng supplementation will improve athletic performance, because the studies researching its effects have not been well designed (26).

Chromium Picolinate

Chromium is an essential mineral that is needed to enhance the effects of the hormone insulin in the body. Although there is no RDA for chromium, there is an Estimated Safe and Adequate Daily Dietary Intake (ESADDI) of chromium, which is 50 to 200 μg/day for individuals 11 years of age and older. Because the main effect of chromium is to enhance the action of insulin—and insulin not only transports glucose into cells but also promotes amino acid uptake and governs protein metabolism—chromium supplementation has been promoted as a possible benefit for body builders and weightlifters who wish to increase their lean body mass and decrease their body fat.

Although chromium is an essential mineral, chromium **picolinate** became popular as an ergogenic aid, because it was thought that the picolinate would enhance chromium's absorption into the body. However, a number of researchers have shown that chromium picolinate does not increase lean body mass or decrease body weight (27).

Even though urinary chromium excretion has been reported to be greater on the days individuals exercise than on the days they do not exercise, chromium supplementation does not seem to be required by athletes (28). In addition, chromium may alter the status of other minerals, like iron; so intakes greater than the ESADDI are not recommended until more studies are completed. Athletes should be encouraged to obtain their chromium through dietary sources instead of chromium picolinate supplementation. Good dietary sources of chromium include whole grains, organ meats, beer, egg yolks, mushrooms, and nuts.

Boron

Boron is a mineral, not yet considered essential for humans, but it may play a role in bone metabolism. Boron became popular, especially among body builders and weightlifters, because it was thought to increase lean body mass and increase bone mineral density; but recent reports have not shown these effects with boron supplementation (29). Thus supplementation does not appear to have any ergogenic benefit. Foods high in boron include fruits, vegetables, nuts, and beans.

Thoughts on Ergogenic Aids

Although not all of the ergogenic aids were discussed in this section, some of the more popular ones were highlighted. Students of exercise science should think about the findings of research studies on nutritional ergogenics to reach a proper interpretation of their alleged benefits. For instance, even though chromium is an essential mineral, does that mean that more of that mineral is better? In fact, more can be harmful. In addition, the placebo effect, often operable in research studies such as these, will cloud any interpretation. If you think something will help you (e.g., athletic performance) quite often it will, purely as a result of your belief. Many people think that supplements help them, but in fact it is their perception that the supplements are helping them that creates the effect. If the supplement is not harmful, the psychological benefit is not so bad. However, a number of supplements can be harmful over time. Athletes need to understand the effects of supplements and understand that they can obtain most things to enhance their performance through real foods, which are healthier and less expensive. Sometimes an athlete who feels tired is not eating breakfast or is hypohydrated, but this same athlete will try a supplement instead of eating breakfast or drinking more fluids. A visit with a registered dietitian can help athletes tremendously.

In addition, the U.S. Food and Drug Administration (FDA) does not regulate the supplement industry. That means that everything that is in a supplement may not necessarily be listed on its label. So, you may actually be purchasing something very different from what you thought. Therein lies another potential hazard of using supplements.

Finally, when you are reading research studies and find that they show mixed results (as discussed in this chapter), you must look cautiously at the risk:benefit ratio and cost of taking a supplement. Different study designs and doses also result in different findings. So take a close look at research studies to evaluate the effectiveness of such supplements. Furthermore, some studies are better designed than others. Reviewing the strength of research studies is also important in evaluating the efficacy of any supplement (see Practical Application 9.2). Box 9.4 presents a number of questions you can ask yourself to ascertain if an ergogenic aid really works and if the research behind it was good.

Practical Application 9.2

TO SUPPLEMENT OR NOT TO SUPPLEMENT?

Dietary supplementation of some form is widespread today; it seems that everyone, from the popular sports hero to the working man or woman is supplementing with everything from vitamin-and-mineral tablets to herbs, creatine, and ginseng. The food supplement industry is a multi-billion-dollar business that actually encourages supplementation for many reasons, including these: to prevent colds and other illnesses, to make up for what is missing in food, and to provide extra energy. But are supplements the way to go for optimal athletic performance and health? Many people who supplement say they perform better; but is this true, given the fact that about 35% of people who take any form of supplementation say they feel or perform better. This is evidence of what science calls the "placebo effect."

Before you recommend supplementation to an athlete, it is important to look at the risks and benefits of supplement use. First, many supplement manufacturers state that "research" has shown their supplement works. However, sometimes there has been no research on the product at all or, if research was conducted, no effects were seen. Many times, supplement manufacturers will misquote scientists' results so that you will buy the product. Some people believe that the soil is being depleted of vitamins and minerals and thus so are the plants we eat. They say we need to supplement to make up for these losses. Plants, however, wouldn't grow without all the necessary vitamins and minerals. So, the next time you think about purchasing a supplement, think about the risk:benefit ratio. Will it really help you and at what cost? Supplements are expensive and they could be harmful to you.

Remember that there are valid reasons to supplement. For instance, women with excessive menstrual bleeding may need iron and women who are pregnant or who are breast-feeding need more of some nutrients. There are other valid reasons for supplementing, but if your nutritionist doesn't recommend it, why not pick up a few apples, bananas, and oranges instead?

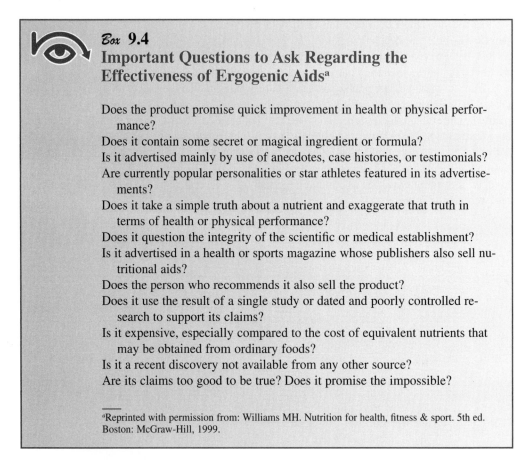

Box 9.4

Important Questions to Ask Regarding the Effectiveness of Ergogenic Aids[a]

Does the product promise quick improvement in health or physical performance?

Does it contain some secret or magical ingredient or formula?

Is it advertised mainly by use of anecdotes, case histories, or testimonials?

Are currently popular personalities or star athletes featured in its advertisements?

Does it take a simple truth about a nutrient and exaggerate that truth in terms of health or physical performance?

Does it question the integrity of the scientific or medical establishment?

Is it advertised in a health or sports magazine whose publishers also sell nutritional aids?

Does the person who recommends it also sell the product?

Does it use the result of a single study or dated and poorly controlled research to support its claims?

Is it expensive, especially compared to the cost of equivalent nutrients that may be obtained from ordinary foods?

Is it a recent discovery not available from any other source?

Are its claims too good to be true? Does it promise the impossible?

[a]Reprinted with permission from: Williams MH. Nutrition for health, fitness & sport. 5th ed. Boston: McGraw-Hill, 1999.

ADVANCES IN SPORTS NUTRITION

There are a number of hot topics in sports nutrition, some of which were addressed: weight loss, weight and muscle gain, and ergogenic aids. This section concentrates on scientific advancement in the assessment of body composition and the use of isotopes to study metabolism.

Body Composition Techniques

Obesity plays a major role in the development of chronic degenerative disease; therefore, accurate knowledge of body composition is an essential tool in the effort to educate the public about risk factors and health. At least since the 1950s, life insurance companies have been interested in linking body weight to actuarial tables to determine the risk associated with overweight clients. Using height and weight tables, however, has the obvious disadvantage of neglecting whether an individual is actually fat (obese) or just heavily muscled.

Today, there are better ways to assess the health risks of being overweight. These focus on estimating actual body fatness, because fatness, not weight per se, is what is really connected to the risk of degenerative diseases. Besides aiding disease prevention efforts, body composition is also a major area of research in exercise science. Athletes of all types are aided by knowing their body composition, which, when combined with proper nutrition, helps them better focus their training methods.

Over the years, methods for assessing body composition have become more accurate, and some methods are more reliable than others. Although I will not offer a comprehensive review of all the methods of assessing body composition, the discussion will help you understand some of the common and popular methods used and pique your interest to study body composition assessment methods even more.

Skinfold Calipers

Skinfold calipers assess the thickness of subcutaneous, or under the skin, fat. Typically, at least three sites are used, but up to eight sites can be measured. These are triceps, biceps, chest, subscapula (under the shoulder blade), abdomen, suprailiac (above the iliac crest), thigh, and calf. When measuring skinfold sites, only the right side of the body is used for all measurements. Once at least three measurements are taken at each site and averaged, they are entered into a regression equation, from which percent body fat can be estimated. Although skinfold measurements are easy to do, they do have a high rate of error and are not widely used in research. If they are used in research, the investigators typically report total sum of skinfold thicknesses and do not estimate percent body fat.

Bioelectrical Impedance Analysis

Another method of estimating body composition is by bioelectrical impedance analysis (BIA). BIA is based on the premise that muscle is a better conductor of electricity than fat. Thus fat will have a greater resistance to electrical conductivity. Usually, four electrodes are placed on the right side of the body: wrist, ankle, top of the hand, and top of the foot. BIA estimates the amount of body water a person has, based on the electrical perturbations of the instrument. From this, lean body mass and percent body fat can be estimated using regression equations. It is important to note that, although BIA is relatively easy to use, it has not been fully validated in a number of populations, such as those who have large variations of total body water (e.g., patients with renal disease). A hand-held BIA instrument can now be purchased in some pharmacies; it is relatively inexpensive and may be a practical method to assess healthy populations.

Total Body Electrical Conductivity

Total body electrical conductivity (TOBEC) is another method of assessing body composition. TOBEC is based on the same premise as BIA, but it uses a more expensive and larger instrument. The person being assessed assumes a supine position inside a cylindrical coil that produces an electrical current. Body composition affects the electromagnetic field within the coil, and calculations are made to estimate percent body fat.

Under Water or Hydrostatic Weighing

Under water or hydrostatic weighing is based on principles defined by the Greek mathematician Archimedes (287—212 B.C.), who discovered that displacement of water could assess the mass of an object. Because water has a density of 1 g/mL and body fat has a density of 0.9 g/mL, a person with a significant amount of body fat will be an effective "floater" in water. Lean tissue, however, has a density of 1.1 g/mL, so leaner individuals will not be effective floaters. Body composition is estimated from density; density equals mass divided by volume ($d = m/v$). Therefore, a person with more girth (volume) than another person of equal mass (weight) will have a lower body density and, therefore, more body fat. Because it has a low measurement error, hydrostatic weighing has for many years been considered the gold standard in assessing body composition.

Dual Energy X-Ray Absorptiometry

Dual-energy x-ray absorptiometry (DEXA) is a common method for assessing bone mineral density. DEXA uses an x-ray source to determine mineral content of bone and percent body fat of individuals. Newer models take about 5 min to scan the entire body (compared to older instruments, which took 20 to 60 min). These are expensive instruments and are typically found in hospitals; physicians who specialize in assessing bone mineral density (e.g., rheumatologists) may have the machines in their offices. DEXA has the potential for becoming the new gold standard for assessing body composition, but many research laboratories will be unable to afford the instrument. The ease of measurement and the low dose of radiation involved (about the same amount that you would get from a cross-country plane flight) make this a highly sought-after method in the research arena.

Air Displacement Plethysmography

Air displacement plethysmography, also known as the "bod pod," was developed to assess body composition. This method uses the same principal as underwater weighing, but air and not water is displaced. A person sits into a chamber (pod) and the displacement of air is measured to assess body composition. This instrument has been validated and is easy to use. Not all laboratories, however, can afford this instrument; it may take some time before it becomes a common method of assessing body composition.

Stable Isotopes

Many scientists use stable isotopes in their research to assess a number of variables when studying metabolism. Isotopes used in this fashion are considered tracers in the body and can be easily detected to determine, for instance, how molecules are split apart and joined together in the complicated processes of metabolism. In this section, I will discuss stable isotopes of minerals.

Stable mineral isotopes are forms of minerals that are not radioactive (unstable). For example, zinc has a number of different forms in nature, such as zinc 70 (^{70}Zn) and zinc 67 (^{67}Zn). In this example, the numbers *70* and *67* are the molecular weights of the zinc isotopes. These isotopes are often used in human research because they are not radioactive and, therefore, are not dangerous. However, stable isotopes are expensive and difficult to obtain, because only a few places in the world can make them.

How Are Stable Isotopes Administered?

Stable isotopes can be administered by either injection or by mouth; and sometimes both methods are used. Basically, think of stable isotopes as labeled markers of the mineral in question. Oral and injected isotopes allow scientists to examine what the mineral does in the body (e.g., they can assess how much of the mineral is absorbed and how much is excreted). When oral isotopes are used, blood, urine, and feces are collected to assess what happened to the mineral; when injected isotopes are used, only blood is collected.

How Are Stable Isotopes Assessed?

Biologic specimens (blood, urine, and feces) are assessed by an inductively coupled plasma mass spectrometer (ICPMS). Other methods, such as thermal ionization mass spectrometry (TIMS) can also be used. Before the samples are analyzed, however, they must undergo a tedious preparation process to get them in the purist form possible. For example, other elements are eliminated so that the spectrometer can be focused on the mineral in question.

Why Use Stable Isotopes?

The use of stable isotopes allows researchers to assess the movement of minerals. If researchers wanted to assess how zinc moves through the body after exercise, they would inject ^{70}Zn into subjects before they exercised and sample the blood after they exercised. With stable isotopes, more than one blood sample is typically needed, because researchers measure the disappearance of that mineral; therefore, multiple (usually 10 or more) blood draws are required to make an accurate assessment of the mineral's movement throughout the body. Usually, when discussing stable isotope movement, researchers use the word *pools*. That is because minerals tend to move through specific areas of the body. Although these pools do not mean the mineral is stored in that area, researchers use the concept to understand how a mineral is used by the body. For example, the major zinc pools are the plasma and the liver. Therefore, zinc isotopes may move from the liver pool to the plasma pool after exercise, or vice versa.

The math used in assessing stable isotopes is quite complicated, yet fascinating. Once a researcher assesses movement of a mineral throughout the body, he or she can begin to make recommendations. Thus stable isotopes allow for focused research that can lead to definitive conclusions.

SUMMARY POINTS

- Nutrition is a multidisciplinary science, and sports nutrition is one facet of nutrition.
- Carbohydrates have 4 kcal/g; 60 to 65% of an athlete's diet should be made up of complex carbohydrates.
- Fats have 9 kcal/g; some fats are healthier than others (monounsaturated and polyunsaturated fats are better than saturated fats).
- Proteins have 4 kcal/g; athletes generally need more protein than do sedentary people.
- Minerals are nutrients required by the body and can be involved in energy-producing reactions but do not provide energy themselves. Some athletes may need higher than normal levels of certain minerals, but generally athletes' mineral needs do not appear to be different from those of nonathletes.
- Vitamins are nutrients required by the body and can be involved in energy-producing reactions but do not provide energy themselves. Some athletes may require higher than normal levels of vitamins, but it appears that most athletes do not require more vitamins than nonathletes.
- Hydration is extremely important for optimal athletic performance and to prevent injury.
- Weight loss practices in athletes are sometimes improper and dangerous. Weight loss of no more than 2 lb per week is safe and minimizes loss of muscle mass and water.
- There are a number of ergogenic aids in the market; it is important to critically review them and to be aware of their side effects.
- There are a number of ways to assess body composition; some are better than others.
- Stable isotopes continue to be a useful research tool for scientists interested in studying metabolism.

REVIEW QUESTIONS

1. What is the main focus of the field of sports nutrition (and hence, a sports nutritionist)?
2. Why are carbohydrates important?
3. List five complex carbohydrates.
4. Why should a person limit his or her saturated fat intake?
5. Do athletes need a higher percentage of fat in their diets than do nonathletes?
6. How much protein do endurance athletes and strength athletes need, respectively?
7. What are some of the roles of minerals in exercise?
8. List the water-soluble and the fat-soluble vitamins.

9. What are some signs of dehydration?
10. What is a safe amount of body weight to lose per week if a person is trying to lose weight?
11. What are the effects of caffeine on endurance performance?
12. Will chromium picolinate increase muscle mass?

References

1. Pike RL, Brown ML. Nutrition: an integrated approach. New York: Wiley, 1975.
2. Williams C, Nicholas CW. Nutrition needs for team sport. Gatorade Sports Sci Inst Sports Sci Exchange 1998;11.
3. Frail H, Burke L. Carbohydrate needs for training. In: L Burke, V Deakin, eds. Clinical sports nutrition, Sydney, Australia: McGraw-Hill, 1994:151–173.
4. Coyle EF. Timing and method of increased carbohydrate intake to cope with heavy training, competition and recovery. J Sports Sci 1991;9:29–52.
5. Burke LM. Nutrition for the female athlete. In: DA Krummel, PM Kris-Etherton, eds. Nutrition in women's health. Gaithersburg, MD: Aspen, 1996:263–298.
6. Brown RC, Cox CM. Effects of high fat versus high carbohydrate diets on plasma lipids and lipoproteins in endurance athletes. Med Sci Sports Exer 1998;30:1677–1683.
7. Lemon PWR. Effects of exercise on dietary protein requirements. Int J Sport Nutr 1998;8:426–447.
8. Heaney RP. 1996. Osteoporosis. In: DA Krummel, PM Kris-Etherton, eds. Nutrition in women's health. Gaithersburg, MD: Aspen, 1996:418–439.
9. Sawka MN, Pandolf KB. Effects of body water loss on physiological function and exercise performance. In: GV Gisolfi, DR Lamb, eds. Perspectives in exercise science and sports medicine: fluid homeostasis during exercise. Vol. 3. Carmel, IN: Cooper, 1990:1–38.
10. Davis JM, Lamb DR, Burgess WA, Bartoli WP. Accumulation of deuterium oxide in body fluids after ingestion of D2O-labeled beverages. J Appl Physiol 1987;63:2060–2066.
11. Clark N. Nancy Clark's Sports nutrition guidebook. 2nd ed. Champaign, IL: Human Kinetics, 1997.
12. Volpe SL. Wrestlers and weight loss: examining nutritional, health, and performance issues. NATA News 1998;Oct:13.
13. Clarkson PM, Levine RE, Volpe SL. Taking it to the mat: the wrestler's guide to optimal performance. National Collegiate Athletic Association, 1998.
14. Spriet LL. Ergogenic aids: recent advances and retreats. In: DR Lamb, R Murray, eds. Optimizing sport performance: perspectives in exercise science and sports medicine. Vol 10. Carmel, IN: Cooper, 1997.
15. Spriet LL. Caffeine and performance. Int J Sport Nutr 1995;5:S84–S99.
16. Burke ER. Nutritional ergogenic aids. In: JR Berning, SN Steen, eds. Nutrition for sport and exercise. 2nd ed. Gaithersburg, MD: Aspen, 1998:119–142.
17. Sandage BW, Sabounjuan LA, White R, et al. Choline citrate may enhance athletic performance. Physiologist 1992;25:236A.
18. Spector SA, Jackman MR, Sabounjian LA, et al. Effects of choline supplementation on fatigue in trained cyclists. Med Sci Sports Exer 1995;27:668–673.
19. Newsholme EA, Actworth IN, Blomstrand E. Amino acids, brain neurotransmitters and a functional link between muscle and brain that is important in sustained exercise. In: G Benzi, ed. Advances in myochemistry. London: Libbey Eurotext, 1989:127–133.
20. Stanko RT, Robertson RJ, Spina RJ, et al. Enhancement of arm-exercise endurance capacity with di-hydroxyacetone and pyruvate. J Appl Physiol 1990;68:119–124.
21. Parry-Billings M, Budgett R, Koutedakis Y, et al. Plasma amino acid concentration in over training syndrome: possible effects on the immune system. Med Sci Sports Exer 1992;24:1353–1358.
22. Varnier M, Leese GP, Thompson J, et al. Stimulatory effect of glutamine on glycogen accumulation in human skeletal muscle. Am J Physiol 1995;269:E309–E315.
23. Montner P, Stark DM, Riedesel ML, et al. Pre-exercise glycerol hydration improves cycling endurance time and testing.. Int J Sports Med 1996;17:27–33.
24. Jeukendrup AE, Saris WH, Schrauwen P, et al. Metabolic activity of medium-chain triglycerides congested with carbohydrates during prolonged exercise. J Appl Physiol 1995;79:756–762.
25. Van Zyl CG, Lambert EV, Hawley JA, et al. Effects of medium chain triglyceride ingestion on carbohydrate metabolism and cycling performance. J Appl Physiol 1996;80:2217–2225.
26. Bahrke MS, Morgan WP. Evaluation of the ergogenic properties of ginseng. Sports Med 1994;18:229–248.

27. Walker LS, Bemben MG, Bemben DA, Knehans AW. Chromium picolinate effects on body composition and muscular performance in wrestlers. Med Sci Sports Exer 1998;30:1730–1737.
28. Anderson RA, Bryden NA, Polansky MM, Deuster PA. Exercise effects on chromium excretion of trained and untrained men consuming a constant diet. J Appl Physiol 1988;64:249–252.
29. Volpe SL, Taper LJ, Meacham SL. The effect of boron supplementation on bone mineral density and hormonal status in college female athletes. Med Exer Nutr Health 1993;2:323–330.

Suggested Readings

Berning JR, Steen SN, eds. Nutrition for sport and exercise. 2nd ed. Gaithersburg, MD: Aspen, 1998.
Clark N. Nancy Clark's sports nutrition guidebook. 2nd ed. Champaign, IL: Human Kinetics, 1997.
Peterson MS. A guide to sports nutrition: eat to compete. 2nd ed. St. Louis: Mosby, 1996.
Ryan MR. Complete guide to sports nutrition. Boulder, CO: Velo, 1999.
Williams MH. Nutrition for health, fitness & sport. 5th ed. Boston: McGraw-Hill, 1999.
Wolinsky I. Nutrition in exercise and sport. 3rd ed. Boca Raton, FL: CRC Press, 1998.

Epidemiology is "the study of the distribution and determinants of health-related states or events in specified populations, and the application of this study to the control of health problems" (1). The science of epidemiology helps us understand how disease spreads through a population (a defined group of individuals). Similar to a detective, the epidemiologist is trained to investigate a specific case (disease or physiologic condition), scientifically gathering the clues to implicate a potential culprit, and then setting out to prove innocence or guilt. The number of situations that warrant the epidemiologic approach is as vast as the multitude of backgrounds from which epidemiologists originate (see Practical Application 10.1).

Physical activity epidemiology involves the specific investigation of the relationship between physical activity and exercise and various diseases and conditions in a population. The diseases and conditions currently thought to be associated with a sedentary lifestyle are listed in Box 10.1. The focus of this chapter is threefold: to discover how physical activity and exercise are measured in population studies, to examine how epidemiology is used as a tool in investigating the associations between physical activity and exercise and health, and to explore current issues in the field of physical activity epidemiology. Figure 10.1 illustrates the way a physical activity epidemiology course or unit may be presented.

DEFINITION, DESCRIPTION, AND SCOPE

Although physical activity epidemiology is one of the newest subdisciplines of exercise science, it has earned national recognition in recent years owing to evidence that physical inactivity is a major **risk factor** for a number of chronic diseases (see Practical Application 10.2). In this section, we examine the nature and scope of physical activity epidemiology.

Major risk factors are separated into biologic, environmental, and behavioral categories.

Practical Application 10.1

HOW EPIDEMIOLOGY IS USED[a]

Epidemiology is used in four ways to better the health of a population. Its first use is to establish cause. It is important to know whether the cause of a disease is related to environmental factors or to genetics. To better understand the causes of chronic diseases such as cardiovascular diseases, epidemiologists use a model called the web of causation, as shown in the figure (see figure on opposite page). Second, epidemiologists trace the natural history of a disease to understand its normal course and how it progresses. Third, epidemiologists describe the health status of a population to determine the total burden of disease in that population. Finally, once an intervention has been tried, epidemiologists evaluate it to determine the success or failure of programs established to prevent or treat the disease. The use of epidemiology in this fourfold fashion helps create the most efficient plan possible for controlling the disease within current fiscal and technological restraints.

---

[a]From Powers SK, Howley ET. Exercise physiology: theory and applications to fitness and performance. Madison, WI: Brown & Benchmark, 1997.

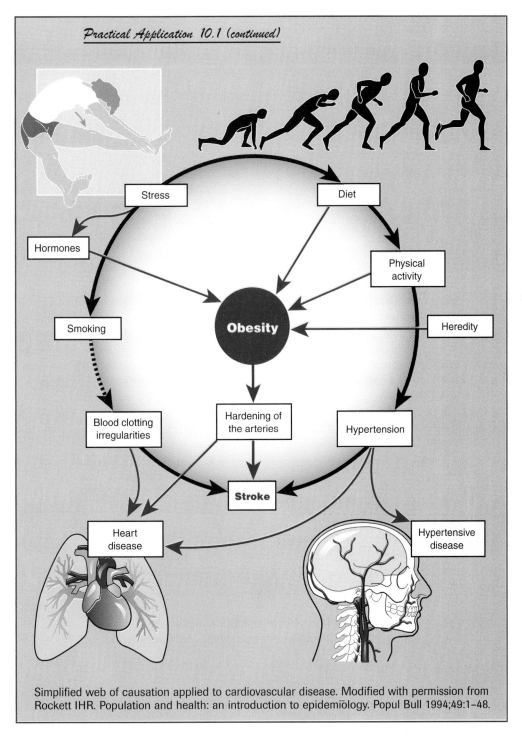

Practical Application 10.1 (continued)

Simplified web of causation applied to cardiovascular disease. Modified with permission from Rockett IHR. Population and health: an introduction to epidemiology. Popul Bull 1994;49:1–48.

Exercise and Physical Activity

Physical activity has been defined as any bodily movement produced by skeletal muscles that results in energy expended (2). Exercise is considered a specific subcategory of physical activity; it is planned, structured, and repetitive and results in the improvement or maintenance of one or more facets of physical fitness (including aerobic power, muscular endurance, muscular strength, body composition, and/or flexibility) (2).

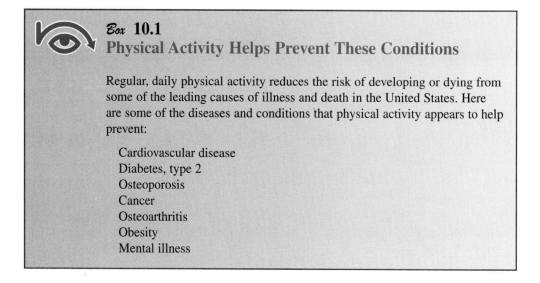

Box 10.1
Physical Activity Helps Prevent These Conditions

Regular, daily physical activity reduces the risk of developing or dying from some of the leading causes of illness and death in the United States. Here are some of the diseases and conditions that physical activity appears to help prevent:

Cardiovascular disease
Diabetes, type 2
Osteoporosis
Cancer
Osteoarthritis
Obesity
Mental illness

Physical activity (which includes exercise) makes up one of the three major components of **total energy expenditure** (3,4); the other two are basal metabolic rate (which typically encompasses 50 to 70% of total energy expended) and the thermic effect of food (which accounts for 7 to 10% of total energy expended) (Fig. 10.2). Total energy expenditure is the total amount of energy, expressed in kilocalories, expended each 24-hr period. Physical activity is the most variable component of total energy expenditure and is divided into two parts: activities of daily living (such as bathing, eating, and grooming) and other activities, such as sports, leisure, and occupational activities. The contribution physical activity makes to total energy expenditure is obviously greater for active individuals than for their sedentary counterparts.

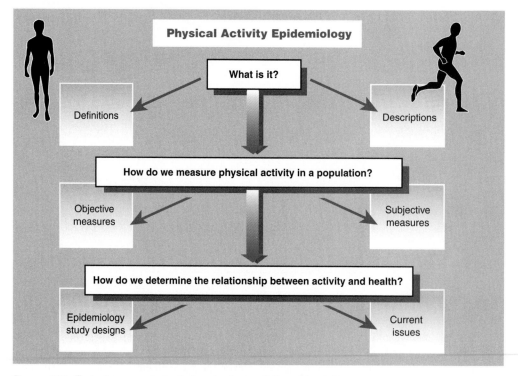

Figure 10.1 Typical course content of a physical activity epidemiology course.

Practical Application 10.2

RISK FACTORS

Chronic diseases (e.g., heart disease and cancer) are the major causes of death in the United States. The causes of these diseases are thought to be the complex interaction of biologic, environmental, and behavioral factors. Finding causal connections among these risk factors and chronic disease has been an extremely difficult task. However, since the 1960s, our understanding of the association between risk factors and disease processes has greatly increased, which has led to public health programs that have been successful in educating the population about this association. Today, many more people are aware of the need to take personal responsibility for their health because of our progress in this area. Becoming personally responsible for one's health is achieved by reducing the influence of chronic disease risk factors in one's lifestyle.

The web of causation is very complex, because the factors that operate in a population interact to a large degree. However, some risk factors work independently (primary risk factors) of others in causing disease, and others work only if the primary factor is present (secondary risk factors). The following table lists factors thought to be associated with coronary heart disease.

Primary Risk Factors		
Cannot Be Changed	**Can Be Changed**	**Secondary Risk Factors**
Heredity	Cigarette smoking	Diabetes
Male sex	High serum cholesterol	Obesity
Aging	High blood pressure	Stress
	Physical inactivity	

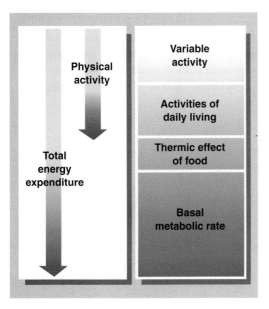

Figure 10.2 Components of total energy expenditure.

Epidemiology Terminology

The two fundamental assumptions of epidemiology are that human disease does not occur at random and that human disease has causal and preventive factors that can be identified through scientific investigation of different populations or subgroups of individuals within a population (5). The primary goal of epidemiology is to identify the determinants of disease to decrease mortality and **morbidity** within a population (6).

Physical activity epidemiology, therefore, involves the specific investigation of the relationship between physical activity (and/or exercise) and health and diseases within a population. These types of epidemiology studies investigate the association of physical activity as a health-related behavior with disease and other health outcomes, the distribution and determinants of physical activity behavior(s) within a given population, and the interrelationship of physical activity with other behaviors (7). Physical activity epidemiology applies the results of scientific research to the prevention and control of diseases and conditions within populations for the purpose of promoting health.

The measurement of the amount of disease in a population is expressed as various rates. A **rate** is a fraction that consists of a numerator (the number of people from a population with the disease) and a denominator (the number of people in the entire population at a given time). Rates of death are known as **mortality rates,** and rates of individuals with the disease (also called cases) are called morbidity rates (8). For example, assume that in a population of 100,000 individuals, 500 are affected with a disease. The measurement of the amount of disease in this population is calculated from these two numbers and may be expressed as a percentage (0.5%) or as a ratio (.005). These figures mean that the morbidity rate is 5 per 1000 people.

Incidence rates are estimates of the number of individuals within a population without a disease who develop that disease during a specific time period. In contrast, **prevalence rates** are estimates of the number of people who already have the disease in a population at a particular point in time or during a given time period (8). Incidence rates inform us of the speed of development of new cases per unit of population compared to prevalence, which estimates the number of existing cases within a population. Prevalence rates are influenced by both the incidence (number of new cases) and the duration of the disease. For example, the incidence rate of first stroke in the United States in 1991 was 220 per 100,000 people. In terms of long-term chronic disease, the prevalence rate would be greater because of the duration of the disease. The opposite would be true for diseases of short duration, like influenza.

> *An increase in the prevalence of a certain disease in a specific population occurs if the number of new cases of the disease increased (incidence), the duration of the disease increased, or both. For example, the prevalence of diabetes would increase if more individuals acquired diabetes, if individuals with diabetes survived longer, or both.*

Early in the research process, it is important to examine if biologic reasons can meaningfully explain the hypothesis of a potential relationship between physical activity and the health outcome of interest. In other words, based on current knowledge about activity and the disease of interest, is it plausible that physical inactivity could cause that specific disease? The fact that the hypothesis and the relationship being proposed are in harmony with existing scientific information is referred to as **biologic plausibility** and is a key piece of sound epidemiology research. For example, in the area of physical activity epidemiology, it has been hypothesized that physical activity and exercise may play a role in the prevention of type 2 diabetes. This causal relationship is biologically plausible and may occur through several known mechanisms and is supported in the clinical literature. Some of these possible physiologic mechanisms include the ability of physical activity to do the following: improve the effectiveness of insulin to regulate blood glucose, better regulate blood glucose levels, decrease overall and central **adiposity,** and cause desirable changes in muscle tissue.

When attempting to determine if an association exists between physical activity and exercise and a disease or health outcome, an epidemiologist often turns to statistical tests to help assess the likelihood that the association is real or is the result of chance. To quantify the degree to which chance may account for an association observed in a particular study, a **p value** is often used. Researchers are bound by certain rules that help them interpret the outcome of their studies. Using statistical procedures, researchers decide when an association between a health outcome and physical inactivity is **statistically significant.** They then are able to quantify the probability that the association could have occurred by chance alone. A statistically significant result is the Holy Grail of research and helps confirm the original hypothesis proposed by the researcher. A statistically significant result does not mean that chance cannot explain the findings, only that such an explanation is unlikely owing to statistical reasoning (see Box 10.2)

In studies designed to determine if an association exists between physical activity and exercise and a disease or health outcome, the study participants often differ by characteristics that may influence the disease outcome. Researchers typically must control for characteristics such as body size, race and ethnic background, and a host of biologic variables. Physical activity epidemiologists adjust for the effects of these characteristics or variables so that the influence of physical activity on the disease or health outcome can be seen more clearly.

A variable with an effect that is *entangled* with the effect of physical activity (i.e., the two variables cannot be easily separated and studied independently) is known as a **confounder,** and it is because of such variables that statistical adjustment of the data is necessary (9). For a variable to be a confounder in physical activity epidemiology, it must be related to the disease or health outcome of interest and be related to physical activity levels. Age is often a potential confounder. As an example, age is directly, or positively, related to the development of diabetes. As age increases, the risk of developing diabetes increases. Similarly, age is often found to be inversely, or negatively, related to physical activity levels. As age increases, physical activity levels are typically found to decrease. Therefore, if a study of the population of the United States shows that diabetes decreases as physical activity increases, age may be a potential confounder, because older individuals tend to get diabetes and tend to be less active then their younger counterparts.

Methods for adjusting for potential confounders (like age) are among the common statistical tools used in epidemiology studies. In the example just cited, adjustment for age would permit researchers to determine whether individuals of the same age with varying levels of physical activity have different diabetes rates.

Box **10.2**
Questions Epidemiologists Ask for Determining Cause

Is there a temporal association between the risk factor and the disease? Does the proposed risk factor precede the disease?

Is there biologic plausibility?

Are the current findings consistent with those of previous studies?

Is the association between cause and effect strong enough?

Is there a dose–response relationship? That is, when exposure to the possible cause is increased is there an associated increase in the effect?

Is the effect reversible when the cause is removed?

Is the study design strong enough to explain the results without equivocation?

Can more than one line of evidence lead to the conclusion?

FOCUS ON SCIENCE

This section centers on the important tools and techniques available to physical activity epidemiologists as they attempt to unravel the clues (data) they have gathered.

Assessment of Physical Activity and Exercise in Epidemiology Studies

When examining the relationships between physical activity and health conditions within a population, the **physical activity survey** (a subjective recall of the activity engaged in over a specific period of time) is usually the method of choice for quantifying physical activity. Reasons for its popularity include its nonreactiveness (lack of alteration of the individual's behavior as a direct result of the assessment technique), its practicality (generally determined by cost and participant convenience), its applicability (ability to modify the instrument to suit the population in question), and its acceptable accuracy (both **reliability** and **validity**) relative to other methods (10,11).

More objective measures of physical activity, such as the doubly-labeled water technique or activity monitors, are not practical in most epidemiologic studies but have been used to validate the physical activity questionnaire (10,11). Examples of objective measures used in epidemiology research for quantifying physical activity include several classes of measurement techniques: *(a)* total energy expenditure (doubly-labeled water technique and the respiratory chamber); *(b)* movement counters, such as activity monitors or accelerometers and pedometers (which initially measured frequency of movement and have been modified to detect differences in speed and direction of movement); *(c)* measures that estimate physical fitness (heart rate monitoring and graded exercise testing); and *(d)* field tests and other observations. (For a comprehensive explanation of the objective measures used to measure physical activity levels, see Suggested Reading.)

The assessment tool must elicit accurate information on the types of physical activity that encompass the greatest proportion of energy expenditure in the study population of interest. The types of activities can range from occupational and leisure activities to transportation and housework activities. The specific types of activities that significantly contribute to an individual's energy expenditure typically varies by age, sex, health status, and culture. Leisure (in particular, sports) and occupational physical activity are important when assessing younger and healthier populations. Some researchers suggest that differences in activities of daily living (bathing and eating) and low-level leisure activities may best represent energy expenditure and physical activity in older or diseased populations (10). In contrast, walking as a form of transportation significantly contributes to total energy expenditure in individuals from developing countries.

In addition, there are different dimensions of physical activity, such as energy expenditure, aerobic intensity, weight bearing, strength, and flexibility. These dimensions of activity relate in varying degrees to different disease and health outcomes (7). As an example, when studying the effects of physical activity on osteoporosis, researchers would be wise to focus their efforts on estimating weight-bearing activities, because weight-bearing activity is the most plausible biologic mechanism through which physical activity can influence osteoporosis development. Therefore, depending on the disease or health outcome of interest, the questionnaire or measurement tool must be able to capture the dimensions of physical activity that most strongly relate to the disease or health outcome of interest.

The survey approaches used to measure physical activity vary from activity diaries to self-administered or interviewer-administered activity questionnaires. The time frame and complexity of the activity questionnaire can range from a single question about usual activity to a recall survey with a time frame of one day, one week, one year, or even a lifetime. The advantage of assessing activity using a survey with a short time frame is that the estimate is easier to validate and less likely to suffer from recall bias (i.e., inaccuracies in remembering exactly what was done). On the other hand, assessment over a short time period is less likely to reflect usual be-havior, because activity may vary with season or as a result of an acute illness.

It is clear that physical activity levels obtained from questionnaires do not reflect total en-ergy expenditure for a particular individual, because they do not consider the energy require-ments of such things as basal metabolic rate and, in most cases, activities of daily living. Determination of total energy expenditure can be obtained only by a more exact measure of en-ergy expenditure, such as the respiratory chamber or the doubly-labeled water technique (3). However, the estimates obtained by the activity questionnaire are valuable in relative terms and can be used to rank individuals or groups of subjects within a population from the least to the most active. The result is a relative distribution of individuals based on their reported levels of physical activity that can then be examined in relation to physiologic parameters and disease out-come. (For a comprehensive look at popular questionnaires used in epidemiology studies, see Suggested Reading.)

Assessment of Exercise and Fitness in Epidemiology Studies

Cardiovascular fitness measured by maximum oxygen uptake ($\dot{V}O_2max$) is often used as an ob-jective measure of physical activity. Individuals who are more active and expend more energy tend to have higher fitness levels. However, when examining population studies, there is only a moderate relationship between physical activity and physical fitness (12,13). This lack of a strong relationship could indicate that there are other factors besides activity, such as genetics, sex, age, and relative weight that influence physical fitness (14,15).

The gold standard for cardiovascular fitness determination is a graded exercise test in which the individual's maximum oxygen uptake is measured (16). A treadmill is usually the preferred ergometer for this type of assessment (16). A maximum test is not practical for use in epidemi-ologic studies, because of the time, personnel, and potential medical risk involved. Alternative assessments of $\dot{V}O_2max$ include a submaximum test (ending the test before the subjects reach their maximum level and then extrapolating—estimating—what their maximal level is likely to be) using the step test or a cycle ergometer. Although the use of a submaximum test in an epi-demiologic study may be more practical than a maximum test, the assumptions made when es-timating $\dot{V}O_2max$ may not be valid (16). A third type of assessment is the field test in which a large group of individuals can be tested simultaneously by one or two technicians. An example is the 12-min run (17). Drawbacks to using a field test include the need for medical screening (for high-risk populations), cooperation, and motivation of the participants (18).

Epidemiology Study Designs

There are two major approaches epidemiologists use to test the hypothesis that physical inactiv-ity may play an important role in the development of a specific disease or condition. The most powerful, most conclusive, but most expensive approach is the **experimental study,** in which the investigator randomly assigns varying levels of the risk factor of interest (physical activity lev-els) to individuals without the disease and then follows these individuals to compare their de-velopment of the disease (8).

A more popular, but less conclusive type of study, is the **observational study,** in which the investigator observes the occurrence of the disease or condition in individuals who differ by the risk factor of interest (in this case, physical inactivity). In these studies, the risk factor of inter-est is self-selected by the individuals themselves and not under the control of the investigator. Another difficulty with these types of studies is that the individuals usually differ by important characteristics other than the one in question (here, physical activity levels), and these charac-teristics may also influence the disease outcome. To attempt to adjust for these potentially con-founding factors, sophisticated statistical methodology is often necessary (8).

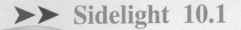

CLINICAL TRIALS

Clinical trials are necessary in research because they yield the best information. A clinical trial, for example, could be set up in which individuals who don't have type 2 diabetes are randomly assigned to either a group that includes a physical activity program or one that does not. After a specified time, data from these groups are reviewed to determine which group has a higher incidence of diabetes. One clinical trial demonstrated that physical activity intervention led to a decrease in the incidence of diabetes over a 6-year period in a Chinese population initially identified with impaired glucose tolerance.[a] At the beginning of the study, 577 individuals with impaired glucose tolerance were picked from a citywide health screening program and randomized into one of four groups: exercise only, diet only, diet plus exercise, and control.

Individuals assigned to the exercise groups were encouraged to increase their daily leisure physical activity by one unit, which was comparable to a 20-min brisk walk. The cumulative incidence of diabetes after 6 years was significantly lower in the intervention groups compared to the control group (exercise only, 41%; diet plus exercise, 46%; diet only, 44%; control, 68%). These group differences remained significant even after adjusting for potential confounding variables (baseline differences in body mass index and fasting glucose level). The conclusion was that individuals assigned to groups that included a physical activity program had a significantly lower risk of developing diabetes than those who were not assigned to the intervention groups (see figure).

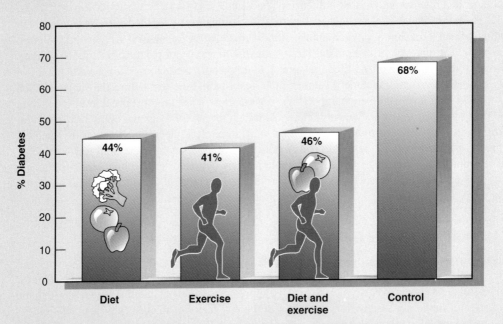

Cumulative incidence of diabetes at 6 years by intervention group. The interventions had about an equal effect on the incidence of diabetes at 6 years. Reprinted with permission from Pan X, Li G, Hu Y. Effects of diet and exercise in preventing NIDDM in people with impaired glucose tolerance: the Da Qing IGT and diabetes study. Diabetes Care 1997;20:537–544.

---

[a]Pan X, Li G, Hu Y. Effects of diet and exercise in preventing NIDDM in people with impaired glucose tolerance: the Da Qing IGT and diabetes study. Diabetes Care 1997;20:537–544.

Detailed descriptions and case examples of the various study designs are provided in this chapter. Because the biologic plausibility of the possible role of physical activity and type 2 diabetes was just presented, we will continue with this example. Therefore, given the hypothesis that physical activity plays a significant role in the prevention of type 2 diabetes, what types of studies could test this hypothesis?

Experimental Study Design

By far, the most powerful and labor-intensive epidemiologic study design is the experimental design or **clinical trial** in which efforts are made to prevent or delay the onset of the disease in question by manipulating the risk factor of interest, in this case, physical activity levels. In this design, individuals free from the disease are randomly assigned to receive either an intervention (the physical activity intervention group) or no intervention (the control group). Subsequent follow-up of the groups help determine if the groups differ, which is revealed by the percent who eventually develop the disease (see Sidelight 10.1).

Observational Study Designs

Cross-sectional studies collect information about the health outcome (e.g., type 2 diabetes) and the potential risk factor (physical inactivity) at the same time within the same group. This type of epidemiologic design is limited, because it is not possible to establish causality: In other words, did inactivity cause the health outcome or did the condition cause the inactivity (see A Case in Point 10.1)?

In **case-control study designs** (also called retrospective studies), individuals with and without the disease or condition of interest are asked questions about their past, particularly their exposure to the specific risk factor in question (i.e., physical activity level). Although this type of study design is valuable in cases in which the disease outcome is rare, it does suffer from potential recall bias, in which the diseased or high-risk individual may remember or recall past events differently (see A Case in Point 10.2).

The strongest of the observational study designs is the **prospective study** design (also called a longitudinal study) (Fig. 10.3). This particular design identifies and follows individuals initially free of the health outcome of interest and seeks to establish if, in our example, initial or subsequent physical activity levels differentiate those who do and do not develop the disease (see A Case in Point 10.3).

ADVANCES IN PHYSICAL ACTIVITY EPIDEMIOLOGY

There has recently been a great deal of attention given to the problem of physical inactivity across all segments of the American population. Major consensus statements have highlighted the importance of getting more people to become physically active. The following advances highlight some of these national efforts and also present research challenges still yet to be met.

Physical Activity and Health: Report of the Surgeon General

In 1996 the publication *Physical Activity and Health: A Report of the Surgeon General* (19) summarized what was then known about activity and health based on decades of research and has helped direct researchers to areas and questions regarding physical activity and health that are not yet known. This landmark review of research on physical activity and health served as a national statement on the importance of physical activity in the realm of public health. Although parts of the surgeon general's report are discussed throughout this chapter, this report is a strongly recommended reading for students and scientists interested in physical activity epidemiology. In addition, students should be aware of the national health promotion and disease

A Case in Point 10.1

CROSS-SECTIONAL STUDIES IN PIMA INDIANS

In this example both diabetes status (and/or glucose or insulin levels) and physical activity levels were determined at the same time and in the same individuals. The relationship between physical activity and diabetes status was examined in the Pima Indians, who have the highest documented incidence of type 2 diabetes in the world. Fasting and 2-hr postload plasma glucose concentrations (based on an oral glucose tolerance test), age, and measures of obesity and fat distribution (body mass index and waist:thigh circumference ratios) were determined in 1054 Pima individuals aged 15 to 59 years. Past year leisure and occupational physical activity were determined by a physical activity questionnaire. The conclusion was that individuals with type 2 diabetes reported being less active than those without diabetes[a] (see figure).

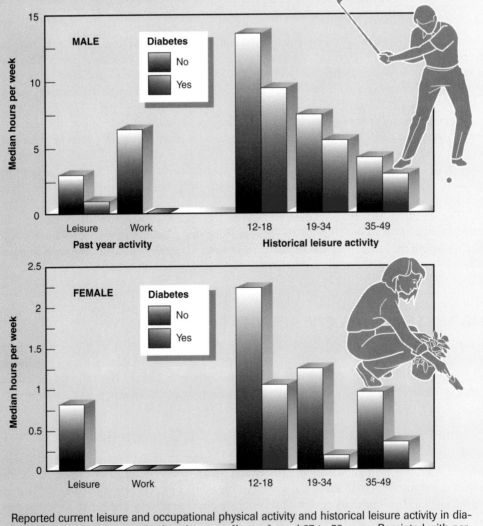

Reported current leisure and occupational physical activity and historical leisure activity in diabetic and nondiabetic men (*top*) and women (*bottom*) aged 37 to 59 years. Reprinted with permission from Kriska A, LaPorte R, Pettitt D, et al. The association of physical activity with obesity, fat distribution and glucose intolerance in Pima Indians. Diabetologia 1993;36:863–869.

A Case in Point 10.1 (continued)

In a second series of cross-sectional analyses, glucose and/or insulin levels and physical activity levels were determined in individuals who did not have diabetes. Current physical activity was found to be negatively related to fasting and 2-hr plasma glucose and insulin concentrations for most sex–age groups in the nondiabetic individuals. Many of these relationships remained significant after controlling for potential confounders (e.g., age, obesity, and fat distribution). The conclusion was that among individuals who do not have type 2 diabetes, those who are physically active have lower glucose and insulin values than those who are not.

———
[a]Kriska A, LaPorte R, Pettitt D, et al. The association of physical activity with obesity, fat distribution and glucose intolerance in Pima Indians. Diabetologia 1993;36:863–869.

A Case in Point 10.2

Retrospective Studies in Pima Indians

In this case, individuals with and without type 2 diabetes were asked questions about their past, specifically, their physical activity levels over their lifetime. A total of 353 individuals aged 37 to 59 years were asked to estimate their levels of physical activity as teenagers (12 to 18 years) and as younger (19 to 34 years) and older (35 to 49 years) adults. The individuals with diabetes reported significantly less leisure physical activity than individuals without diabetes. Even after controlling for body mass index, sex, age, and waist:thigh ratio, subjects who had type 2 diabetes reported lower levels of historical leisure activity than those who did not have diabetes.[a] The conclusion was that individuals with type 2 diabetes reported less physical activity over their lifetime than individuals without diabetes.

———
[a]Kriska A, LaPorte R, Pettitt D, et al. The association of physical activity with obesity, fat distribution and glucose intolerance in Pima Indians. Diabetologia 1993;36:863–869.

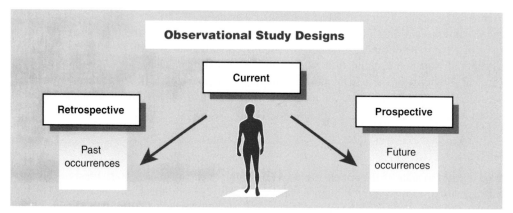

Figure 10.3 Observational study designs.

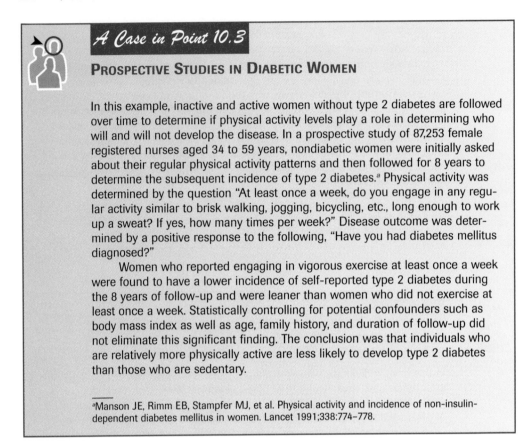

A Case in Point 10.3

PROSPECTIVE STUDIES IN DIABETIC WOMEN

In this example, inactive and active women without type 2 diabetes are followed over time to determine if physical activity levels play a role in determining who will and will not develop the disease. In a prospective study of 87,253 female registered nurses aged 34 to 59 years, nondiabetic women were initially asked about their regular physical activity patterns and then followed for 8 years to determine the subsequent incidence of type 2 diabetes.[a] Physical activity was determined by the question "At least once a week, do you engage in any regular activity similar to brisk walking, jogging, bicycling, etc., long enough to work up a sweat? If yes, how many times per week?" Disease outcome was determined by a positive response to the following, "Have you had diabetes mellitus diagnosed?"

Women who reported engaging in vigorous exercise at least once a week were found to have a lower incidence of self-reported type 2 diabetes during the 8 years of follow-up and were leaner than women who did not exercise at least once a week. Statistically controlling for potential confounders such as body mass index as well as age, family history, and duration of follow-up did not eliminate this significant finding. The conclusion was that individuals who are relatively more physically active are less likely to develop type 2 diabetes than those who are sedentary.

[a]Manson JE, Rimm EB, Stampfer MJ, et al. Physical activity and incidence of non-insulin-dependent diabetes mellitus in women. Lancet 1991;338:774–778.

prevention objectives as outlined in *Healthy People 2000* (20). The objectives specifically related to exercise are listed in Box 10.3.

The Prevalence of Sedentary Behavior in the United States

One of the most troublesome findings in public health today is the extremely large number of individuals who continue to lead a sedentary lifestyle (19). As cars, elevators, and TV sets replace human effort, incorporating physical activity into a typical day's activity has become less of an automatic occurrence and more of a planned behavior.

National surveys of physical activity in the United States, such as the Behavioral Risk Factor Surveillance System (BRFSS), identify that at least 25% of U.S. adults do not engage in any leisure-time physical activity at all (21). Unfortunately, the prevalence of sedentary behavior is even higher in the U.S. minority populations. Results of the third National Health and Nutrition Examination Survey showed that the prevalence of reporting no leisure physical activity over the past month in individuals 20 years or older was higher for African-American and Mexican-American men and women than their non-Hispanic white counterparts (21) (Fig. 10.4).

National Efforts

In an attempt to address the critical problem of a high prevalence of sedentary lifestyle throughout the nation, experts were brought together in early 1993 by the U.S. Centers for Disease Control and Prevention (CDC) and the American College of Sports Medicine (ACSM) to review the pertinent scientific evidence and develop a clear, concise public health message regarding

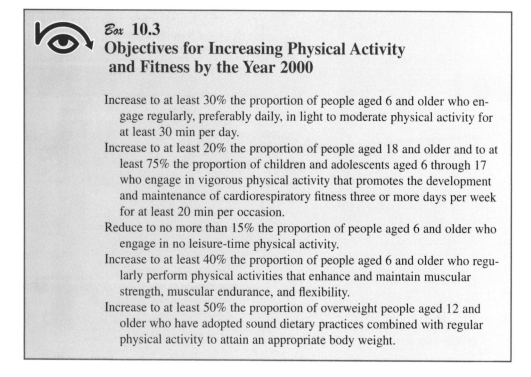

Box **10.3**

**Objectives for Increasing Physical Activity
and Fitness by the Year 2000**

Increase to at least 30% the proportion of people aged 6 and older who engage regularly, preferably daily, in light to moderate physical activity for
at least 30 min per day.

Increase to at least 20% the proportion of people aged 18 and older and to at
least 75% the proportion of children and adolescents aged 6 through 17
who engage in vigorous physical activity that promotes the development
and maintenance of cardiorespiratory fitness three or more days per week
for at least 20 min per occasion.

Reduce to no more than 15% the proportion of people aged 6 and older who
engage in no leisure-time physical activity.

Increase to at least 40% the proportion of people aged 6 and older who regularly perform physical activities that enhance and maintain muscular
strength, muscular endurance, and flexibility.

Increase to at least 50% the proportion of overweight people aged 12 and
older who have adopted sound dietary practices combined with regular
physical activity to attain an appropriate body weight.

physical activity. One of the important concerns identified at this meeting was the public misconception that to gain any health benefits from physical activity one must engage in vigorous,
continuous exercise (22). The most valuable message that came out of this meeting was the re-
vision of the old exercise recommendations in an attempt to clear up this public misconception
(Fig. 10.5).

The old exercise prescription was a structured, inflexible series of criteria designed for the
athlete. As with any prescription, one had to follow this set of criteria religiously or the effort

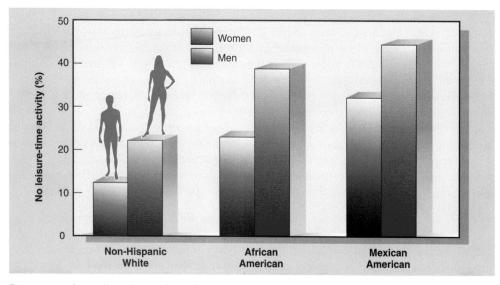

Figure 10.4 Age-adjusted prevalence (per 100) of no leisure-time physical activity in the U.S. popu-
lation, 20 years of age and older, 1988 to 1991. Reprinted with permission from Crespo C, Keteyian
SJ, Heath GW, Sempos CT. Leisure-time physical activity among US adults. Results from the Third
National Health and Nutrition Examination Survey. Arch Intern Med 1996;156:93–98.

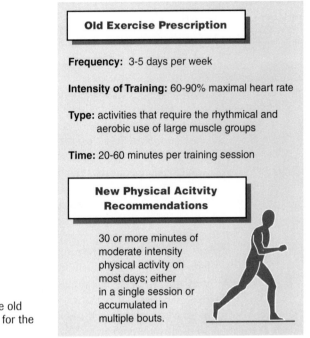

Old Exercise Prescription

Frequency: 3-5 days per week

Intensity of Training: 60-90% maximal heart rate

Type: activities that require the rhythmical and aerobic use of large muscle groups

Time: 20-60 minutes per training session

New Physical Acitvity Recommendations

30 or more minutes of moderate intensity physical activity on most days; either in a single session or accumulated in multiple bouts.

Figure 10.5 Comparison of the old and new exercise prescription for the general population.

"didn't count." Exercise meant high levels of intensity and was associated with gyms, exercise equipment, and sweat. In contrast, the new public health recommendations were designed for the general public with the message that each and every individual could be more active. The major thrust of the effort was to encourage sedentary individuals to increase their levels of moderate, feasible physical activity, such as walking.

How Much Physical Activity Is Enough?

The physiologic, clinical, and epidemiologic evidence suggests that many of the overall health benefits from physical activity can be gained by performing activities that are not necessarily of high intensity (22). In fact, research to date suggests that individuals engaging in a moderate level of physical activity have a lower risk of many chronic diseases compared to sedentary individuals (22).

In examining some of the prospective data, significant differences in risk of diabetes and coronary heart disease (CHD) appear to occur between individuals who report relatively no physical activity or exercise and those who report doing something. For example, when examining the association between frequency of reported vigorous activity per week in nurses, most of the difference in incidence of diabetes occurred between those who reported less than one time per week of activity and those who were active a minimum of once per week (23). A prospective study of physical fitness and mortality mirror these findings, demonstrating a decrease in mortality rates in originally healthy individuals as you move from the least fit to the most fit groups; the largest gain in health benefits is observed between the least fit and those somewhat fitter (24). For more information on the right amount of physical activity see A Case in Point 10.4.

Physical inactivity has been shown to be an independent risk factor for the development of CHD. The relative risk of CHD owing to inactivity is 1.9 (sedentary individuals are almost twice as likely to develop CHD than physically active people). This risk is similar to that of high blood pressure (2.1) and high cholesterol (2.4). A change in activity status, however, is likely to have an enormous effect on the nation's health because 59% of the population is inactive, contrasted with 10% who have high blood pressure and 10% who have high cholesterol.

A Case in Point 10.4

MORTALITY RATES AND CORONARY HEART DISEASE

Coronary heart disease and overall mortality were examined in 12,138 middle-aged men participating in the Multiple Risk Factor Intervention Trial.[a] Although at high risk for CHD, these men were all free of disease at the baseline of the study. At baseline, researchers obtained the subjects' levels of leisure physical activity. Based on these reported activity levels, men were divided into three groups (low, moderate, and high physical activity) and then followed for 7 years. CHD mortality rates by tertiles (thirds) of physical activity (low, moderate, and high activity) were recorded (see figure).

Examining the results at the 7 year follow-up, the researchers noted that the major decrease in mortality rates existed between the men who were part of the low activity group at baseline and the two more active groups (low activity group compared to moderate and high activity groups). In this study, there did not appear to be any apparent difference between the two more active groups of men (moderate and high activity groups). The conclusion was that data from this study suggest that most of the protective effect of physical activity in the prevention of CHD occurs between those engaged in moderate to high levels of physical activity and those that are the least active.

[a]Leon AS, Connett J, Jacobs DR, Rauramaa R. Leisure-time physical activity levels and risk of coronary heart disease and death: the Multiple Risk Factor Intervention Trial. JAMA 1987;258:2388–2395.

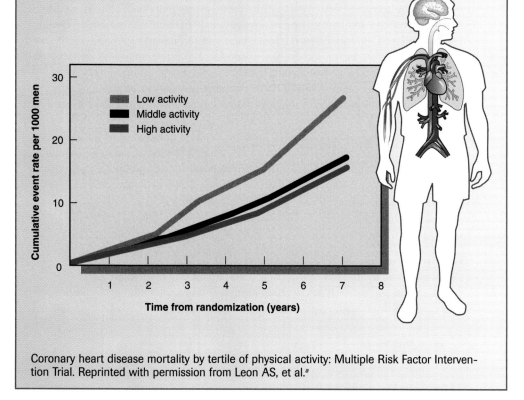

Coronary heart disease mortality by tertile of physical activity: Multiple Risk Factor Intervention Trial. Reprinted with permission from Leon AS, et al.[a]

The Challenge

In 1993, a physical activity and health workshop was held at a conference sponsored by the National Institutes of Health (NIH) titled "Disease Prevention Research at NIH: An Agenda for All." At this workshop, recommendations were made regarding future physical activity research directions. Three of the key recommendations for activity research were as follows (25):

"The type, pattern, intensity, frequency, and total amount of physical activity required to provide . . . physical health benefits should be clarified and specified". And we should "identify variations in dose-response relationships between different populations."
"Develop strategies to promote long-term increases in physical activity throughout the U.S. population."

These three challenges are still the most important issues in the field of physical activity epidemiology today. Although progress is being made in these areas, we are only beginning to understand how much physical activity or exercise is enough to gain health benefit, and we still have tremendous difficulty helping the sedentary to become more active and maintain that active behavior. Additional research is needed in these areas to properly address these issues.

SUMMARY POINTS

- Physical activity epidemiology is a field of research that investigates the relationship between physical activity (and/or exercise) and health and diseases in a population.
- A variety of assessment tools are used in physical activity epidemiology to study the relationship between physical activity and health conditions within populations. Some of the most frequently used methods are the physical activity survey, the doubly-labeled water technique, and activity monitors.
- In physical activity epidemiology, the experimental study design is favored because it is the most powerful and most conclusive. The investigator can manipulate the risk factor of interest (e.g., physical activity levels) by randomizing individuals free from disease into an intervention and control groups. Because experimental studies are expensive, observational studies (e.g., cross-sectional, case-control, cohort) are more widely used to observe the occurrence of the disease or condition in individuals who differ by the factor of interest (e.g., physical activity).
- Recently, there was a major national focus on the positive effect of physical activity on public health. The importance of this area was exemplified by the surgeon general's report of 1996.
- Three of the most important issues for future research in the field of physical activity epidemiology are to *(a)* clarify and specify the amount of physical activity required to provide physical health benefits, *(b)* identify variations in dose-response relationships between different populations, and *(c)* develop strategies to promote long-term increases in physical activity throughout the U.S. population.

REVIEW QUESTIONS

1. Why are surveys a popular measure of physical activity?
2. What objective measures of physical activity are used in epidemiologic studies?
3. What are the two major types of study designs used in epidemiologic studies?
4. What are the three major types of observational studies?

Acknowledgments

The authors would like to acknowledge the helpful comments of Dr. Edward Gregg and Annette Rexroad in preparing this chapter.

References

1. Last JM, ed. A dictionary of epidemiology. New York: Oxford University Press, 1988.
2. Caspersen CJ, Powell KE, Christenson GM. Physical activity, exercise and physical fitness: definitions and distinctions for health-related research. Pub Health Rep 1985;100:126–131.
3. Ravussin E, Rising R. Daily energy expenditure in humans: measurements in a respiratory chamber and by doubly labeled water. In: JM Kinney, HN Tucker, eds. Energy metabolism: tissue determinants and cellular corollaries. New York: Raven, 1992:81–96.
4. Ravussin E, Bogardus C. A brief overview of human energy metabolism and its relationship to essential obesity. Am J Clin Nut 1992;55(suppl):242S–245S.
5. Hennekens CH, Buring JE. Definition and background. In: SL Mayrent, ed. Epidemiology in medicine. Boston: Little, Brown, 1987:3–15.
6. Kuller LH. Relationship between acute and chronic disease epidemiology. Yale J Biol Med 1987;60:363–377.
7. Caspersen CJ, Powell KE, Merritt RK. Measurement of health status and well being. In: C Bouchard, RJ Shephard, T Stephens, eds. Physical activity, fitness, and health: international proceedings and consensus statement. Champaign, IL: Human Kinetics, 1994:180–202.
8. Mausner JS, Bahn AK. Epidemiology: an introductory text. Philadelphia: Saunders, 1974.
9. Kahn HA, Sempos CT. Statistical methods in epidemiology. New York: Oxford University Press, 1989.
10. LaPorte RE, Montoye HJ, Caspersen CJ. Assessment of physical activity in epidemiologic research: problems and prospects. Pub Health Rep 1985;100:131–146.
11. Montoye HJ, Taylor HL. Measurement of physical activity in population studies: a review. Hum Biol 1984;56:195–216.
12. Jacobs DR Jr, Ainsworth BE, Hartman TJ, Leon AS. A simultaneous evaluation of 10 commonly used physical activity questionnaires. Med Sci Sports Exer 1993;25:81–91.
13. Siconolfi SF, Lasater TM, Snow RCK, Carleton RA. Self-reported physical activity compared with maximal oxygen uptake. Am J Epidemiol 1985;122:101–105.
14. Bouchard C, Boulay MR, Simoneau JA, et al. Heredity and trainability of aerobic and anaerobic performance: an update. Sports Med 1988;5:69–73.
15. Leon AS, Jacobs DR Jr, DeBacker G, Taylor HL. Relationship of physical characteristics and life habits to treadmill exercise capacity. Am J Epidemiol 1981;113:653–660.
16. Wilmore JH. Design issues and alternatives in assessing physical fitness among apparently healthy adults in a health examination survey of the general population. In: T.F. Drury, ed. Assessing physical fitness and physical activity in population-based surveys. DHHS Pub. No. (PHS) 89-1253. Washington, DC: GPO, 1989:107–153.
17. Cooper KH. A means of assessing maximal oxygen intake: correlation between field and treadmill testing. J Am Med Assoc 1968;203:201–204.
18. Montoye HJ. Lessons from Tecumseh on the assessment of physical activity and fitness. In: T.F. Drury, ed. Assessing physical fitness and physical activity in population-based surveys. DHHS Pub. No. (PHS) 89-1253. Washington, DC: GPO, 1989:349–376.
19. U.S. Department of Health and Human Services, Centers for Disease Control and Prevention, National Center for Chronic Disease Prevention and Health Promotion, President's Council on Physical Fitness and Sports. Physical activity and health: a report of the surgeon general. Atlanta, GA, 1996.
20. U.S. Department of Health and Human Services. Healthy People 2000: national health promotion and disease prevention objectives. Publication number 91-50212. Washington, DC: DHHS, 1991.
21. Crespo CJ, Keteyian SJ, Heath GW, Sempos CT. Leisure time physical activity among U.S. adults: results from the third National Health and Nutrition Examination Survey. Arch Int Med 1996;156:93–98.
22. Pate RR, Pratt M, Blair SN, et al. Physical activity and public health: recommendation from the Centers for Disease Control and Prevention and the American College of Sports Medicine. JAMA 1995;273:402–407.
23. Manson JE, Rimm EB, Stampfer MJ, et al. Physical activity and incidence of non-insulin-dependent diabetes mellitus in women. Lancet 1991;338:774–778.
24. Blair SN, Kohl HW, Paffenbarger RS, et al. Physical fitness and all-cause mortality: a prospective study of healthy men and women. JAMA 1989;262:2395–2401.
25. Blair SN, Wood PD, Sallis JF, et al. Workshop E: Physical activity and health. Preventive Medicine 1994;23:558–559.

Suggested Readings

Montoye HJ, Kemper HCG, Saris WHM, Washburn RA, eds. Measuring physical activity and energy expenditure. Champaign, IL: Human Kinetics, 1996.
Pereira MA, Fitzgerald SJ, Gregg EW, et al. A collection of physical activity questionnaires for health-related research. Med Sci Sports Exer 1997;29(suppl):S1–S205.

Clinical Exercise Physiology

W. Guyton Hornsby, Jr, and Randall W. Brynar

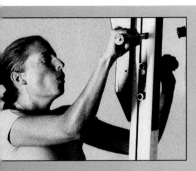

Objectives

1. Identify unique contributions of the clinical exercise physiologist in preventive, therapeutic, and rehabilitative healthcare.
2. Describe how a clinical exercise physiologist would be trained to work with patients in a medical setting.
3. Explain the similarities and differences between diagnostic and functional exercise tests.
4. List the types of measurements that are made during exercise tests to clear patients for safe participation in physical activity and to develop the exercise prescription.
5. Demonstrate a basic understanding of how exercise prescription is used in the clinical setting to prevent or delay chronic diseases or to treat patients that are already afflicted.
6. Describe the role of the clinical exercise physiologist in the treatment of selected chronic diseases and conditions.
7. Explain how advances in basic research can lead to important clinical applications in the treatment of chronic disease.

- **Definition, Description, and Scope**
- **Focus on Science**
  Clinical Testing and Evaluation Principles
  Exercise Prescription Applied to Preventive, Therapeutic, and Rehabilitative Practice
  Special Populations and Clinical Exercise Physiology Practice
- **Advances in Clinical Exercise Physiology**
  Heart Transplantation
  Molecular Basis of Obesity

Summary Points
Review Questions
References
Suggested Readings

Clinical exercise physiology is a rapidly evolving field that is becoming increasingly important in the delivery of healthcare. Physical activity plays a vital role in the prevention, treatment, and rehabilitation of a variety of disease states and physical disabilities. With a thorough understanding of exercise science and a knowledge of how performance may be altered by disease and disease management, the clinical exercise physiologist is now recognized as a valuable member of the healthcare team who works together with physicians, nurses, dietitians, pharmacists, physical therapists, occupational therapists, and psychologists to improve the overall health and functional status of an individual. Unique contributions of the clinical exercise physiologist in preventive, therapeutic, and rehabilitative care include using exercise as a means of evaluating functional capacity and assisting physicians in diagnostic testing; prescribing exercise based on individual patient needs and abilities; and instructing, supervising, and monitoring exercise programs in clinical settings.

This chapter presents a definition and description of clinical exercise physiology; describes principles of clinical screening, evaluation, and exercise testing; introduces the concept of **exercise prescription** in the clinical setting; presents major disease states served by clinical exercise physiologists; and describes important advances in the field.

DEFINITION, DESCRIPTION, AND SCOPE

Clinical exercise physiology involves the application of exercise science to prevent or delay the onset of chronic disease in healthy participants or provide therapeutic or functional benefits to patients with underlying pathologies. Clinical exercise physiologists are healthcare professionals who use fundamental principles of exercise physiology (see Chapter 8) in clinical settings to minimize the risk of chronic diseases associated with physical inactivity and to treat those already afflicted. Services may be offered in a variety of medical settings, such as hospitals, rehabilitation centers, and outpatient clinics. Services are also offered in community, corporate, commercial, and university fitness and wellness centers, nursing homes, and senior citizen centers (Fig. 11.1). The scope of practice ranges from apparently healthy individuals with no known medical problems to patients with documented cardiovascular, pulmonary, metabolic, rheumatologic, orthopedic, and/or neuromuscular diseases and conditions.

The clinical exercise physiologist is responsible for pre-exercise screening (Fig. 11.2), exercise testing and evaluation (Fig. 11.3), development of exercise prescriptions, instruction of training techniques, and supervision of safe and effective exercise programs in the healthcare setting. A knowledge of normal physiologic responses to acute and chronic exercise is essential before attempting to use exercise to prevent, manage, or rehabilitate disease. It is also important to understand pathophysiology and how functional capacity and responses to exercise may be affected by different disease states and their medical management.

Exercise therapy may be altered by specific treatments such as drugs and medications; surgical procedures; radiation therapy; orthopedic bracing, casting, or splinting; dialysis; and diet therapy. For example, heart rate and blood pressure responses to exercise can be reduced signif-

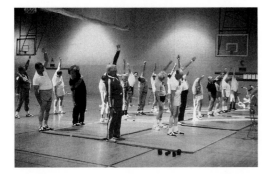

FIGURE 11.1 Group exercise in an adult fitness program.

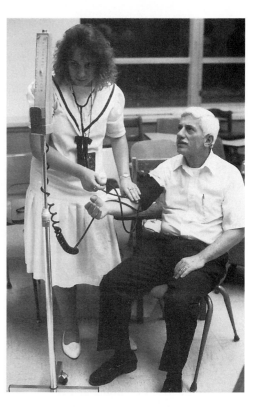

FIGURE 11.2 Pre-exercise screening.

icantly by **beta adrenergic blocking agents** commonly used in the management of angina or hypertension and must be considered when developing exercise prescriptions for patients taking these medications. Exercise itself may produce effects requiring alterations in other therapies. For example, it is often necessary for insulin dosages to be reduced in patients with **type 1 diabetes** because exercise changes the **pharmacokinetics** of subcutaneously injected drugs.

Clinical exercise physiologists should be well prepared in the exercise sciences with a solid background in basic exercise physiology combined with more advance training, including pathophysiology of chronic diseases, pharmacology of drugs and medicines, medical terminology, medical record keeping and charting, electrocardiographic interpretation, exercise testing for special populations, business management and marketing, and nutrition and diet therapy. It would also be helpful to complete a clinical internship, which would allow the exercise physiologist to work with patients in a medical setting and to interact with a variety of healthcare professionals. Figure 11.4 presents the general course of study in clinical exercise physiology.

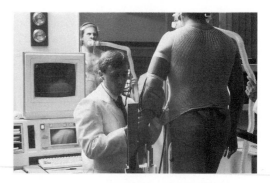

FIGURE 11.3 Graded exercise testing.

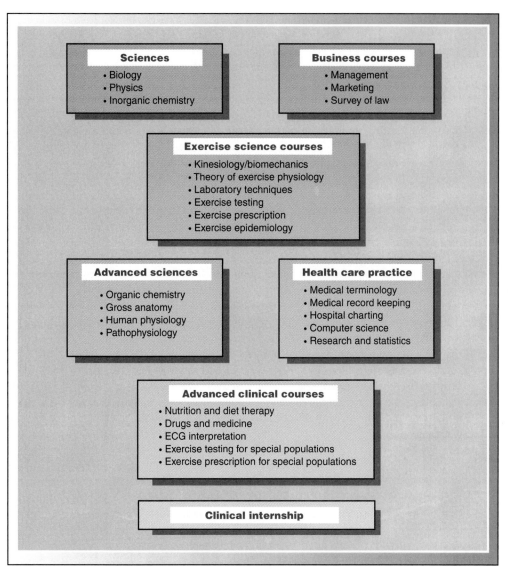

FOCUS ON SCIENCE

The clinical exercise physiologist must be able to apply his or her training in the basic and clinical sciences in healthcare settings by using exercise to prevent or delay disease or to provide therapeutic care to patients. It is vital that scientific principles of exercise testing and evaluation and exercise prescription be understood so that the best possible care can be provided to patients with cardiovascular disease, pulmonary disorders, metabolic disorders, rheumatologic diseases, and orthopedic and neuromuscular diseases and conditions.

Clinical Testing and Evaluation Principles

Exercise testing by an exercise physiologist has become an important tool in the clinical setting to clear individuals for safe participation in physical activity and as a basis for exercise prescription. The two broad classifications of exercise testing are diagnostic and functional capacity testing. Simply, diagnostic testing is performed to see how sick someone is and functional capacity testing is performed to see how well someone is. In other words, the diagnostic test is performed to uncover underlying disease and the functional test is performed to determine the capacity for exercise.

The primary reason for performing a diagnostic test is to assess heart or pulmonary disease. This type of test may be indicated if a patient is found to have symptoms of heart disease, a history of a possible cardiac event, electrocardiographic abnormalities, or a high probability of underlying disease. The diagnosis of heart disease after an exercise test relies primarily on the basis of abnormal electrocardiographic changes. However, although the exercise physiologist may play a major role in conducting the test, a medical diagnosis of disease can be made only by a physician.

A functional test gives information about a person's capacity for exercise and can be used to prescribe an appropriate exercise program to enhance fitness. Functional capacity is usually determined by a direct or estimated measurement of the maximum volume of oxygen consumed (Vo_2max) during exercise. The functional test may also be used to determine if an individual has normal cardiovascular responses to exercise. In most clinical situations, both diagnostic and functional information contribute to the overall interpretation of the test result.

In general, an exercise test will give the cardiopulmonary response of an individual to a standard exercise workload. Exercise tests, whether for diagnostic or functional purposes, are usually incremental in nature and as such are referred to as graded exercise tests (GXT). *Graded* means that the exercise is progressed in a stepwise fashion from light to maximum levels. Also, these progressive steps in exercise intensity are measurable and repeatable. A number of **exercise protocols,** usually performed on a treadmill or cycle ergometer, are available to the examiner, depending on the purpose of the test and the population being tested. The same GXT would not be used to evaluate the capacity of a healthy young adult as would be chosen for a 70-year-old cardiac patient.

Screening

The determination of an individual's suitability for exercise and exercise testing is important at the start of any exercise program. For most healthy individuals, exercise does not pose a safety risk if proper training techniques are followed. However, exercise may not be safe for everyone, especially if pre-existing medical conditions, such as coronary artery disease (CAD), are present. For a limited number of individuals, exercise testing may even be contraindicated (should not be done for medical reasons). Each year, many people suffer heart attacks and die suddenly, some while overexerting themselves doing things like shoveling snow and other forms of yard work. The safety of exercise must be determined before the start of any program. See Sidelight 11.1 for a brief look at the risks associated with exercise testing and the complications that may arise.

Physical Examination

Many patients require a physician's referral before they can undergo exercise testing or enter into an exercise program. The American College of Sports Medicine (ACSM) has developed guidelines to aid the healthcare professional in determining the safety of exercise for individuals (1). These guidelines suggest that it is unnecessary for men under the age of 40 and women under the age of 50 who have no symptoms of heart disease, are apparently healthy, and have fewer than two risk factors for CAD to have a medical evaluation by a physician before starting an exercise program (see Practical Application 10.2). However, many exercise programs are conducted in nonmedical settings and thus require a physician's referral for anyone over the age of 35.

Health History

An important component of the prescreening phase of an exercise program is the assessment of an individual's personal health history and risk factors for CAD. The purpose of this assessment is to *(a)* identify and exclude individuals with medical **contraindications** to exercise, *(b)* identify individuals with clinically significant disease conditions who should be referred to a medically supervised exercise program, *(c)* identify individuals with symptoms and risk factors for a disease who should receive further medical evaluation before starting an exercise program, and *(d)* identify individuals with special needs for safe exercise participation (e.g., elderly persons, pregnant women) (1). A useful instrument for recording clients' health histories and for guiding their programs is the Physical Activity Readiness Questionnaire (PAR-Q).

The exercise physiologist should assess the behavior-dependent risk factors for CAD for each participant before beginning any exercise testing or program. Items that should be included are the history of high blood pressure, high serum cholesterol, chest discomfort, lightheadedness, shortness of breath, **diabetes mellitus,** smoking, poor nutrition, alcohol consumption, inactivity, high stress levels, and history of coronary or other atherosclerotic disease in parents or siblings before age 55. The level of physical activity at which the individual normally engages should also be determined.

Informed Consent

All of the procedures involved in the test should be thoroughly explained to the client before he or she is tested. In addition, potential risks or benefits of the exercise test need to be discussed. Participants should be encouraged to ask questions to clarify and resolve uncertainties about the procedures. A signed consent based on this information is then obtained from the participant.

Informed consent is an "active" procedure involving a dialogue between the patient and the healthcare professional. Properly done, the patient has ample time to read, ask questions, and understand his or her role and the role of the technicians carrying out the procedure.

Physiologic Measurements

The final phase of the screening process involves the collection of pertinent physiologic measurements. Resting heart rate and blood pressure are always taken before a GXT, whether the test is considered functional or diagnostic. All diagnostic tests are also preceded by a resting **electrocardiogram** (ECG).The measurement of blood glucose and serum cholesterol are often performed as part of the screening process. Abnormal findings for any of these indices may indicate an underlying problem such as heart disease, hypertension, or diabetes, which may warrant further medical evaluation before proceeding with the actual test. Findings such as these are often expected during the course of a diagnostic test at which physicians are present, because of the nature of the subject being tested. However, in exercise facilities where there are no medical personnel present, abnormal resting values should not be ignored. The participant needs to be referred for further medical evaluation.

Exercise Testing

Once participants have completed the pre-exercise screening, they usually undergo the exercise test. As stated, the purpose of an exercise test is either to determine the functional capacity of the individual or to diagnose the presence of heart or pulmonary disease. In its simplest form, a fitness test measures resting and exercise heart rate and blood pressure as well as a person's functional capacity and is usually performed on a treadmill or cycle ergometer. Additional parameters often measured during both fitness and diagnostic tests include the **rating of perceived exertion** (RPE), ECG, and $\dot{V}O_2$max. Both submaximum and maximum GXTs are used for exercise evaluations, depending on the information that needs to be obtained.

HEART RATE   The resting heart rate is usually measured for at least 60 sec after the individual has been sitting quietly for 5 min or more. Methods used to measure both resting and exercise heart rate include chest auscultation with a sensitive stethoscope or radial pulse palpation. At times it becomes difficult to obtain an accurate heart rate by either of these methods during exercise. In such cases, carotid artery palpation may be attempted if the examiner has clear access to the neck region of the subject. In some exercise facilities and in all clinical settings, the heart rate is determined through readings obtained from ECG recordings and directly off the digital display of the **oscilloscope.**

The fitness professional should understand that many factors can influence the resting heart rate; smoking, caffeine ingestion, fever, high humidity, stress, food digestion, certain medications, and acute exercise can result in higher than normal recordings. Other medications have the opposite effect and depress resting and exercise heart rate. In addition, exercise training can also cause the resting heart rate to be lower than would be normally observed in someone who is deconditioned.

BLOOD PRESSURE   Arterial blood pressure is a function of the arterial blood flow each minute (cardiac output) and the resistance offered by the vasculature to that flow. When the heart contracts and pushes blood into the arterial vasculature, the vessels do not permit the blood to instantaneously flow to all areas of the arterial system as fast as it is being ejected from the heart. This creates a pressure throughout the arterial vasculature, which can be recorded. The highest pressure recorded during a heart beat occurs during the contraction (**systole**) of the left ventricle and is called the **systolic blood pressure.** This provides an estimation of the work of the heart as well as the pressure exerted against the walls of the arteries. During the relaxation phase of the heart (**diastole**) the pressure decreases. The pressure measured at this time is called the **diastolic blood pressure.** This pressure gives an indirect indication of total peripheral resistance or the ease with which blood flows from the arterioles into the capillaries. Blood pressure, therefore, is the product of cardiac output and peripheral resistance. The magnitude of a person's blood pressure is an important indicator of his or her general health. Resting blood pressure that is chronically elevated is a diseased condition called hypertension. People with hypertension have an increased risk of stroke and of developing CAD. In most clinical exercise settings blood pressure can be estimated by the use of a sphygmomanometer (blood pressure cuff) and a stethoscope. The normal blood pressure for an adult male is approximately 120/80 mm Hg and for adult females is 110/70 mm Hg.

Exercise will result in an increased cardiac output causing an increase in the arterial blood pressure. An important component of the GXT is to evaluate the blood pressure response to increasing workloads and to determine any abnormal responses that may occur. Blood pressure is normally taken every 1 to 3 min during the test. After an initial rapid rise from resting values, systolic blood pressure increases linearly with increasing exercise intensity. Failure to do so indicates a significant problem with the heart. Systolic blood pressure can increase to approximately 200 mm Hg in healthy, fit men and women during maximum exercise, despite large acute reductions in total peripheral resistance. Systolic blood pressure multiplied by the heart rate is called the **double product** (also referred to as the rate pressure product), which provides an estimate of the myocardial (heart tissue) oxygen demand.

RATING OF PERCEIVED EXERTION   During the course of a GXT, it is important to determine the participant's psychological perception of the intensity of the exercise. A measurement tool commonly used to determine this is called the RPE; psychologist Borg (2) developed the original scale. The numerical RPE scale of 6 to 20 relates closely to the heart rates from rest to maximum exercise when multiplied by a factor of 10 (60 to 200 beats/min) (Fig. 11.5). This scale provides a fairly accurate measure of how the subject feels in relation to the level of exertion. It also allows the person conducting the test to know when the subject is nearing exhaustion. A revised scale has recently been adopted that attempts to provide a ratio scale of the RPE values (ranging from 0 to 10). The Borg scale can also be used for exercise prescription, because individuals can easily learn to exercise at a particular RPE that corresponds to a given exercise intensity.

ELECTROCARDIOGRAM   Heart rate, blood pressure, and an electrocardiographic recording are typically measured during tests used for diagnostic purposes. Similar to all nerve and muscle cells,

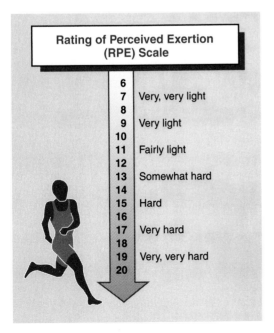

FIGURE 11.5 Rating of perceived exertion.

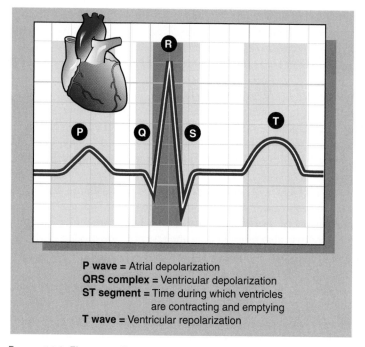

P wave = Atrial depolarization
QRS complex = Ventricular depolarization
ST segment = Time during which ventricles
                 are contracting and emptying
T wave = Ventricular repolarization

FIGURE 11.6 Electrocardiogram: waveforms in lead II.

the outer surface of myocardial (heart) cells is positive and the inner surface is negative. This electrical condition of the cell is referred to as being *polarized.* Immediately before contraction, the cell receives a jolt of electrical activity, which causes a complete reversal of the cells' polarity, meaning the positive charge is now on the inside of the cell. This process, called **depolarization,** produces an **action potential.** During the diastolic phase of the cardiac cycle, the polarity is reversed back to the original resting state. The electrical activity of the heart can be recorded from electrodes placed on the surface of the chest, because of the electrolytic (containing charged particles, such as sodium and potassium ions) nature of body fluids. The graphic tracing of the heart's electrical activity is called the electrocardiogram (Fig. 11.6).

The ECG is a valuable component of the exercise test because of its use in determining the presence of heart problems. The ECG is important for diagnosing problems associated with abnormal cardiac electrical conductivity and rhythm, insufficient supply of oxygen to the myocardium, and the presence of damage to the myocardium. Many of these conditions do not become a problem until the heart is forced to work above resting levels. Because exercise makes the heart work harder, a GXT is an excellent tool for the initial diagnosis of heart disease.

PHYSICAL WORK CAPACITY   Numerous laboratory and field tests (e.g., 1-mile walk, 12-min run) have been used to determine functional capacity. Functional capacity is the extent to which a person can increase exercise intensity and maintain this increased level. It is related to the maximum ability of an individual to convert chemical energy into mechanical energy. A major part of one's functional capacity is the fitness level of the cardiorespiratory system. The measurement of $\dot{V}O_2$max is the best estimate of cardiorespiratory fitness. $\dot{V}O_2$max may be defined as the maximum rate at which oxygen can be taken up, distributed, and used by the body in the performance of exercise that uses a large muscle mass (3).

One of the primary purposes of a GXT is to gradually increase the load until the maximum capacity of the cardiorespiratory system has been reached. $\dot{V}O_2$max is represented by the oxygen consumption measured at this point. Criteria have been established to ensure that a real maximum has been reached. These include a respiratory exchange ratio (RER) of more than 1.1, the attainment of an age-predicted maximum heart rate (e.g., 220 − age), and a leveling off of the oxygen consumption even with an increase in the workload.

SUBMAXIMUM GXT   A submaximum GXT is used to evaluate the cardiorespiratory response to a standard submaximum exercise bout and to give an estimate of one's maximum fitness level. Often an estimate of $\dot{V}O_2$max is all that is needed in an exercise facility to determine the exercise prescription. Submaximum tests that give an estimate of $\dot{V}O_2$max are less expensive to perform and may be safer for the participant. $\dot{V}O_2$max can be estimated from equations that either calculate $\dot{V}O_2$max from the last work achieved on the GXT, from the oxygen requirement for horizontal and grade walking on a motor-driven treadmill, or from the subject's heart rate response to a series of submaximum work rates. For a test using the latter method, the heart rate is plotted against workload until the subject reaches a predetermined submaximum heart rate, at which time the test is terminated (Fig. 11.7). Physiologic variables that are normally recorded at each stage are the heart rate, blood pressure, and ECG (when appropriate). The test is usually taken to a workload that elicits 70 to 85% of the age-predicted maximum heart rate. Any abnormal response in the heart rate, blood pressure, or ECG is a reason to stop the test and seek further medical opinion.

MAXIMUM GXT   There are times when it is important to assess the maximum exercise capacity of an individual and the use of a submaximum test is inappropriate. A maximum GXT is used for many reasons, ranging from the measurement of $\dot{V}O_2$max in world-class athletes to the diagnosis of abnormal cardiorespiratory function in cardiac patients. The test is not terminated at a predetermined workload (i.e., 70 to 85% of the age-predicted maximum heart rate) but is taken to the point of volitional exhaustion or to the point at which abnormal physiologic responses occur (called a symptom-limited stress test). These abnormal signs and symptoms may include blood pressure and ECG changes as well as chest pain (**angina pectoris**), shortness of breath (**dyspnea**) or lightheadedness. It is often important to be able to take clients to their maximum, because many abnormal symptoms do not occur until the workload is at a high intensity. The obvious problem associated with a maximum test is the stress placed on the participants, especially those who are normally sedentary. For this reason, it may be prudent to use a submaximum test at the start of a fitness program, except if the goal is to diagnose heart disease.

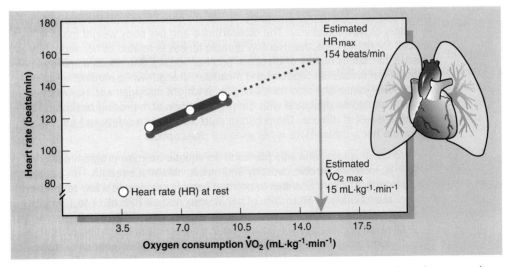

FIGURE 11.7 Estimate of aerobic capacity from heart rates obtained during a submaximum exercise test. Owing to the linear relationship between heart rate and $\dot{V}O_2$max, the line formed by obtaining heart rates at three submaximum intensities can be extrapolated to the age-predicted maximal heart rate. A vertical line to the $\dot{V}O_2$max scale provides an estimate of $\dot{V}O_2$max.

is caused by chemical (e.g., products found in cigarettes) or mechanical (e.g., high blood pressure) factors. The injury leads to fibroblast proliferation in the inner lining (intima) of the artery. Lipids are then able to accumulate between the junction of the inner and middle linings of the artery, resulting in the obstruction of blood flow. Calcium deposits accumulate in the intima area where degeneration and hyalin formation have occurred.

In the beginning stages of the process of atherosclerosis, few symptoms are usually present, and the person may feel completely fine. As the disease progresses and the artery becomes filled with plaque, limiting blood flow, the patient begins to notice specific symptoms that normally progress in severity. The progression of the disease may take several decades, with the gradual onset of symptoms in the latter stages. The first sign that something is wrong is often when a patient complains of pain or tightness in the chest area (angina pectoris). The ability of the person to do even modest-intensity work or exercise is usually compromised and brings on the clinical symptom of angina. The pain is sometimes felt in the neck, upper back, or jaw or as a radiant pain down the left arm. In limited situations, an individual may have CHD and experience no pain at all. This latter condition is a major concern for the clinician, because if undiagnosed the patient may experience a silent heart attack. If the condition is more severe, the patient may also experience anxiety, nausea, vomiting, and dyspnea. If untreated, this can lead to the myocardium becoming weak and eventual heart failure, which results in a heart that is unable to meet the metabolic demands of the body.

Pulmonary Disorders

Chronic pulmonary disease affects an estimated 19.5 million Americans, and pulmonary disorders account for 25% of all physician visits (9). These diseases are commonly separated into three groups: obstructive (e.g., asthma, chronic bronchitis, and emphysema), restrictive (e.g., pulmonary fibrosis, chest wall deformity, and neuromuscular weakness), and disordered control of breathing (e.g., sleep apnea and obesity hypoventilation). Patients with chronic pulmonary diseases suffer from dyspnea (difficult breathing) and are subject to **hypoxemia** (deficiency of oxygen in arterial blood). Depression, anxiety, and fear are common in these patients, and exercise capacities are often dramatically reduced.

Pulmonary rehabilitation typically combines exercise therapy, education, smoking cessation, nutrition, breathing retraining, chest physiotherapy, and optimization of medications. Exercise can be an important component of pulmonary rehabilitation; the goals are increasing physical activity, producing more efficient breathing, and reducing dyspnea (10,11). Exercise training has been shown to produce important physiologic and psychological benefits for patients with chronic pulmonary diseases (see Box 11.1).

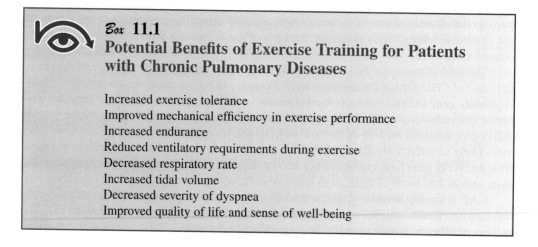

Box **11.1**

Potential Benefits of Exercise Training for Patients with Chronic Pulmonary Diseases

Increased exercise tolerance
Improved mechanical efficiency in exercise performance
Increased endurance
Reduced ventilatory requirements during exercise
Decreased respiratory rate
Increased tidal volume
Decreased severity of dyspnea
Improved quality of life and sense of well-being

Metabolic Disorders

Metabolism refers to all the chemical changes that occur within the body. An increase in physical activity requires an increase in chemical reactions that can support the energy demands of exercise. Any defect in the metabolic processes that allow for fuels to be properly stored in the body, delivered to active muscles, and oxidized for energy can interfere with exercise performance.

DIABETES   Diabetes mellitus is a serious health problem in the United States resulting in significant morbidity and mortality in approximately 16 million Americans (12). This condition is actually a heterogeneous collection of metabolic diseases, all characterized by blood glucose values above the normal range. Diabetes is caused by inadequate secretion of the pancreatic hormone insulin, by problems related to the inadequate action of insulin, or by a combination of both defective insulin action and impaired insulin secretion. The overwhelming majority of diabetes cases fall into two broad categories, classified by their cause and pathogenesis. Type 1 diabetes (also referred to as insulin-dependent diabetes mellitus; IDDM) occurs primarily as a result of a defect in which the immune system mistakenly turns on its own body and destroys the insulin-producing b-cells of the islets of Langerhans. After the autoimmune destruction of the b-cells, little or no endogenous insulin is produced, and the body is unable to move glucose from the bloodstream into body cells to be used for energy or to be stored as glycogen. Although normal blood glucose values in healthy people are less than 110 mg/dL in the fasting state and less than 140 mg/dL after a meal, blood glucose values in untreated type 1 diabetics can range anywhere from 200 to 1800 mg/dL.

Symptoms of untreated type 1 diabetes include frequent urination (polyuria), unusual thirst (polydipsia), weight loss (often despite excessive eating; polyphagia), blurred vision, extreme fatigue, and increased susceptibility to infection (13). Patients are usually thin at the onset of this disease. Symptoms usually appear rapidly and dramatically in type 1 diabetes, most often in children and young adults. It is important to be aware, however, that the autoimmune destruction of b-cells can sometimes proceed slowly and, in rare cases, may appear in older adults and in obese individuals.

Because the defect in type 1 diabetes is an inability to produce insulin, the focus of therapy in this form of the disease is to control blood glucose by adequate insulin replacement. In healthy individuals, blood glucose remains fairly constant while insulin levels vary considerably throughout the day in response to food intake, physical activity, and psychological and physical stress. It is virtually impossible to match the physiologic insulin profile of a healthy person with insulin that's delivered by subcutaneous (underneath the skin) injections. The attempt to normalize blood glucose in type 1 diabetes requires frequent glucose monitoring and multiple insulin injections. The clinical exercise physiologist is an important member of the healthcare team in helping to make decisions on insulin and diet adjustments to allow patients with type 1 diabetes to exercise safely (14).

Type 2 diabetes (also referred to as noninsulin-dependent diabetes mellitus; NIDDM) occurs as a result of **insulin resistance** and accounts for 90 to 95% of the total number of all diabetes cases. Insulin resistance is strongly associated with physical inactivity. There is a strong genetic predisposition for developing type 2 diabetes. Most of these patients are obese and those that are not obese are found to have a large amount of fat stored in the abdominal region. It is much more common in people who have a family history of the disease, in individuals with high waist:hip ratios, and in women who have delivered babies weighing more than 9 lb.

Patients with type 2 diabetes have a relative deficiency of insulin rather than the absolute deficiency found in type 1 diabetes. These patients do produce insulin, sometimes in large amounts, but it is not enough to overcome their insulin insensitivity. Type 2 diabetes is usually diagnosed after the age of 30, but can appear in children and adolescents. Symptoms of type 2 diabetes can be the same as those for type 1 diabetes, but they are often more subtle, appear much more gradually, and are many times overlooked. It is thought that there are about 5.4 million people with undiagnosed type 2 diabetes in the United States.

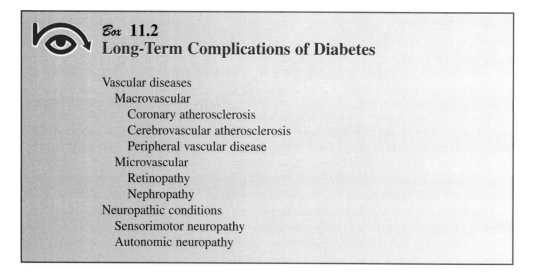

Box 11.2
Long-Term Complications of Diabetes

Vascular diseases
    Macrovascular
        Coronary atherosclerosis
        Cerebrovascular atherosclerosis
        Peripheral vascular disease
    Microvascular
        Retinopathy
        Nephropathy
Neuropathic conditions
    Sensorimotor neuropathy
    Autonomic neuropathy

The focus of therapy in type 2 diabetes is to reduce insulin resistance. Sensitivity to insulin can be improved by oral medications, by diet and weight loss, and by exercise. Oral medications include biguanides (metformin), alpha-glucosidase inhibitors (acarbose), thiazolidinediones (troglitazone), meglitinides (repaglinide), and sulfonylureas (all other diabetes pills). If insulin resistance cannot be improved satisfactorily by any combination of diet, weight loss, exercise, or oral medication, insulin injections may be required. Exercise therapy has been specifically recommended to improve blood glucose for patients with type 2 diabetes by both the American Diabetes Association (ADbA) and the ACSM (15,16). The clinical exercise physiologist can, therefore, play a major role in the management of this disease.

Patients with diabetes are at risk for several acute life-threatening complications related to dangerously high (hyperglycemia) or low (hypoglycemia) blood glucose levels. In addition, a number of serious long-term complications can be linked to chronic hyperglycemia (see Box 11.2). Acute **hyperglycemic** emergencies include **diabetic ketoacidosis** in patients with type 1 diabetes and **hyperglycemic hyperosmolar nonketotic syndrome** in those with type 2 diabetes. If not treated promptly, these conditions can lead to coma, shock, respiratory distress, and death.

Medications used to control diabetes can sometimes cause blood glucose levels to fall too low. The central nervous system relies almost totally on glucose for energy, and hypoglycemia is a hazardous medical emergency that can rapidly result in unconsciousness and death. Anyone working with patients with diabetes, especially those taking hypoglycemic medications should know how to accurately monitor blood glucose values and must know appropriate responses for blood glucose emergencies (see Practical Application 11.1).

Chronic hyperglycemia is associated with long-term complications affecting the eyes (retinopathy), kidneys (nephropathy), nerves (neuropathy), blood vessels, and heart. Diabetes is the leading cause of adult blindness and increases the risk of end-stage renal disease by 20 times. Nerve damage affects at least half of those with diabetes and places patients at risk for foot injuries and amputations and results in gastrointestinal, genitourinary, cardiovascular, and sexual dysfunction. Patients with diabetes have an increased risk of atherosclerotic cardiovascular, cerebrovascular, and peripheral vascular disease. It is not uncommon for 40% or more of patients being treated in cardiovascular rehabilitation programs to have diabetes as the underlying disease.

Results of a large-scale clinical study known as the Diabetes Control and Complications Trial convincingly demonstrated that the long-term complications of type 1 diabetes can be significantly reduced by controlling blood glucose (17). The ADbA position statement on diabetes mellitus and exercise provides clinical practice recommendations for the care of patients with diabetes and states that the healthcare team "will benefit from working with an individual with knowledge and training in exercise physiology" (15). Clinical exercise physiologists have important roles in diabetes management, prevention of type 2 diabetes in people at risk, and rehabilitation of chronic complications of diabetes such as CHD and stroke.

It is important to understand the role of exercise in diabetes therapy, to know the effects of exercise in patients with diabetes, and to be able to determine the risks and benefits of exercise in patients with a variety of complications and different drug and diet management plans. The goals of therapy for both type 1 and type 2 diabetes include keeping blood glucose levels as close to normal as possible and reducing risk factors for cardiovascular disease, such as hypertension, cigarette smoking, lipid abnormalities, and sedentary lifestyle. Treatment to normalize blood glucose in type 1 diabetes is an attempt to adequately replace insulin. Although exercise can play an important role in reducing cardiovascular risk factors, it does not help replace insulin. The clinical exercise physiologist must understand the effects of exercise in type 1 diabetes and be able to work with the healthcare team so that proper adjustments can be made to the diet and insulin therapy to allow these patients to exercise safely. Controlling blood glucose in type 2 diabetes is an attempt to reduce insulin resistance. Because exercise has been shown to directly improve insulin sensitivity and to reduce insulin resistance by assisting in weight loss, exercise therapy is an extremely important component of treatment for type 2 diabetes.

Practical Application 11.1

HYPOGLYCEMIC EFFECTS OF EXERCISE

A 42-year-old white male who experienced an inferior wall myocardial infarction 12 weeks earlier has just completed his first workout in a phase III cardiac rehabilitation program. His medical history includes hypertension, mild background retinopathy, and a 25-year course of type 1 diabetes (currently treated with a split/mixed regimen of regular and neutral protamine Hagedom insulin). As his recovery heart rate and blood pressure are being monitored, the exercise physiologist explains that she will monitor his blood glucose before he leaves. Although he willingly had his blood glucose checked when he arrived for the exercise session (it was 144 mg/dL), the patient now refuses to let his glucose level be tested and aggressively argues that he is in this exercise program for his heart and says that he will control his own diabetes. The exercise physiologist is aware that hypoglycemia often leads to belligerent behavior. She calmly explains that she will be happy to allow him to do the monitoring himself and that it is in his best interest to know what his blood glucose is before he drives home. She also explains that all patients with diabetes on any hypoglycemic medication are required to have their blood glucose monitored both before and after their exercise sessions.

The patient finally agrees to check his blood glucose level and finds that the value is 37 mg/dL. He is treated with 6 oz of a nondiet soft drink, and after 20 min his blood glucose is 82 mg/dL. The exercise physiologist instructs the patient to be aware that the hypoglycemic effects of physical activity may continue for many hours after the exercise session has ended and explains that he should be prepared to monitor his blood more frequently and to adjust his diet accordingly. The patient is also directed to discuss this episode with his physician to see if any changes in his insulin therapy should be made.

OBESITY   Obesity, or the excess accumulation of body fat, is an important health problem in the United States (18). It is estimated that approximately 58 million American adults (33%) are currently overweight. Obesity is associated with an increased frequency of atherogenic risk factors, including hypertension, hyperinsulinemia, type 2 diabetes mellitus, and reduced HDL. This metabolic disorder is also associated with an increased risk of osteoarthritis and various types of cancer.

Substantial weight loss in adults is difficult to achieve and even more difficult to maintain. A negative energy balance must develop for weight loss to occur. In other words, more calories must be expended than are consumed. Exercise is an important component of clinical weight management programs, because physical activity expends energy and can help maintain muscle mass. Another added benefit is that exercise decreases certain atherogenic risk factors associated with fat distribution by reducing abdominal obesity, also known as central body fat (19).

The ACSM has provided guidelines for safe, effective weight-loss programs for healthy adults (19). This plan recommends that caloric intake should be no less than 1200 kcal per day and that energy expenditure through exercise should not exceed more than 500 to 1000 kcal per day. The maximum weight loss in 1 week should be no more than 1 kg (2.2 lb) unless the diet is medically supervised.

Because 1 lb of body fat contains approximately 3500 kcal of energy, a person would have to create a negative caloric balance equivalent to 1000 kcal per day to lose 2 lb of fat in 1 week. This could be done by increasing daily physical activity by 1000 kcal, by reducing daily intake of food and drink by 1000 kcal, or by simultaneously increasing daily energy output by 500 kcal and reducing daily energy intake by 500 kcal.

To help clients increase energy expenditure, exercise prescriptions should include aerobic activity that is well tolerated. The exercise plan may also include resistance exercise, because it may be especially effective in maintaining muscle mass during weight loss. Exercise physiologists working in clinical weight management programs should be familiar with cardiovascular disease risks associated with obesity and with training techniques to reduce orthopedic injuries, which are common in this population. It is also important to be familiar with behavioral management strategies to maximize patient compliance.

Rheumatologic Diseases

Rheumatologic diseases encompass disorders of the musculoskeletal system, including osteoarthritis and rheumatoid and other inflammatory arthritides, such as gout and lupus (20,21). These disorders are typically chronic and often lead to disability. The clinical exercise physiologist can play a role in minimizing disability through appropriate evaluation and exercise prescription.

Osteoarthritis, also known as degenerative joint disease, is the most common form of arthritis and is characterized by local deterioration of cartilage, leading to joint space loss and new bone formation (**osteophytes**). Osteoarthritis typically affects weight-bearing joints, especially the knees and hips. Common risk factors are advanced age, obesity, genetic factors, and trauma and repetitive use. Osteoarthritis is usually manifested as local joint pain after use, which can be relieved by rest. Medical treatment often includes analgesics to minimize pain, weight reduction in the obese, protection of joints from overuse, range of motion exercises, and passive and assistive exercises.

Rheumatoid arthritis, which is an inflammatory joint disease, is present in approximately 1% of the population. It is a systemic **autoimmune disease** of unknown cause whose major features are redness, swelling, warmth, and significant stiffness of the joints. Predisposing factors include age, female sex, lower socioeconomic status, and genetics. It commonly affects the small joints of the hands and feet but can also involve the cervical spine and large joints, such as the shoulders, hips, and knees. The heart, lungs, eyes, skin, and nervous system may also be affected by this systemic disease. Patients with rheumatoid arthritis frequently experience muscle wasting owing to inflammation and physical inactivity (22). Aerobic fitness is typically quite poor. People with rheumatoid arthritis have been reported to have increased mortality rates, and patients with severe forms of this disease may die 10 to 15 years earlier than expected. Medical treatment includes anti-inflammatory drugs such as aspirin, corticosteroids, and antirheumatic agents such as gold injections.

Patients with rheumatologic diseases are typically found to be unfit owing to their inactivity and can benefit from individually prescribed exercise programs. It is important that patients with both degenerative and inflammatory arthritis be evaluated to determine the severity of joint involvement so that appropriate activity can be performed to improve function within the limitations of the disease. Aquatic exercise programs in a warm-water environment may be especially well tolerated, and therapeutic effects have been demonstrated. Low to moderate conditioning programs with gradual progression have the potential to improve muscle strength and endurance, to increase joint flexibility, to prevent muscle wasting, to maintain or improve aerobic fitness, and to lessen depression and boost psychological well-being (23).

Orthopedic and Neuromuscular Diseases and Conditions

The clinical exercise physiologist is frequently asked to assist patients with a wide variety of orthopedic and neuromuscular diseases and conditions in rehabilitation settings and in general wellness programs. These range from relatively rare diseases affecting the central nervous system and/or muscle cells, to the widespread occurrence of pain affecting the neck and back. In many of these cases, psychological issues are an important consideration in management and effective exercise programming. Depending on the specific orthopedic or neuromuscular disease or condition, exercise may be used to enhance fitness within the limitations of the ailment, return the individual to normal functioning, provide for functional maintenance, or delay the rate of disease progression.

Low back pain is the most frequent musculoskeletal complaint for all people at all ages (24). Although many persons believe that muscular weakness in the low back and abdominal region, inadequate flexibility in the low back, obesity, and physical inactivity may directly contribute to low back pain, there is little scientific evidence supporting a therapeutic or preventive effect of exercise. Acute low back pain is typically first treated with a mild analgesic, such as acetaminophen, along with a warm shower. Other medications, such as nonsteroidal anti-inflammatory drugs (NSAIDs), muscle relaxants, and other pain medications may be indicated.

Bedrest is usually not effective in managing low back pain. It is important to educate patients about postures that may aggravate the condition and to teach them modifications of postural positions and correct biomechanical techniques. If exercise is begun within the first 2 weeks of acute pain, it should be extremely mild with minimal stress on the back. Exercise intensity should progress gradually and only as pain allows. Specific exercises for strengthening and increasing flexibility are usually not begun for at least 2 weeks after the acute episode.

Muscular dystrophy is the most common muscle disease of children (25). It is actually a collection of hereditary conditions that lead to biochemical and structural changes within the muscle cell. The changes result in progressive degeneration of the contractile elements, which are subsequently replaced with fibrous tissue. Types of muscular dystrophy include facioscapulohumeral, limb-girdle, and pseudohypertrophic or Duchenne. Although the different forms of the disease progress at different rates and have unique anatomic distributions and genetic abnormalities, they all result in gradual muscle wasting with an incremental decrease in muscle strength, leading to disability, deformity, and (often) premature death.

Duchenne muscular dystrophy is the most common and destructive form of the disease. It is caused by a sex-linked recessive genetic defect and affects young boys at a rate of 1 out of every 3500 live births (26). Symptoms of muscle weakness such as having difficulty climbing stairs or rising from a sitting or lying position usually appear between the ages of 2 and 6 years. This condition is also known as pseudohypertrophic muscular dystrophy, because harmful fibrous changes lead to an increase in the size of the calves and sometimes the forearms and thighs, giving the appearance of strong, healthy muscles. The muscles are actually weakening dramatically and this typically leads to paralysis and joint contracture. It is common for these patients to be in wheelchairs by 9 years of age. Patients with Duchenne muscular dystrophy typically die from infections, respiratory problems, or heart failure before they reach their early 20s.

There is no cure for muscular dystrophy. Exercise therapy may be useful in maintaining mobility for as long as possible and in improving the patient's psychological outlook (27). The clinical exercise physiologist may work closely with physical and occupational therapists to achieve the best outcome. It is important to focus on preserving independent daily activity, because these children seem to deteriorate more rapidly once they are in a wheelchair. The exercise prescription should focus on maintaining muscle strength and endurance, enhancing energy expenditure, and preventing contracture. It is important to set realistic goals, and physical activity should be planned to allow patients to feel some degree of success and enjoyment while undergoing exercise therapy, especially in the face of this tragic, fatal disease.

Multiple sclerosis is the most common neurologic disease in early to middle adulthood (28). The average age of diagnosis is between 20 and 40 years of age, and it is approximately twice as common in women. This disease can place significant limitations on the ability to carry out daily tasks and is especially devastating in that it typically affects people just when they should be in their prime productive period. Multiple sclerosis is a disease of the central nervous system characterized by loss of the myelin sheath, a fatty substance that encases nerve fibers. The destruction of myelin is eventually followed by scarring and formation of numerous sclerotic (hard) plaques throughout the white matter of the brain and spinal cord. Thus the name multiple sclerosis.

The initial damage is brought on by the body's own immune system as it mistakenly attacks the myelin sheath. It is, therefore, described as an autoimmune disease. **Demyelinization** interferes with rapid, smooth conduction of nerve impulses from the brain to various parts of the body. Eventually, the associated scarring further obstructs the body's ability to send messages via the nervous system and produces a variety of symptoms that differ in the extent and location of central nervous system damage (29). Symptoms can range from minimal involvement to severe disability (see Box 11.3). It is common for multiple sclerosis symptoms to intensify (exacerbations) and then diminish (remissions), producing progressive functional impairment.

Patients with multiple sclerosis have a reduced life span, but most will survive at least 25 years after diagnosis. Although exercise therapy is believed to have no effect on the course of the disease, for many patients it is possible to improve muscular strength and endurance, joint

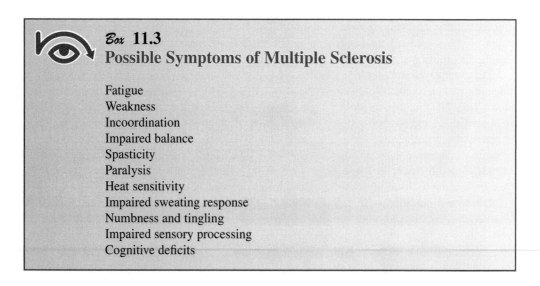

Box 11.3
Possible Symptoms of Multiple Sclerosis

Fatigue
Weakness
Incoordination
Impaired balance
Spasticity
Paralysis
Heat sensitivity
Impaired sweating response
Numbness and tingling
Impaired sensory processing
Cognitive deficits

flexibility, aerobic fitness, and improve efficiency of performing work-related activities and self-care tasks, thus improving the quality of life. The exercise prescription must take into consideration the specific type and degree of impairments as well as fluctuations associated with periods of exacerbation and remission. As the disease progresses, it is important to work closely with other members of the healthcare team, including neurologists, physical therapists, and occupational therapists, to plan appropriate levels of activity and to adapt exercise performance and exercise equipment to allow patients with multiple sclerosis to maintain their highest level of functional ability.

ADVANCES IN CLINICAL EXERCISE PHYSIOLOGY

Important breakthroughs in basic research have led to meaningful applications in the treatment of chronic diseases. New scientific and medical advances have brought about new opportunities and challenges for the clinical exercise physiologist. Physical activity is now considered to have a critical role in therapies that at one time could not have even been imagined. As scientific discoveries lead to a better understanding of chronic diseases, advances will continue to be made in the field of clinical exercise physiology. Many advances could be mentioned. The two discussed here are particularly timely.

Heart Transplantation

Approximately 2800 heart transplants are performed each year, and the procedure is now recognized as an established treatment for advanced heart disease (30). Much has changed since the first experimental heart transplant was conducted in December 1967. The discovery of immunosuppressant drugs has helped overcome critical problems associated with rejection of a donor heart and 1-year survival rates are now greater than 80%. Heart transplantation is a difficult procedure, and there are many dangers and discomforts that must be faced, but exercise appears to have a crucial role in post-transplant therapy.

The surgery to replace a patient's diseased heart with a healthy donor heart begins with the removal of the patient's heart, except for the back walls of the atria. The backs of the atria of the donor heart are opened and then sewn to those of the patient. The blood vessels are connected, allowing blood to flow into the transplanted heart; but currently, there is no way to establish nervous system connections between the patient and the new heart.

The transplanted heart functions differently because it is **denervated.** The heart beats faster at rest, typically from 100 to 110 beats/min, and responds more slowly to exercise. Because heart rate is no longer controlled by the nervous system, the only way it can increase is by humeral factors (circulating hormones called catecholamines). This results in a sluggish exercise response and reduces the peak heart rate. For some patients, the maximal heart rate may be only 20 to 40 beats above the resting rate.

Patients receive immunosuppressive medications to prevent rejection of the new heart. The most common drugs used are cyclosporine, azathioprine, and prednisone. The most common causes of death in transplant patients are rejection of the heart and infections. There must be a careful balance between providing appropriate medications to prevent rejection and dangerously suppressing the immune system. Side effects of immunosuppressive therapy include hypertension, obesity, hyperlipidemia, diabetes, kidney damage, lymphoma, and advanced osteoporosis.

Clinical exercise physiologists working with heart transplant patients must be aware of the complications of immunosuppressive therapy as well as the altered exercise responses produced by this surgical procedure. Safety precautions with exercise have been developed specifically for heart transplant patients (31). These include attempts to avoid hypotensive episodes, conservative approaches to prevent bone fractures when using resistance training, discontinuing exercise therapy during periods of acute rejection that require enhanced immunosuppression, and general guidelines for prescribing appropriate exercise intensities.

Molecular Basis of Obesity

The recent isolation of the *ob* gene in mice has renewed interest in the pathophysiology of human obesity (32). Leptin, a protein encoded by this gene, is secreted from the white adipose tissue and is believed to regulate energy balance through its effects on receptors in the central nervous system. Most of the existing research has been conducted in rodents. In *ob/ob* mice, a mutation of the leptin gene causes leptin deficiency and results in overeating, decreased energy expenditure, severe obesity, and insulin resistance. Administration of leptin to these mice causes acute decreases in food intake, increases in energy expenditure, and marked reductions in body fat. Research has shown that leptin interacts with the hypothalamus to decrease neuropeptide-Y expression, a potent central appetite stimulant (33).

The role of leptin in the pathogenesis and treatment of obesity in humans is unclear. Most obese persons do not appear to have abnormalities in the coding sequence for leptin and, in fact, secrete elevated amounts in direct proportion to body fat mass. Some suspect obesity may be linked to a failure of leptin to act on its target in the hypothalamus (neuropeptide-Y), leading to excess food consumption. Others have suggested that the primary role of leptin may be to indicate whether somatic fat stores are sufficient for growth and reproduction. Little data are available about the effect of exercise training on leptin levels. Prolonged endurance training does appear to reduce leptin levels independent of changes in body fat or insulin sensitivity, and the effect may be more prominent in women than men.

The identification and sequencing of the *ob* gene and its product, leptin, have led to a surge in basic research examining the mechanisms that control body weight. Although studies in humans have just begun, it is exciting to think that these advances in molecular biology may one day have direct applications to patient care. Clinical exercise physiologists should attempt to keep up with these findings because they could have important implications for the management of obesity and its associated health risks.

SUMMARY POINTS

- Clinical exercise physiologists are healthcare professionals who use scientific knowledge in clinical settings to minimize the risk of chronic disease in individuals and provide rehabilitation for affected patients.
- The clinical exercise physiologist is responsible for pre-exercise screening, exercise testing and evaluation, development of exercise prescriptions, and supervision of safe and effective exercise programs.
- Clinical exercise physiologists use diagnostic and functional exercise testing in a wide variety of individuals to uncover underlying disease and to determine exercise capacity.
- Common physiologic measurements collected during exercise testing include the resting and exercise ECG, blood pressure, heart rate, RPE, and $\dot{V}O_2$max.
- Clinical exercise physiologists work with patients who have chronic diseases, such as cardiovascular diseases, pulmonary disorders, metabolic disorders, rheumatologic diseases, and orthopedic and neuromuscular diseases.
- Scientific advances in basic and applied research are being used by clinical exercise physiologists in the treatment of chronic diseases.

REVIEW QUESTIONS

1. What role does a clinical exercise physiologist play in healthcare?
2. List three unique contributions of the clinical exercise physiologist in healthcare.
3. How does a diagnostic exercise test differ from a functional exercise test?
4. What physiologic measurements are taken during an exercise test?

5. What chronic diseases and conditions are commonly treated by clinical exercise physiologists.

6. Give two examples of how basic research may be applied in a clinical setting.

References

1. Franklin BA, ed. ACSM's guidelines for exercise testing and prescription. 6th ed. Baltimore: Lippincott Williams & Wilkins, 2000.
2. Borg G. Perceived exertion as an indicator of somatic stress. Scand J Rehabil Med 1970;2:92–98.
3. Roitman, JL, ed. ACSM's resource manual for guidelines for exercise testing and prescription. 3rd ed. Baltimore: Williams & Wilkins, 1998.
4. U.S. Department of Health and Human Services, Centers for Disease Control and Prevention, National Center for Chronic Disease Prevention and Health Promotion, President's Council on Physical Fitness and Sports. Physical activity and health: a report of the surgeon general. Atlanta: DHHS, 1996.
5. American Heart Association, 1998.
6. Roman O. Do randomized trials support the use of cardiac rehabilitation? J Cardiac Rehabil 1985;5:93–96.
7. Tas J. Genetic predisposition to coronary heart disease and gene for apolipoprotein CIII. Lancet 1991;337:113–114.
8. Nishina PM, Johnson JP, Naggert JK, et al. Linkage of atherogenic lipoprotein phenotype to the low density lipoprotein receptor locus on the short arm of chromosome 19. Proc Natl Acad Sci U S A 1992;89:708–712.
9. Fishman AP, ed. Update: pulmonary diseases and disorders. New York: McGraw-Hill, 1992.
10. AACP/AACVPR Pulmonary Rehabilitation Guidelines Panel. Pulmonary rehabilitation: joint AACP/AACVPR evidence-based guidelines. J Cardiopulm Rehabil 1997;17:371–405.
11. Ries AL. Position paper of the American Association of Cardiovascular and Pulmonary Rehabilitation. J Cardiopulm Rehabil 1990;10:418–441.
12. American Diabetes Association. Report of the expert committee on the diagnosis and classification of diabetes mellitus. Diabetes Care 1998;21:S5–S19.
13. American Diabetes Association. American Diabetes Association complete guide to diabetes. Alexandria, VA: ADA, 1996.
14. Ruderman N, Devlin JT, eds. The health professionals guide to diabetes and exercise. Alexandria, VA: American Diabetes Association, 1995.
15. Diabetes mellitus and exercise. Diabetes Care 1998;21:S40–S46.
16. Diabetes mellitus and exercise. Med Sci Sports Exer 1997;29:i–vi.
17. The effect of intensive treatment of diabetes on the development and progression of long-term complications in insulin-dependent diabetes mellitus. N Engl J Med 1993;329:977–986.
18. Bouchard C, Depres J-P, Tremblay A. Exercise and obesity. Obesity Res 1993;1:133–147.
19. Position stand: proper and improper weight loss programs. Med Sci Sports Exer 1983;15:ix–xiii.
20. Kelley WN, Harris ED, Ruddy S, Sledge CB. Textbook of rheumatology. 4th ed. Philadelphia: Saunders, 1993.
21. Rall LC, Roubenoff R. Body composition, metabolism, and resistance exercise in patients with rheumatoid arthritis. Arthritis Care Res 1996;9:151–156.
22. Schumacher HR, ed. Primer on the rheumatic diseases. 10th ed. Atlanta: Arthritis Foundation, 1993.
23. Minor MA. Arthritis and exercise: the times they are a changing. Arthritis Care Res 1996;9:79–81.
24. Gordon CY, Schanzenbacher KE, Case-Smith J, Carrasco RC. Diagnostic problems in pediatrics. In: J Case-Smith, AS Allen, PN Pratt, eds. Occupational therapy for children. 3rd ed. St. Louis: Mosby, 1996:113–164.
25. Wong DL. Whaley and Wong's essentials of pediatric nursing. 4th ed. St. Louis: Mosby, 1993.
26. Bar-Or O. Muscular dystrophy. In: JL Durstine, ed. ACSM's exercise management for persons with chronic disease and disabilities. Champaign, IL: Human Kinetics, 1997:180–184.
27. Hauser SL. Multiple sclerosis and other demyelinating diseases. In: KJ Iselbacher, E Braunwald, JD Wilson, et al., eds. Harrison's principles of internal medicine. 13th ed. New York: McGraw-Hill, 1994:2287–2295.
28. Ponichtera-Mulcare JA. Exercise and multiple sclerosis. Med Sci Sports Exer 1993;25:451–465.
29. Mulcare JA. Multiple sclerosis. In: JL Durstine, ed. ACSM's exercise management for persons with chronic disease and disabilities. Champaign, IL: Human Kinetics, 1997:189–193.
30. Keteyian SJ, Brawner C. Cardiac transplant. In: JL Durstine, ed. ACSM's exercise management for persons with chronic disease and disabilities. Champaign, IL: Human Kinetics, 1997:54–58.
31. Braith RW. Exercise training in patients with CHF and heart transplant recipients. Med Sci Sports Exer 1998;30:S367–S378.

32. Zhang Y, Proenca R, Maffei M, et al. Positional cloning of the mouse obese gene and its human homologue. Nature 1994;372:425–432.
33. Zukowska-Grojec Z. Neuropeptide-Y: a novel sympathetic stress hormone and more. Ann NY Acad Sci 1995;771:219–233.

Suggested Readings

Durstine JL, ed. ACSM's exercise management for persons with chronic disease and disabilities. Champaign, IL: Human Kinetics, 1997.
Hasson SM. Clinical exercise physiology. St. Louis: Mosby, 1994.
Robergs, RA, Roberts SO. Exercise physiology: exercise performance and clinical applications. St. Louis: Mosby, 1997.
Roitman, JL, ed. ACSM's resource manual for guidelines for exercise testing and prescription. 3rd ed. Baltimore: Williams & Wilkins, 1998.
Ruderman N, Devlin, JT, eds. The health professionals guide to diabetes and exercise. Alexandria, VA: American Diabetes Association, 1995.

Sports Medicine and Kinesiologic Knowledge Base

To explain how and why one moves is to go beyond a purely physiologic understanding of human movement. The title of this section intends to convey the idea that the fields of clinical (Chapter 12) and sports (Chapter 13) biomechanics originated from the kinesiologic study of movement. Historically, the study of kinesiology in exercise science academic programs coupled anatomy with principles and concepts from physics. Currently, the twin fields of clinical and sports biomechanics are enjoying an unprecedented growth, as can be seen by the increase in the number of academic courses devoted to this knowledge base. These courses are not only important to the sibling disciplines of exercise science and physical education but also to the professional preparation of physical and occupational therapists, ergonomists, and athletic trainers.

Section 5 focuses on the kinesiologic and sports medicine foundations of movement by first investigating biomechanics, which is the study of biologic phenomena (e.g., processes, function, and structure) using the methods of Newtonian mechanics and mathematics. Chapter 12 focuses on the concept of force and discusses biomechanics in the clinical setting, with special reference to functional anatomy. Chapter 13 discusses other important mechanical concepts and applies them to sports and exercise performance. Chapter 14 introduces the field of athletic training, which is an allied health profession closely aligned to kinesiology and sports medicine.

12

Clinical Biomechanics

BARNEY F. LEVEAU

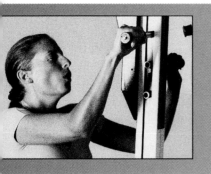

Objectives

1. Describe how clinical biomechanics is integrated into the greater discipline of exercise science.
2. Identify the characteristics of force.
3. Describe several basic biomechanical principles.
4. Explain the effects of forces on biologic tissues.
5. Describe how electromyography is being incorporated into clinical practice.
6. Define the scope of ergonomics and its relationship to clinical biomechanics.

Clinical biomechanics applies concepts and principles that are important to the discipline of exercise science, yet it is also closely related to a variety of other academic disciplines and professions. Orthopedists, physical therapists, occupational therapists, and athletic trainers are health professionals who use biomechanical concepts to evaluate and treat patients. In addition, professionals such as bioengineers, ergonomists, and human factors specialists use biomechanical concepts to understand how individuals physically interact with their environment (e.g., in the workplace, in vehicles, and when using tools) and explore the efficiency and safety with which such interaction takes place. Physical educators also use biomechanical principles to teach basic and advanced sports and physical activity skills.

Research in clinical biomechanics has broadened our understanding of human movement, and has application to the clinical setting: It helps physical therapists rehabilitate injured patients, it helps orthopedic physicians repair broken limbs or ruptured ligaments, it instructs workers in proper lifting techniques, and it helps individuals who suffer physical disabilities adjust to perform activities of daily living.

The study of biomechanics involves both **statics** and **dynamics.** This chapter emphasizes primarily the static, or stationary, concepts, but makes some reference to dynamics, which is the study of a body (or body parts) undergoing accelerations. The chapter begins with an explanation of basic mechanical principles and shows how these principles are related to clinical aspects of exercise science. A more detailed description of dynamic principles and mechanical analysis of movement, especially as applied to sports and exercise, is provided in Chapter 13. In addition, because anatomy is central to understanding biomechanics, this chapter introduces important principles and concepts in human anatomy and kinesiology.

DEFINITION, DESCRIPTION, AND SCOPE

Clinical biomechanics is the study of forces and their effect on living organisms. It is basic to the understanding of human movement; mechanics of injury; and the principles of prevention, evaluation, and treatment of musculoskeletal problems. Concepts of clinical biomechanics are not limited to the study of range of motion of joints, posture, and analysis of locomotion or gait. Everything we do involves biomechanics in some form or degree. The principles of biomechanics are at work in the couch potato as well as the elite athlete. Biomechanical principles apply to disabled as well as able-bodied individuals. They are employed throughout the life span, from the womb until death. Because biomechanics is the study of the effect of forces on the human body, whenever a **force** is present, biomechanical principles are involved.

The Scope of Clinical Biomechanics

Clinical biomechanics is based on the content areas of anatomy, mathematics, physics, and clinical sciences. The career goals of the student determine the depth and breadth of study in these areas. Figure 12.1 illustrates how a course in biomechanics is typically organized. In this scheme, after the foundational principles are set, other important concepts are introduced. The basic knowledge level allows the student to understand how forces and anatomy interrelate. A general course in biomechanics can serve as a foundation for both clinical and sports-related biomechanics. Box 12.1 presents key questions that are answered by the study of clinical biomechanics.

After an introductory course in biomechanics students may choose more advanced topics. Box 12.2 lists some advanced biomechanical topics that may be presented in units within a single course or as free-standing college courses. Individuals with more advanced knowledge will be able to analyze and evaluate how forces act on the body and how the body exerts forces on other objects. They will also be able to research and establish programs to enhance rehabilitation and prevent injuries. The advanced clinical biomechanist will be able to design an environment that allows disabled individuals to live an efficient and safe lifestyle, and possibly to participate

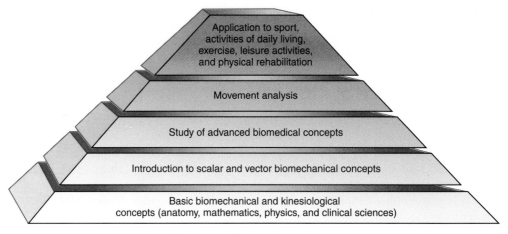

FIGURE 12.1 Course sequence in clinical biomechanics.

in recreational and competitive sporting activities. Box 12.3 lists some of the many questions that can be addressed by the advanced clinical biomechanist.

Additional content areas in clinical biomechanics include specific rehabilitation techniques, wheelchair design, anthropology, specific tissue repair, surgical techniques, and architecture. Because force is everywhere, the scope of clinical biomechanics is limited only by the professional's imagination and the needs of specific populations.

Clinical biomechanists not only deal with abnormal conditions but also must know how the body responds in normal situations so they can set goals for injured or disabled individuals. Clinical biomechanists must understand the specific activities of individuals to help prevent injuries from happening. Normal patterns of movement and their variations for healthy individuals must be understood so the movement pattern of an injured or disabled individual can be directed toward a more normal pattern. If movement cannot return to normal, the movement pattern must be directed toward the most efficient and safe pattern for that individual. To analyze these movement patterns, the clinical biomechanist uses instrumentation and techniques such as video analysis, electromyography, force plate, and force transducer analysis (discussed in Chapter 13).

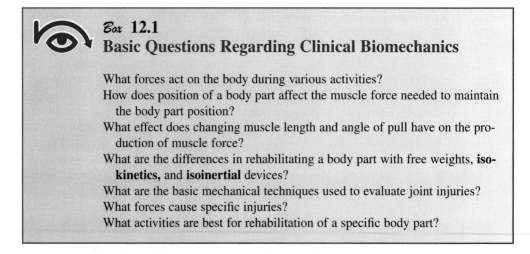

Box **12.1**
Basic Questions Regarding Clinical Biomechanics

What forces act on the body during various activities?
How does position of a body part affect the muscle force needed to maintain the body part position?
What effect does changing muscle length and angle of pull have on the production of muscle force?
What are the differences in rehabilitating a body part with free weights, **isokinetics,** and **isoinertial** devices?
What are the basic mechanical techniques used to evaluate joint injuries?
What forces cause specific injuries?
What activities are best for rehabilitation of a specific body part?

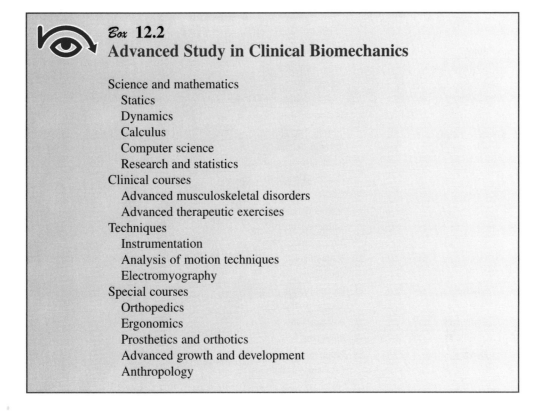

Box **12.2**
Advanced Study in Clinical Biomechanics

Science and mathematics
    Statics
    Dynamics
    Calculus
    Computer science
    Research and statistics
Clinical courses
    Advanced musculoskeletal disorders
    Advanced therapeutic exercises
Techniques
    Instrumentation
    Analysis of motion techniques
    Electromyography
Special courses
    Orthopedics
    Ergonomics
    Prosthetics and orthotics
    Advanced growth and development
    Anthropology

Kinesiology

Kinesiology, the study of movement, is an important content area within clinical biomechanics, because a sound grasp of functional anatomy is basic to an understanding, from a mechanical standpoint, of how and why we move. Kinesiology involves the study of the skeletal system, including its major joint articulations and the major muscles and muscle groups that are the **prime movers** during various kinds of joint movements. The specific terminology of kinesiology can be complex, yet it is essential for students of exercise science to learn which muscles produce which movements and why. The major joints along with their prime movers and the specific actions are given in Table 12.1. The table is not meant to be an exhaustive list of all the

Box **12.3**
Advanced Questions Regarding Clinical Biomechanics

What are the differences in the sequence of muscle activity in abnormal and
    normal gaits?
How do biologic tissues respond to various magnitudes of loads?
How do tissues react to repetitious or prolonged loads?
How can injuries be prevented?
How can activities be made more efficient and safe?
What are the forces that cause a deformity of a body part, such as clubfoot?
How can forces be used to treat and reverse the deformities caused before
    and after birth?
What implant materials respond best to loading?

Table 12.1	MAJOR JOINTS, PRIME MOVERS, AND ACTIONS	
Joint	**Prime Mover**	**Action**
Shoulder girdle	Serratus anterior	Abduction
	Rhomboids	Adduction; elevation
	Trapezius, upper and lower fibers	Upward rotation
	Trapezius, lower fibers	Depression
	Levator scapulae	Downward rotation
Shoulder	Anterior deltoid	Flexion
	Pectoralis major, sternal portion	Extension
	Pectoralis major, both portions	Horizontal flexion
	Latissimus dorsi	Hyperextension
	Middle deltoid	Abduction
	Latissimus dorsi	Adduction
	Infraspinatus	Lateral rotation
	Teres major	Medial rotation
	Latissimus dorsi	Horizontal extension
Elbow	Biceps brachii	Flexion
	Triceps brachii	Extension
Radioulnar	Pronator teres	Pronation
	Supinator	Supination
Wrist	Flexor carpi ulnaris	Flexion
	Extensor carpi ulnaris	Extension
	Flexor carpi radialis	Radial flexion
Lumbosacral	Iliopsoas	Anterior pelvic tilt
	Rectus abdominus	Posterior pelvic tilt
Spine (thoracic and lumbar)	Rectus abdominus	Flexion
	Spinae group	Extension
	Internal and external obliques	Rotation; lateral flexion
Hip	Iliopsoas, pectineus	Flexion
	Gluteus maximus	Extension; lateral rotation
	Gluteus medius	Abduction
	Adductor brevis	Adduction
	Gluteus minimus	Medial rotation
Knee	Biceps femoris	Flexion
	Rectus femoris	Extension
Ankle	Gastrocnemius	Plantar flexion
	Tibialis anterior	Dorsiflexion
Intertarsal	Tibialis anterior	Inversion
	Extensor digitorum longus	Eversion

muscles involved at each joint. Exercise science students will be exposed a more complete list in a kinesiology course. Box 12.4 defines the joint actions listed in Table 12.1.

In studying kinesiology, exercise science students typically memorize the muscles, their **proximal attachments,** their **distal attachments,** their nerves, and their specific actions (how they move bones at specific joints) as well as the anatomic landmarks on the surfaces of the major bones that serve as attachment locations for the tendons. By convention, joint movements are studied within the major planes of the body. Figure 12.2 shows a person in the anatomic position with palms facing forward. The midline of the body is the sagittal plane, which divides the body into right and left halves.

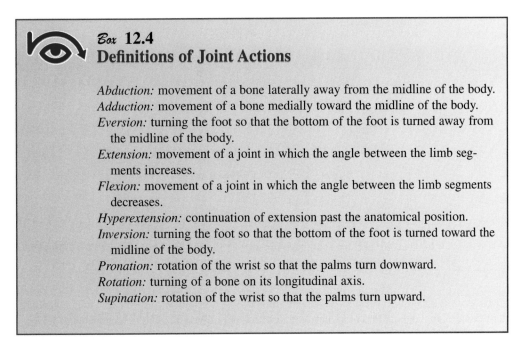

𝓑𝓸𝔁 **12.4**
Definitions of Joint Actions

Abduction: movement of a bone laterally away from the midline of the body.
Adduction: movement of a bone medially toward the midline of the body.
Eversion: turning the foot so that the bottom of the foot is turned away from the midline of the body.
Extension: movement of a joint in which the angle between the limb segments increases.
Flexion: movement of a joint in which the angle between the limb segments decreases.
Hyperextension: continuation of extension past the anatomical position.
Inversion: turning the foot so that the bottom of the foot is turned toward the midline of the body.
Pronation: rotation of the wrist so that the palms turn downward.
Rotation: turning of a bone on its longitudinal axis.
Supination: rotation of the wrist so that the palms turn upward.

FOCUS ON SCIENCE

Force is an important concept to grasp in studying biomechanics. Forces can be separated, combined, and manipulated. An understanding of how force acts on objects and what can result when forces are applied to various materials is central to the study of clinical biomechanics.

Force

Force can be defined simply as a push or a pull. A force that is applied externally to an object is called a **load.** When motion occurs, force is the factor that causes a **mass** to accelerate. This relationship is

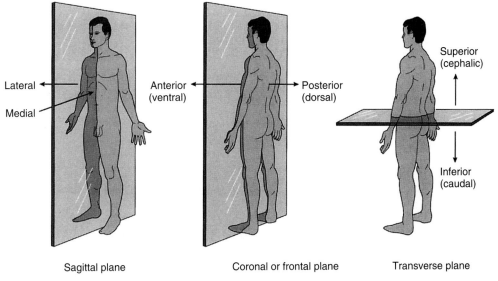

FIGURE **12.2** The major planes of the body are shown in respect to the anatomic position. Reprinted with permission from Willis MC. Medical terminology: the language of health care. Baltimore: Williams & Wilkins, 1996.

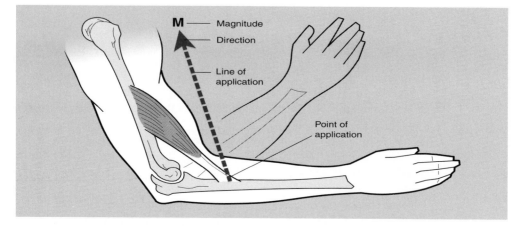

FIGURE 12.3 A force vector and the four characteristics of force. Reprinted with permission from LeVeau BF. Williams and Lissner's biomechanics of human motion. 3rd ed. Philadelphia: Saunders, 1992.

given by the equation $F = ma$. An exact definition of force, however, must include four characteristics: point of application, line of application, direction of pull or push, and magnitude (Fig. 12.3).

Force must have a point of application. Examples of points of application are attachments of muscles to bones, the center of mass of a limb, and the point of contact of a dumbbell. Force acts anywhere along a line of application, but this line can be redirected by a fixed pulley. For example, the peroneus longus (a leg muscle) tendon traversing behind the lateral malleolus (ankle bone) is a fixed pulley that changes the line of application for the force produced by a muscle.

The third characteristic of force is its direction of pull or push. In Figure 12.3, an arrow placed at the end of the line of application shows the direction of the force. The force of gravity,

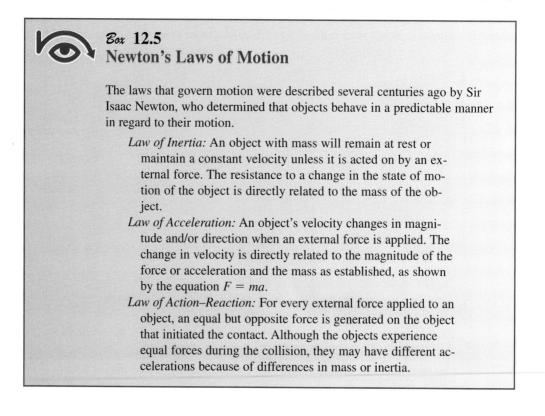

Box **12.5**
Newton's Laws of Motion

The laws that govern motion were described several centuries ago by Sir Isaac Newton, who determined that objects behave in a predictable manner in regard to their motion.

Law of Inertia: An object with mass will remain at rest or maintain a constant velocity unless it is acted on by an external force. The resistance to a change in the state of motion of the object is directly related to the mass of the object.

Law of Acceleration: An object's velocity changes in magnitude and/or direction when an external force is applied. The change in velocity is directly related to the magnitude of the force or acceleration and the mass as established, as shown by the equation $F = ma$.

Law of Action–Reaction: For every external force applied to an object, an equal but opposite force is generated on the object that initiated the contact. Although the objects experience equal forces during the collision, they may have different accelerations because of differences in mass or inertia.

for example, acts in a downward direction on the human body. Magnitude, which is the quantity of force, is the fourth characteristic of force. The forces involved are also governed by Newton's laws of motion (Box 12.5).

Gravity

The force of gravity, usually considered the most common force, is the mutual attraction between two objects. The magnitude of the force of gravity is directly proportional to the mass of each object and inversely proportional to the distance between the objects. Because the mass of the earth is extremely large, the earth dominates over the negligible attraction between other objects. The magnitude of the earth's gravity on an object is called its weight (W). The following equations define the relationship between weight and mass:

$$F = ma$$
$$W = mg$$

where m is the mass of the object, and g is the **acceleration** of the object caused by the earth's gravitational force.

The line of application of the gravitational force is a straight line between the center of mass of the two objects. For the earth, this line is vertical. Of the two objects attracting each other, the one that can more easily move travels toward the less moveable object. Hence, on earth, all objects are directed toward the center of the earth, which we consider "down." Although objects are usually made up of several small components, the point of application is considered to be the center of mass of the object. The weight of the arm or leg, for example, is considered to be concentrated at the center of mass of the body part.

Contact

Whenever two objects are in contact, a force exists between them. A contact force is the result of an outside or external force. Contact forces are related to Newton's third law, i.e., for every action there is an equal and opposite reaction.

An important, but often overlooked, contact force is the joint reaction force. Forces acting on bones can set up contact forces in the joints that can cause **compression** of the articular cartilage and underlying ends of the involved bones. In some situations, distraction (pulling apart) occurs at the joint. Hence, ligaments and other soft tissues are placed under **tension** while the compression on the cartilage and bone is reduced. If movement occurs between two objects in contact, friction develops. The magnitude of frictional force (F_s) depends on the composition of the adjacent surfaces. The two surfaces establish the coefficient of friction (μ), which is the ratio between the force of friction and the normal force. The greater the force of contact (N) during the movement, the greater the frictional force. A high contact force with movement can produce tissue damage. Examples of such damage are degenerative joint disease of the hip, patellofemoral (knee) joint syndrome, and lacerations of the hands in gymnastics. Contact forces are common, existing in all postures and movements. They always exist in a gravitational system but are of major importance in a reduced-gravity environment (i.e., space).

The force created by friction equals the coefficient of friction times the normal force of contact between the two surfaces: $F_s = \mu N$.

Muscle

An important force for maintenance of body posture and movement is muscle force. In general, muscles function as motors, providing the forces that move our appendicular skeleton (our limbs). The muscular system is associated with other structures that form the musculotendinous unit, which consists of units that are organized in the following order: bone, tendon, muscle, tendon, and bone.

Skeletal muscles are arranged in four architectural shapes, which affect both appearance and function, based on how the muscle fibers are aligned to the direction of pull of the whole musculotendinous unit:

Spindle shape: in line to the direction of pull.

Fan shape: in line to the direction of pull; more flared (wider) than the spindle shape.

Bipennate shape: at an angle to the direction of pull; fibers converge on both sides of the tendons.

Unipennate shape: at an angle to the direction of pull; fibers converge on only one side of the tendons.

Muscles have the properties of excitability, conductivity, contractility, extensibility, and elasticity and are capable of producing force under the control of the nervous system (see Sidelight 8.1). The property of excitability gives muscles the ability to respond to a stimulus. Conductivity gives it the ability to propagate an electrical current. Contractility is the ability of the muscle to shorten and generate force when an adequate stimulus is received. The muscle can be stretched (extensibility) and then returned to its original resting length (elasticity) when the stretching force is removed. The magnitude of force that a muscle can produce depends on its contractile ability, its structure, and its biomechanical and biochemical characteristics.

The contractile ability and structure of the muscle influence the magnitude of force that a muscle can produce. The contractile ability of the muscle depends on the rate of **motor unit** firing, the number of motor units firing, and the size of the motor units. A motor unit consists of the nerve and all the muscle fibers it connects to. The muscle's contractile ability and the magnitude of force it can develop also depends on its physiologic cross-sectional area, the length of the muscle, its type of contraction, and its rate of contraction. The physiologic cross-sectional area is the sum of the cross-sectional areas of all muscle fibers within the muscle, excluding noncontractile connective tissue within the muscle (1).

A direct relationship exists between the length of a muscle and the magnitude of force it can produce. The position of the actin and myosin filaments of the muscle fibers helps determine the amount of force generated. Muscle develops maximal force when the actin and myosin filaments (the contractile protein of muscle) are arranged to form the maximum number of connections, or cross-bridges. If the muscle is made longer or shorter than this optimal length, fewer cross-bridges are formed and less force develops. When the muscle is overly stretched, actin and myosin filaments are positioned sufficiently apart so that all connections or cross-bridges cannot form. As the muscle is shortened, the actin and myosin filaments overlap, and additional cross-bridges are formed. At the position where the greatest overlapping region for filaments is obtained (optimal length), the greatest magnitude of force occurs. As the muscle is placed in increasingly shorter positions, the actin and myosin filaments overlap too much, resulting in less tension development.

The velocity of muscle shortening has a predictable effect on the force that a muscle can produce. Because cross-bridges require a minimum time to attach and develop force, their function depends on the rate of shortening. As the filaments slide past each other at a faster rate, fewer cross-bridges can be formed at a specific instant. Thus the faster a muscle shortens, the less magnitude of force is produced.

Force is produced by a muscle whenever cross-bridges are formed. If the muscle force developed is equal to the resistance offered at the attachments of the muscle, and no change in length of the total muscle occurs, the muscle contraction is **isometric.** If the muscle force results in a change in length of the total muscle, the contraction is either concentric or eccentric.

A **concentric contraction** occurs if the muscle force exceeds the resistance offered at the muscle attachments and the distance between the attachments decreases. In this situation, the actin filaments are being pulled toward the myosin filaments. An **eccentric contraction** occurs when the resisting force at the muscle attachments exceeds the muscle force produced by the muscle, and the muscle lengthens. In this situation, the actin filaments are being pulled away from the myosin filaments.

An eccentric contraction can control a greater magnitude of external force than an isometric contraction. In turn, an isometric contraction can hold a greater magnitude of external force than a concentric contraction. The number of motor units that are active in the different types of contractions shows the reverse order. If the same resistance is applied, the concentric contraction requires a greater number of active motor units than an isometric contraction. An isometric contraction uses more active motor units than an eccentric contraction.

Inertia

Whether an object is stationary or moving, it has the property of inertia. As stated in Newton's First Law, an object at rest tends to remain at rest, and an object in motion tends to remain in motion at a constant velocity unless acted on by an external force. This law indicates that inertia is a force that resists an object's change in movement status. A force external to the object must be applied to a stationary object to make it move or to a moving object to make it stop. An object that is stationary resists changing position if an external force acts on it. In such a situation, the magnitude of inertial force is equal to the external force applied to the stationary object along the same line as the external force. Inertial force responds whenever any external force is applied to an object.

A force external to the object must be applied to a moving object to make it change directions. The change in velocity can be positive or negative and is called acceleration or deceleration, respectively. The magnitude of the external force needed to cause an object to start, stop, or change its direction is determined by the equation $F = ma$. The line of application of the inertial force for a moving object is along its straight path of motion. The force is directed along the same line as the moving object. The point of application is considered to be at the object's center of mass. Here are some examples of inertia.

The motion of a passenger's head when his or her automobile stops, starts, or is hit from the rear (Fig. 12.4).

A heavily loaded truck starting, stopping, or changing direction.

The starting, stopping, or changing direction of an exercise weight.

Elasticity

Some materials have the capacity to reform to their original size and shape once they have been deformed. This type of force is called **elastic** force. The magnitude of the force depends on the type of material and the amount of deformation:

$$F = -kl$$

where k is a constant value for the specific type of material and l is the amount of deformation that has occurred. The line of application is along the line of the deforming force but in the opposite direction. The point of application is the point of contact between the elastic material and the external force.

When muscles (including connective tissue) are stretched, they react in a manner similar to that of other materials with elastic properties. Some other body tissues have elastin and collagen fibers, which provides for a **viscoelastic** response when they are stretched by a force. When the force is released, the tissue rebounds to its previous shape. The property of viscoelasticity combines the elastic reaction with a dashpot- or syringe-type of reaction. The elastic property allows

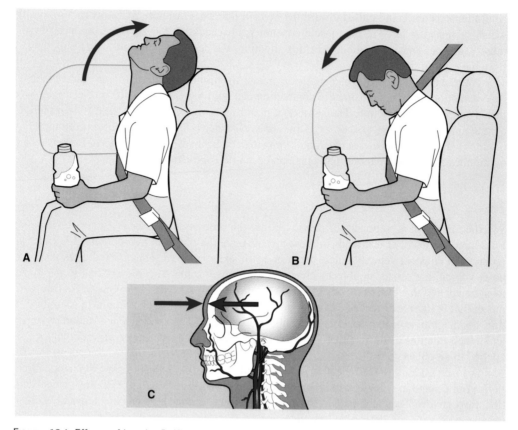

FIGURE 12.4 Effects of inertia. **A,** If an automobile starts rapidly or is hit from behind, the head of the passenger tends to remain at rest as the body is moved forward. **B,** If an automobile stops rapidly, the head tends to continue moving as the body stops (note the fluid in the cup). **C,** The inertia of the brain can cause brain and vessel damage if the head is hit or stopped suddenly. Reprinted with permission from LeVeau BF. Williams and Lissner's biomechanics of human motion. 3rd ed. Philadelphia: Saunders, 1992.

deformation of the tissue in a direct proportion to the applied force and then an immediate return to its original size and shape when the force is released. The dashpot effect resists the rapid rate of change in length of a tissue.

This effect is similar to what happens when a fluid is forced through a syringe. The small opening at the end of a syringe retards the rapid rate of plunger motion. The combined viscoelastic response of the tissue allows for a slow return of the material to its original size and shape. The viscoelastic property of the muscle aids in the smooth control of human movement and may protect the muscle from injury. Strengthening devices, such as elastic bands, sponge balls, and bending rods, have been developed that use elastic force as the resisting force.

Buoyancy

An upward, buoyant force acts on an object when that object is immersed in a fluid, with the magnitude of the force being equal to the weight of the fluid displaced by the object (Fig. 12.5). The line of application of the buoyant force is vertical, and the effective point of application is at the object's center of mass. Because of the buoyant force of water, pool therapy is often used to reduce the force of gravity on the lower limbs. While an individual is standing in the pool, the force (F) on the individual's feet is equal to the body weight (W) minus the weight of the displaced water (B), or $F = W - B$.

Composition and Resolution of Forces

Once we know the types and characteristics of the forces involved, we can determine how these forces affect and react to the human body. Forces can be combined to provide a single resulting force. The process of combining forces is called the **composition** of forces. A single force can also be separated into two perpendicular components. The process of breaking one force into two is called **resolution** of forces. These two processes are very important for understanding how forces affect various objects (see A Case in Point 12.1).

Composition

Often a set of several forces acts simultaneously on an object. These forces, arriving from different directions, may be replaced by a single force that will have the same effect as that of the set of forces. This single force is called the **resultant** of the forces. The process of composition of forces can be shown either graphically or algebraically.

Because forces are **vectors** (quantities with both magnitude and direction), the graphic method uses precise measurements of magnitude and direction of the involved forces to obtain the resulting force (Fig. 12.6). The forces are represented by arrows: The length of the arrow indicates the magnitude of the force, the shaft shows its line of action, and the arrowhead illustrates its direction. The arrows are drawn end to end. The first arrow begins at a point representing the point of application. The tail of each successive arrow is placed at the head of the preceding arrow. When all the arrows are drawn, the resultant is determined by an arrow with its tail at the point of application and its head at the tip of the last connected arrow. If the individual arrows are drawn precisely, the magnitude and direction of the resultant are displayed.

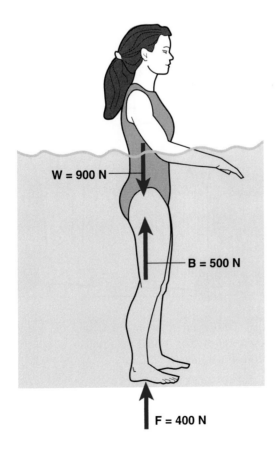

FIGURE 12.5 Buoyant force (*B*) acts on an individual standing in a pool so that the lower limbs bear less (*F*) than the total body weight (*W*).Reprinted with permission from LeVeau BF. Williams and Lissner's biomechanics of human motion. 3rd ed. Philadelphia: Saunders, 1992.

A Case in Point 12.1

PAIN AROUND THE PATELLA

A 22-year-old female was complaining of pain on the lateral aspect of her knee joint (see figure). She stated that the knee felt like it was "going out of joint." She felt pain, especially when she went up or down stairs or inclines. The problem had existed for a few months and the pain was becoming more severe.

The clinical biomechanist determines what forces are acting on the patella (see the figure below). All the forces and their characteristics are considered. Resolution of some of these forces may indicate that the patella is being pulled laterally (away from the midline of the body; see the figure). As a result, there is a tendency for the patella to dislocate (sublux). The lateral part of the patella is being forced against the lateral condyle of the femur. How can the total force be made to pull less laterally?

The clinical biomechanist may want to strengthen the vastus medialis muscle to create a greater medial (toward the midline of the body) pull. How can this be done? Maybe strengthening the entire quadriceps muscle group would help. An orthopedic surgeon decided to direct the patellar tendon force more medially by moving the tibial tuberosity medially. This eliminated the pain on the lateral side, but then the patella began to dislocate medially. The patient again had an unstable situation. The forces involved must be analyzed as accurately as possible to allow for the best results.

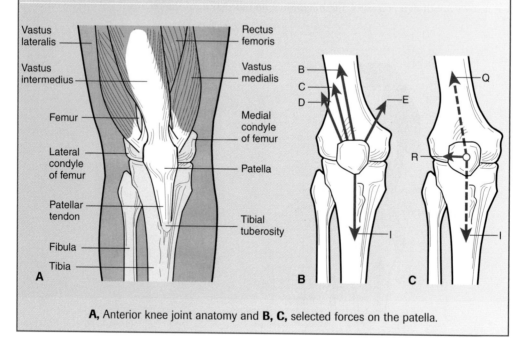

A, Anterior knee joint anatomy and **B, C,** selected forces on the patella.

The resultant can also be determined by use of algebra and trigonometry. If only two forces are acting on the object, the cosine law can be used (Fig. 12.6). To find the resultant of several forces, the equation may be used by taking two forces at a time.

Resolution

The process of resolution separates the force into two perpendicular components (Fig. 12.7). This process can also be presented graphically or mathematically. The selection of the line of ap-

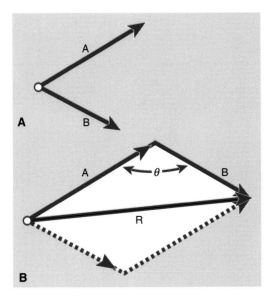

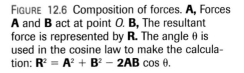

FIGURE 12.6 Composition of forces. **A,** Forces **A** and **B** act at point *O.* **B,** The resultant force is represented by **R.** The angle θ is used in the cosine law to make the calculation: $\mathbf{R}^2 = \mathbf{A}^2 + \mathbf{B}^2 - \mathbf{2AB} \cos \theta$.

plication for the components is important for determining the effects of the acting force. An important example is the resolution of muscle force as it acts on the body (Fig. 12.8). The lines of application should be perpendicular and parallel to the bone on which the muscle is acting. The perpendicular component (*R*) is the force component that tends to cause the bone to rotate around the adjacent joint. The parallel component (*NR*) determines the magnitude of force directed toward or away from the adjacent joint. In Figure 12.8, this parallel component is directed toward the adjacent joint, or the elbow.

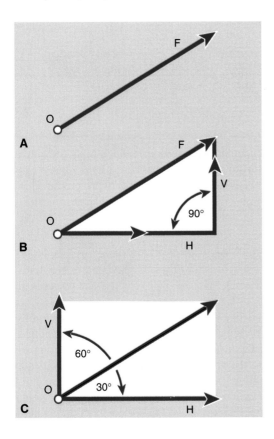

FIGURE 12.7 Resolution of forces. **A,** Force *F* is acting at point *O.* **B,** Perpendicular components *H* and *V* are drawn end to end from the point of application to the tip of *F.* **C,** The force components are placed at the point of application *O.*

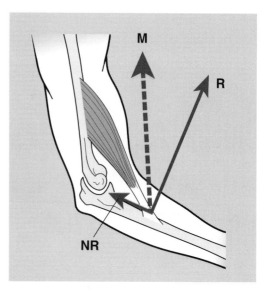

FIGURE 12.8 Components of muscle force *M*. The rotatory component *R* is perpendicular to the bone and tends to cause rotation. The nonrotatory component *NR* is parallel to the bone and tends to compress (in this case) or distract the joint.

In the graphic method, the components should be drawn perpendicular to each other along the appropriate lines of application directed from the point of application. Once this graphic display is made, one of the component force arrows should be constructed so that its arrowhead is placed at the head of the original force and its tail at the head of the other component. This construction produces a right triangle in which the lengths of the sides represent the magnitude of force components. The hypotenuse represents the magnitude and direction of the original force (Fig. 12.7). The mathematical determination of these force components uses the right triangle approach.

> *The relationship of the forces is demonstrated by the trigonometric functions of sine (sin = opp ÷ hyp), cosine (cos = adj ÷ hyp), tangent (tan = opp ÷ adj), and the cosine law (hyp² = opp² + adj² − (2opp × adj cos θ).*

Equilibrium

A force is a push or pull that causes a body to change its state of motion. For a body to be in a state of equilibrium, the sum of the forces and **torques** (forces that tend to rotate a body segment) acting on the body must equal zero. The two conditions of equilibrium are presented in this section.

First Condition

An object is considered to be in equilibrium when it acts according to the first part of Newton's first law, i.e., when it is in rest or when it is in motion with a constant velocity. The object is in static equilibrium when it is at rest.

The first condition of static equilibrium states that the sum of the forces acting on an object equals zero ($\Sigma F = 0$), where the summation sign Σ signifies the addition of the quantity. This equation is often used to determine the magnitude and direction of the forces acting on an object. If the forces are **collinear** or **concurrent,** the graphic and mathematical solutions are similar to the processes of resolution and composition. In the graphical method, instead of ending with a resultant, the arrows are placed head to tail beginning and ending at the graphic point of application.

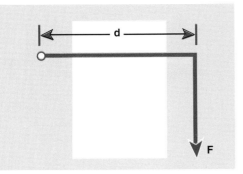

FIGURE 12.9 Application of a force (F) at a distance (d) from the axis of rotation (O). The moment equals force times distance ($F \times d$).

Second Condition

In many situations, the acting forces are not concurrent. In these situations, the forces tend to cause the object to rotate around a pivot point, or axis. For the object to remain at rest without rotating, it must adhere to the second condition of equilibrium. The sum of the torques acting on an object must equal zero ($\gamma M = 0$), where M is the **moment** or the application of a force at a distance from a point of pivot for the object (Fig. 12.9). The distance (d) from the point of application of the force to the pivot point can be called the lever arm, or moment arm. Because the force is not acting through the pivot point, it tends to turn the object around this point.

To remain in static equilibrium, another moment or moments must tend to turn the object in the opposite direction (Fig. 12.10). The directions for moments are not up, down, right, and left, but are clockwise and counterclockwise. Engineers have established the convention for mathematical analysis that counterclockwise moments are positive and clockwise moments are negative. To determine the actual moment applied to an object, the force component that is perpendicular to the lever arm must be used. Therefore, the definition of a moment is often stated as the force times its perpendicular distance from the axis. The ability to determine force components is essential to evaluate the effects of moments on an object. Because a moment is the product of force and lever length, a predictable relationship for lever systems can be determined. If one lever arm is twice as long as a second lever arm, the perpendicular force component applied to the first lever arm must be one half the magnitude of that applied to the second.

FIRST-CLASS LEVERS   Levers are classified simply as first class, second class, and third class. A first-class lever, designated *EOR,* has the pivot point or axis (O) between the two forces, called the effort (E) and the resistance (R). With this lever, a greater resistance can be moved a short distance, or a small resistance can be moved a great distance. If the point of application for the effort is placed four times the distance from the axis as the distance for the point of application for the resistance, the effort will need only one quarter the magnitude of force to hold the resistance. One of the forces will tend to cause the lever to rotate clockwise around the axis, while

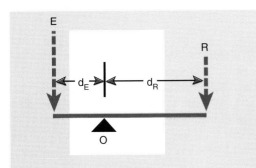

FIGURE 12.10 Clockwise force (R) and counterclockwise force (E) acting on a lever with the axis at $O.$ The moment arm for the counterclockwise (positive) force is d_E and the moment arm for the clockwise (negative) force is $d_R.$

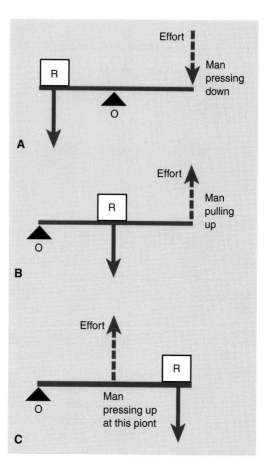

FIGURE 12.11 Three classes of levers. **A,** A first-class lever. **B,** A second-class lever. **C,** A third-class lever.

the other will tend to rotate it counterclockwise. With movement, the effort must move four times the distance of the resistance. The point of effort application will move four times faster than the point of application of the resistance. But the force at the axis must not be forgotten. In this situation, the force on the axis will be five times greater than the force of the effort. The axis force will equal the sum of the effort plus the resistance. A teeter-totter, or seesaw, is an example of a first-class lever (Fig. 12.11*A*).

SECOND-CLASS LEVERS   A second-class lever, designated *ORE,* has the resistance (*R*) between the axis (*O*) and the effort (*E*). In this case, the magnitude of the effort is always less than the resistance. The distance moved and the speed of the effort point of application will always be greater than those of the resistance. The magnitude of force at the axis will always be less than the resistance in this simple situation. A wheelbarrow is an example of a second-class lever (Fig. 12.11*B*).

THIRD-CLASS LEVERS   A third-class lever, designated *OER,* has the effort (*E*) between the resistance (*R*) and the axis (*O*). In this situation, the magnitude of the effort is always greater than the resistance. However, the resistance will always move farther and faster than the effort. Such an arrangement works well for throwing a baseball, kicking a football, and lifting weights. Because only three forces are involved, the force at the axis will be less than that of the effort.

The human body is composed of many lever arm situations, and many lever situations are imposed on the body. Refer to Practical Application 12.1 for an example of how these principles may work in a real situation.

Practical Application 12.1

HIP JOINT PAIN AND MUSCLE WEAKNESS

A 50-year-old female who is 162 cm tall and weighs 91 kg has hip pain and weak hip abductor muscles on her right side. The treatment goal is to allow the patient to walk more normally with little or no pain. To do this she needs to decrease the load that she puts on her right hip. This can be done in at least three ways:

- She may use an antalgic gait (limp) in which she tilts her trunk over her hip while standing on the right foot. This is done to compensate for the weak abductors on that side.
- She may use a cane in the left hand, which increases the lever arm of the muscle–bone attachment, giving her increased leverage and taking stress off the weak side, thus reducing her pain.
- She may also decrease her body weight.

The third option is the best choice, because it is a long-term solution. Until her body weight is reduced, however, the use of the cane in the left hand would be better than the limp. She must also do exercises to strengthen her right hip abductor muscles.

A clinical biomechanist can calculate the magnitude of muscle force needed for the woman to walk unassisted in a normal manner. An exercise program can be implemented to improve her right hip abductor muscle strength. Several different devices may be used, such as cuff weights, a pulley system, or specific hip abduction machines. The target load would be different for each device and should be determined as a goal for which she should strive. A weight loss program that does not overload the hip should also be instituted. The buoyancy force of water during exercise in a pool would be appropriate, because it would lessen the force of gravity and her own body weight, allowing her to workout without pain.

The pull by the triceps muscle is an example of a first-class lever. The gastrocnemius acts as a second-class lever when it lifts the heel. The pull by the biceps muscle represents a third-class lever.

Strength of Materials

Biologic materials are often affected by external forces. As a load is imposed on the material, it tends to deform (change in size or shape) the material. In turn, the material tends to resist this deformation. The amount of deformation depends on the magnitude of the load and the ability of the material to resist the deformation. The ability of the material to resist deformation is often referred to as the strength of the material.

As the load acts on the material and the material tends to resist, a change in size and shape may occur. This change can often be determined by measuring the change in length of the object or the change in an angle within the body. This change in dimensions is called **strain.** The property of a material to resist the deformation caused by forces acting on it is called mechanical **stress.** The units for stress are force per unit area.

Three principal strains and stresses exist (Fig. 12.12). Tension occurs when two or more external forces act on the material along the same line of application (collinear) in opposite directions

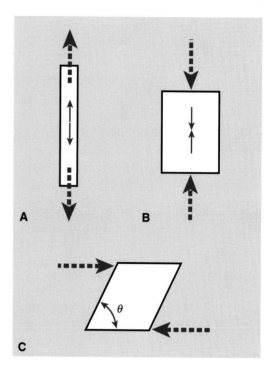

FIGURE 12.12 Three principal strains. **A,** Tension. **B,** Compression. **C,** Shear. *Arrows,* direction and points of application of the forces.

(away) from each other. The material tends to be pulled apart. Compression occurs when two or more forces act on the material along the same line of application in opposite directions directed toward each other. In this case the material tends to be pressed together. The third strain or stress is shearing. Shearing occurs when two or more parallel, but noncollinear forces pointed in opposite directions act on the material. The adjacent surfaces of the material tend to slide past each other.

These three stresses may arise within the body by **axial loading** (or direct, linear loading) or by loads acting at a distance, such as bending or **torsion.** Axial, bending, and torsion loading may occur alone or in combination. In all instances, tension, compression, and **shear** occur in some degree when the material is loaded. The resulting stress and strain are related to the force components applied to the material.

Axial Load

Loading along the axis of an object is referred to as axial loading. An object, such as an intervertebral disk, that is loaded by collinear forces acting toward each other will obviously have compressive stress (Fig. 12.13). The height of the disk will tend to decrease, and the disk will get wider. The widening of the disk illustrates that tension stresses are also operating perpendicular to the line of application of the loads. Shear stresses will be produced at 45° angles to the loads. Similarly, a ligament, tendon, muscle, or other soft tissue that is stretched by tension-producing loads will become narrower. This narrowing of the tissue shows that compression stress is also involved. Shear stresses will also develop at 45° to the load in this situation.

Bending Loads

Objects bend when forces or force components act in a **coplanar manner,** but are not collinear. These forces lie in the same plane, but do not have the same line of application or point of application.

A beam that is supported at both ends with a load between the ends demonstrates a **bending loading** situation (Fig. 12.14). The load can be the force of gravity, which causes contact

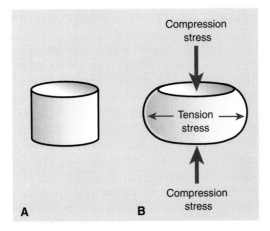
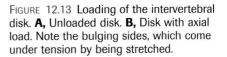

FIGURE 12.13 Loading of the intervertebral disk. **A,** Unloaded disk. **B,** Disk with axial load. Note the bulging sides, which come under tension by being stretched.

forces to develop at the supporting ends. The greater the gravitational force, the greater the supporting contact forces. These forces tend to cause the beam to bend or curve. Compression stress will arise in the concave (top) side of the beam, and tension stress develops in the convex (bottom) side of the beam. Shearing stresses in a homogenous material are present within the beam perpendicular and parallel to the forces. The amount of bending and stress depend on the magnitude and the location of the forces. Greater bending and related stresses develop if the magnitude of the forces is increased or the distance between the supporting forces is increased. This loading system is often referred to as the three-point principle, which is used by healthcare professionals when creating many braces, casts, and splints.

Figure 12.14*C* demonstrates how a weight-bearing foot acts as a loaded beam. As an individual stands, the heel and the ball of the foot are the supporting surfaces. The gravitational force is the weight of the body. Tension stresses develop in the ligaments and plantar fascia along the plantar surface (sole) of the foot. Compression stresses act between the bones of the foot. Shearing occurs parallel to the surfaces of the bones. Because the foot is not a homogenous ma-

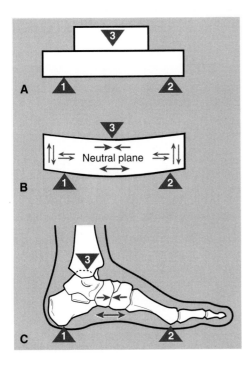

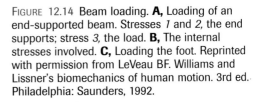

FIGURE 12.14 Beam loading. **A,** Loading of an end-supported beam. Stresses *1* and *2,* the end supports; stress *3,* the load. **B,** The internal stresses involved. **C,** Loading the foot. Reprinted with permission from LeVeau BF. Williams and Lissner's biomechanics of human motion. 3rd ed. Philadelphia: Saunders, 1992.

terial, these lines of stress are not at exactly 45° angles to the forces. Numerous other examples exist within and in relation to the human body.

An eccentrically loaded beam is considered to be a cantilever, and loading in this case is referred to as **cantilever loading.** In the simplest situation, a horizontal beam is supported and anchored at one end while the free end is loaded (Fig. 12.15*A*). The loaded beam tends to bend, producing stresses and strains (Fig. 12.15*B*). Tension stress and strain will occur in the upper, convex, side of the beam. Compression stress and strain will occur in the lower, concave, side of the beam. Shearing stress and strain will be perpendicular and parallel to the applied forces.

The magnitudes of the stress and resulting strain depend on the magnitude of the load and the point at which the load is applied to the beam. The greater the magnitude, or the greater the distance of the load from the supported end, the greater the bending.

In the human body, the proximal end of the femur represents an eccentrically loaded cantilever (Fig. 12.15*C*). The body weight loads the head of the femur so that the neck of the femur tends to bend. Tension stress is developed in the upper part of the femoral neck. Compression stress is produced in the lower aspect of the femoral neck. Shearing occurs along the epiphyseal plate. Other examples include a diving board, a baseball bat, and some splints.

Torsion Loads

When a rod or shaft is loaded so that it will twist around its long axis, torsion develops (Fig. 12.16). Forces on one end of the rod tend to rotate it clockwise, and forces on the other end of the rod tend to rotate it counterclockwise. When torsion occurs, tension, compression, and shearing stresses and strains are produced. Tension and compression stresses are located along spiraling lines along the length of the rod. Shearing stresses occur perpendicular and parallel to the rod. The magnitude of the stresses depends on the magnitude of the applied loads and the location of the application points on the long axis of the rod.

Forces overcoming the friction resistance when removing a lid from a jar illustrate the perpendicular shearing stress of torsion. A spiral fracture of the tibia is an example of a bone failing because of torsion loading (Fig. 12.16*C*). The spiral fracture line indicates the failure of tension stress to resist the breaking of the bone. A spiral fracture of the humerus can also occur. The muscle forces of the rotator cuff (the area of the scapula) hold the proximal end (near the shoulder) of the humerus, while the inertial forces of the forearm and hand act on the distal end (near

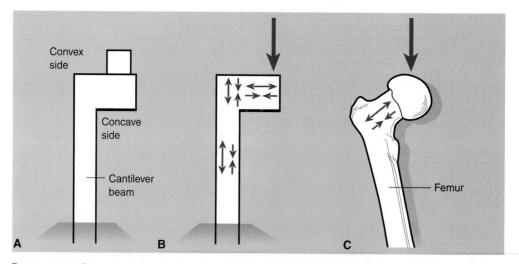

FIGURE 12.15 **A,** Loading of a cantilever beam. **B,** Location of internal stresses (*arrows*). **C,** Proximal end of the femur. Reprinted with permission from LeVeau BF. Williams and Lissner's biomechanics of human motion. 3rd ed. Philadelphia: Saunders, 1992.

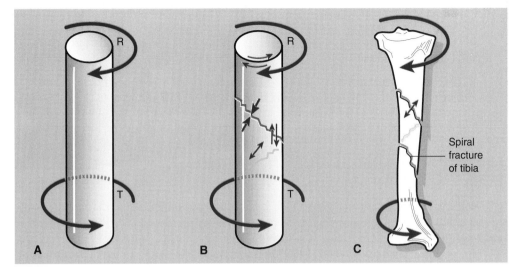

FIGURE 12.16 Torsion loading. **A,** Forces *R* and *T* act in opposite directions, causing twisting. **B,** Stresses during torsion. **C,** Spiral fracture resulting from torsion. Reprinted with permission from LeVeau BF. Williams and Lissner's biomechanics of human motion. 3rd ed. Philadelphia: Saunders, 1992.

the elbow) of the bone. Occasionally, splints are placed on the legs of children in an attempt to correct torsional growth deformities.

Effects of Loading on Biologic Tissue

Biologic tissues are living materials that readily respond to the presence and absence of loads. The enhancement or deprivation of stresses within a tissue reacting to a load influence the tissue's structure and mechanical characteristics. When muscle is not used, it becomes smaller and weaker, but a muscle that is used becomes larger and stronger.

Loads can greatly modify the size, shape, and strength of bone, cartilage, ligaments, and tendons. The ability of bone to adapt by changing its size, shape, and internal structure depends on the mechanical stresses established by the load. This ability is referred to as **Wolff's law.** Early in life, tissue differentiation and growth seem to follow loading of muscle contraction of the embryo and fetus, and the muscular activity of the mother (2). Mechanical stresses are important for early skeletal development. The type of loading has effects on the type of tissues developed and the amount and direction of tissue growth (3). In general, large loads (within limits) increase the size and strength of tissues. Zero load or low loads lead to a decrease in the size and strength of the tissues. Weight-bearing activity (e.g., walking or running) and muscle-strengthening exercises can increase bone mass, direct trabecular growth, and retard tissue atrophy, because these types of activities place loads on the body. Would non-weight-bearing activity, likewise, increase bone mass (Fig. 12.17)?

Many examples of the effect of loads on growth exist. Tennis players have greater bone cortex thickness of the upper limb on the playing side than on the nonplaying side. Individuals who take part in weight-training exercises have denser bones than those who don't. Disabled children who stand have more normally developed hips and femurs than those who do not stand. Exercise has been shown to increase the strength of ligaments and tendons. Early passive motion after injury appears to increase the strength of damaged fibrous tissues and accelerate tissue healing. Studies, however, have also provided a warning about forces on tissues. After prolonged immobilization, improvement in tissue strength with exercise will take a long time. Too much force or force applied too early may cause increased damage. The clinician must be cognizant of the magnitude of force necessary for the most efficient rehabilitation of the patient.

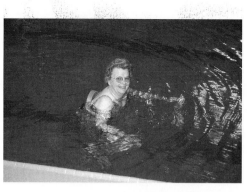

FIGURE 12.17 Deep-water walking or running is a non-weight-bearing activity.

Decrease in tissue mass and strength can occur during immobilization of a body or body part. Immobilization may be imposed by such situations as prolonged bedrest or casting of a limb. Most individuals readily notice muscle atrophy; however, they rarely realize that other tissues have also been similarly affected. Bone, cartilage, ligaments, and tendons also tend to atrophy and lose strength. Bone mineral loss because of immobilization has been seen in patients with paralysis or fractures. Space travel may be limited because of loss of bone minerals brought about by weightlessness. Articular cartilage and ligaments deteriorate with immobilization. Sufficient loads, but not too much, are needed to retard or eliminate tissue atrophy.

Prolonged loading may also have adverse effects on tissues. Constant loading may cause breakdown of the material by mechanical means of **creep** or by restricting blood flow and nutrition to the area. Early prolonged loading may create deformities of bone and cartilage, such as club foot or hip dysplasia. Such problems must be corrected at an early age.

The size, shape, strength, and health of tissues are determined by the characteristics of the loads applied to them. An exercise science professional can have influence on what the characteristics of these forces will be.

ADVANCES IN CLINICAL BIOMECHANICS

The previous section demonstrated that the study of force is basic to the study of clinical biomechanics. This section introduces readers to the interactions of forces in specific situations related to exercise science.

The Use of Electromyography

Electromyography (EMG) is an established technique that records the electrical signal emanating from muscle motor units as the muscle is stimulated. The technology is increasingly being used in the clinic to understand the function of muscles. EMG is often used with indwelling needles to assist in the diagnosis of a disease process. Surface electrodes and electrical stimulation combine to determine the conduction velocity of peripheral nerves. Surface and fine-wire electrodes are used to evaluate the function of muscles in a variety of situations, including workplace activities, strengthening and endurance exercises, and locomotion. It can also be used for evaluating pain, comparing different activities, and assessing relaxation.

Clinical biomechanics does not deal with needle EMG or nerve conduction studies; rather, it uses the surface and fine-wire electrode techniques that monitor the state of activation of the muscle. The most common characteristics of the EMG signal are its amplitude, timing, and frequency. The amplitude of the signal is generally related to the force of the muscle contraction. If no signal is present, the muscle is not contracting and, therefore, is not producing any active force. If the amplitude is maximal, the muscle is producing a maximal force. The timing is often associated with the initiation and termination of the muscle contraction. Often, however, the timing can be related to the points of peak amplitude. The combination of amplitude and timing provides a pattern of muscle contraction for a specific activity. The frequency, commonly referred to as spectral analysis, provides information related to the state of fatigue of the muscle.

EMG has been used in recent years for biofeedback, to assess muscle function in various exercises and activities, and to identify pathologic status. Newer electronic and computer technologies have enhanced these applications by allowing more direct subject viewing of the biologic signal, and offer the possibility of additional uses for EMG.

EMG biofeedback can involve training an individual to relax the muscle so that no signal is present or to selectively contract the muscle to enhance muscle strength or coordination. Several clinical protocols exist to reduce the pain of headaches and neck and shoulder tension and to control muscle spasm (4,5). Other protocols have been developed to train the vastus medials, to strengthen the bladder muscles to overcome incontinence, and to strengthen weakened muscles such as the peroneus longus (6–8). Research is continuing to improve these protocols and to develop new ones for other disorders.

Muscle function is commonly assessed when analyzing the gait of children with cerebral palsy. The assessment is focused on determining if there is any abnormal firing of the muscles during the walking cycle. Such studies can help physicians ascertain the need for surgery (9). EMG can also be used to assess muscle recruitment patterns in various exercises to determine the value of the exercise (10).

If one knows the specific muscle activity that occurs during particular exercises, it is possible to select the most appropriate training and rehabilitation program for an individual client. EMG can also be used to determine the effect of an exercise device or machine. The clinician uses the EMG data to develop a progressive exercise program based on that specific machine (11).

The function of individual parts of a muscle has been studied. For instance, the gluteus medius muscle has three sections that act somewhat independently from the others, and the lateral gastrocnemius has three independently functioning heads. Functional subdivisions were also found in the upper trapezius muscle (12). More investigation is needed to determine the functions of specific parts of the muscles.

Identification of pathologic status of a muscle has been performed for peripheral arterial disease, soft tissue damage, and back muscle impairment (13–15). Surface EMG has shown that patients may often alter their motor strategy after a painful injury (16). The muscle pattern may change because of excessive fatigue or because of inhibition of muscle activity owing to pain. Compensatory muscle activity may occur, which then becomes a source of pain. Researchers have found that surface EMG using spectral parameters has merit in distinguishing individuals with low back pain from those without it (15,17).

EMG does have some limitations. Researchers, however, are developing reliable and valid procedures for its use. Advances in electronics and computers continue to be made. EMG is a valuable tool, although the clinical biomechanist must be aware of the technology's limitations and should be familiar with the nuances of interpretation of the signal.

Ergonomics

Ergonomics is similar to clinical biomechanics in that it includes physiology, anatomy, medicine, physics, and engineering. Ergonomics includes the prevention of injuries and the capacity for the individual to return to work after an injury has occurred. The discipline of ergonomics also includes design of equipment and the environment for special populations, such as the disabled. Ergonomists focus on the workplace, home, recreational sites, vehicles, schools, clinics, and other human-built environments. The definition of *ergonomics* then, is the study of the interaction between humans, the objects they use, and the environments in which they function (18).

Several risk factors identified by ergonomists can cause, maintain, or worsen musculoskeletal injury and pain, including factors related to force. Forceful exertions and postures, localized contact loads, and repetitive motion may lead to musculoskeletal disorders caused by **mechanical fatigue.** The characteristics of force must be considered with these factors.

▶▶ Sidelight 12.1

LOAD ON THE LUMBAR SPINE CAUSES PAIN

Pain in the low back or lumbar region of the spine is a common problem that can occur in individuals of almost any age but is most often encountered in people between the ages of 30 and 60. Low back pain is commonly the result of lifting a heavy load (see the figure below.) When added to the weight of the upper body, the heavy load produces forces that must be counterbalanced in the opposite direction by the musculature of the lumbar spine (lower back). However, the length of levers involved in this lift puts the muscles of the lumbar spine at a great disadvantage. For example, the lever arm of the combined weight of the trunk and load could be 15 to 20 in., whereas the lever arm for the muscles is 1 to 1.5 in. This means that the muscles must exert a force 10 to 20 times the weight of the combined trunk and load to move the body frame.

Several problems can occur when lifting excessive loads. First, attempting to lift the load with less-than-adequate muscle force may result in sprained ligaments of the back. Second, the muscles could be strained if the load is too great for the muscle force available. Third, the muscles may be sufficiently strong to lift the load, but the load may place too much stress within the lumbar disk, damaging it. When treating the individual, the clinician should address these important questions:

- What exercise would be best for rehabilitation of the injury?
- What activities should the individual have restricted?
- When should this individual be allowed to return to work?

Injuries of this type should be prevented before they happen. The entire situation related to low back pain could be addressed by the clinical biomechanist, who should do the following:

- Establish the cause of the injury.
- Evaluate the injury.
- Determine short- and long-term treatment procedures.
- Evaluate the environment and make recommendations to eliminate or reduce the possibility of such accidents occurring.
- Devise preventative measures so that future incidences will be eliminated or their incidence reduced.

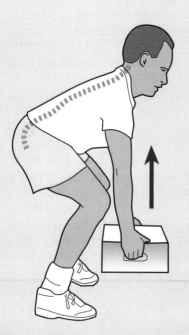

Lifting a heavy load.

Forceful exertions refer to activities that require a large magnitude of force to perform a task. The use of excessive forces may easily lead to an injury. For example, the National Institute of Occupational Safety and Health has noted that handling heavy weights is a risk factor for the development of back pain (see Sidelight 12.1) (19). Standards have been set to reduce the incidence of excessive force injuries. Many of these standards were devised based on the two conditions of equilibrium presented in this chapter and the principles of kinetics presented in Chapter 13.

Occasionally, awkward postures are necessary to perform certain tasks. Using these postures often or for a prolonged period of time can produce disabling injuries. Musculoskeletal tissues may be sufficiently stressed to result in injury. Supporting muscles may become overly fatigued. The task can be analyzed using the conditions of equilibrium. The activity can then be designed to reduce or eliminate the stressful posture.

Localized contact loads can occur between body tissue and an object in the environment. For example, thin individuals sitting on a hard bench for a long period of time can feel the effect of localized contact on their ischial tuberosities. Localized contact loads can cause increased compression or shearing on the tissues. Compression nerve injuries, fractures, contusions, lacerations, and blisters are examples of localized contact injuries.

Repetitious motions are a common cause of injury and discomfort. Some tasks require thousands of repetitions during the day, and may result in significant injury. Repetitious friction force of a tendon moving through its tendon sheath can cause inflammation of the tissues. Carpal tunnel syndrome (wrist, finger, and hand pain involving weakness and inflammation) is an example of a repetitive-motion disorder. Repetitive bending of the trunk can create low back pain. Runners and joggers may develop a stress fracture in the foot as a result of repetitive motion. Stress fractures occur in regions that experience high stress concentration brought about by repetitive loading. The repeated loading may trigger an adaptive response, which accelerates the remodeling of the bone. As the bone begins to remodel, the first step of the process is resorption of existing bony material. This step in the process reduces the bone mass and weakens the bone. Repeated overuse without allowing the progression of the adaptive process toward development of a strong bone may lead to a fracture.

Analysis of the task and redesign of the object or environment using biomechanical principles can reduce the risk of injury. Forces, often with motion, are involved in all activities, whether they occur in the workplace, at home, or in the recreational setting.

Athletic training and sports medicine reflect an ergonomic approach to the special population of athletes (see Chapter 14). Individuals knowledgeable in biomechanical and physiologic principles can be highly effective consultants for reducing and eliminating injuries. They may also help provide safe and efficient living, working, and playing environments for individuals from special populations.

SUMMARY POINTS

- Clinical biomechanics is the science of how forces act on the body and how the body exerts forces on other objects.
- Clinical biomechanics covers the entire life span.
- Forces are always present and are always described by four characteristics: point of application, line of application, direction, and magnitude.
- The amount of force a muscle produces depends on a variety of factors, including its cross-sectional area, its length, the speed of contraction, the type of contraction, and the motor unit firing situation.
- The greater the mass of an object, the greater the force needed to change its velocity.
- The angle between concurrent forces plays a major role in the resulting force obtained.
- In lever systems, what is gained in force is lost in speed and range of motion, and vice versa.

- The amount of torque depends on the magnitude of force and its location from the axis of rotation.
- The mechanical characteristics of an object determine how it will respond when a force is applied or removed.
- The amount of force produced by a muscle is related to the magnitude of its electrical signal.
- Ergonomics relates to the efficiency and safety of an individual within the environment.

REVIEW QUESTIONS

1. Explain the effects of a muscle that pulls perpendicular to the bone to which it is attached compared to a muscle that pulls more parallel to the bone.
2. Explain the effect of a load applied to the limb when the limb is positioned at 0°, 30°, 45°, 60°, and 90° to the horizontal.
3. How does the resultant change as the angle between two concurrent forces decreases?
4. What type of lever is the most common in the human body? What are the advantages and disadvantages of this anatomic arrangement?
5. Discuss the importance of Wolff's law and how an exercise professional can use this law.

References

1. Patel TJ, Lieber RL. Force transmission in skeletal muscle from actomyosin to external tendons. Exerc Sport Sci Rev 1997;25:321–363.
2. Carter DR. Mechanical loading histories and cortical bone remodeling. Calcif Tissue Int 1984;36:519–524.
3. LeVeau BF, Bernhardt DB. Developmental biomechanics: effect of forces on the growth, development, and maintenance of the human body. Phys Ther 1984;64:1874–1882.
4. Bussone G, Grazzi L, D'Amico D, Leone M, Andrasik F. Biofeedback-assisted relaxation training for young adolescents with tension-type headache: a controlled study. Cephalalgia 1998;18:463–467.
5. Wong AM, Lee MY, Chang WH, Tang FT. Clinical trial of cervical traction modality with electromyographical biofeedback. Am J Phys Med Rehabil 1997;76:19–25.
6. Ingersoll CD, Knight KL. Patellar location changes following EMG biofeedback or progressive resistive exercises. Med Sci Sports Exerc 1991;23:1122–1127.
7. McKenna PH, Herndon CD, Connery S, Ferrer FA. Pelvic floor muscle retraining for pediatric voiding dysfunction using interactive computer games. J Urol 1999;162:1056–62.
8. Larsen E, Lund PM. Peroneal muscle function in chronically unstable ankles—a prospective preoperative and postoperative electromyographic study. Clin Orthop 1991;272:219–226.
9. DeLuca PA, Davis RB III, Ounpuu S, et al. Alterations in surgical decision making in patients with cerebral palsy based on three-dimensional gait analysis. J Pediatr Orthop 1997;17:608–614.
10. Plamondon A, Marceau C, Stainton S, Desjardins P. Toward a better prescription of the prone back extension exercise to strengthen the back muscles. Scand J Med Sci Sports 1999;9:226–232.
11. Mayer JM, Graves JE, Robertson VL, et al. Electromyographic activity of the lumbar extensor muscles: effect of angle and hand position during Roman chair exercise. Arch Phys Med Rehabil 1999;80:751–755.
12. Jensen C, Westgaard RH. Functional subdivision of the upper trapezius muscle during low-level activation. Eur J Appl Physiol 1997;76:335–339.
13. Casale R, Buonocore M, Di Massa A, Setacci C. Arch Phys Med Rehabil 1994;75:1118–1121.
14. Bauer JA, Murray RD. Electromyographic patterns of individuals suffering from lateral tennis elbow. J Electromyogr Kinesiol 1999;9:245–252.
15. Hodges PW, Richardson CA. Altered trunk muscle recruitment in people with low back pain with upper limb movement at different speeds. Arch Phys Med Rehabil 1999;80:1005–1012.
16. Headley BJ. Surface EMG: New rehab horizons. Phys Ther Products 1994;5:30–34.
17. Greenough CG, Oliver CW, Jones AP. Assessment of spinal musculature using surface electromyographic spectral color mapping. Spine 1998;23:1768–1774.

18. Pulat BM. Fundamentals of industrial ergonomics. 2nd ed. Prospect Heights, IL: Waveland Press, 1997.
19. NIOSH. Work practice guide for manual lifting. Technical report. DHHS (NIOSH) publication no. 81-122. Washington DC: DHHS, 1981.

Suggested Readings

Bernstein AH, Wright TM. Fundamentals of orthopedic biomechanics. Baltimore: Williams & Wilkins, 1994.
Bridger RS. Introduction to ergonomics. New York: McGraw-Hill, 1995.
Kumar S. Perspectives in rehabilitation ergonomics. Bristol, TN: Taylor & Francis, 1997.
LeVeau BF. Williams and Lissner's biomechanics of human motion. Philadelphia: Saunders, 1992.
Lieber RL. Skeletal muscle structure and function. Baltimore: Williams & Wilkins, 1992.
Rice VJB. Ergonomics in health care and rehabilitation. Boston: Butterworth-Heinemann, 1998.

13

Sports Biomechanics

BENJAMIN F. JOHNSON

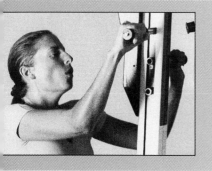

Objectives

1. Define sports biomechanics.
2. Distinguish between the biomechanical concepts of kinematics and kinetics.
3. Explain the kinetic link principle and correctly list activities into the sequential or simultaneous category.
4. Discuss how instrumentation has advanced the science of sports biomechanics.

- **Definition, Description, and Scope**
  To Minimize, Maximize, or Optimize Effort
  Instrumentation—The Key to Measuring Human Motion
- **Focus on Science**
  Basic Biomechanical Concepts
  Advanced Biomechanical Concepts
  Basic Biomechanical Analysis of Movement Activities
- **Advances in Sports Biomechanics**
  Stretch–Shortening Cycle
  Kinetic Link Principle
  Instrumentation—Computer Modeling

Summary Points
Review Questions
References
Suggested Readings

Sports biomechanics is a subdiscipline of exercise science that provides insight into human movement associated with sports and exercise. Research in sports biomechanics provides direct measures of human motion that can be used to improve athletic performance. This information often affects how a coach instructs an athlete, and it may also help dictate how a physical education teacher instructs a young student in a basic locomotor skill. In conjunction with Chapter 12, this chapter offers an overview of the science of biomechanics and provides descriptions of movement activities explained from a biomechanical standpoint.

DEFINITION, DESCRIPTION, AND SCOPE

Sport biomechanics combines the study of applied human anatomy with that of mechanical physics. These combined sciences allow for detailed descriptions of how and why the human body moves the way it does and why individuals perform at varying levels of success in sports endeavors. Understanding the neuromuscular and mechanical factors associated with human movement allows the sports biomechanist to describe the requirements necessary for performing at an elite level. These biomechanical descriptions influence coaches and athletes to refine their knowledge and approach to training, as well as consider new and innovative techniques for improved sport performance (see Practical Application 13.1). In addition, this information provides insight into the mechanical causes of sport-related injuries, potentially leading to safer sport participation.

To Minimize, Maximize, or Optimize Effort

Sports biomechanists determine how an athlete should generate the mechanical techniques necessary for successful performance in particular events. There are many possible anatomic movements and muscular levels of effort available to the athlete, and the sports biomechanist can advise the coach or athlete whether it is necessary to maximize, minimize, or optimize the effort and the best movement patterns for success. For example, when performing a standing vertical jump, it is necessary to exert a maximum amount of muscular effort to generate large vertical forces on the ground. This maximum force applied to the ground as a result of the athlete's muscular effort enables the athlete to overcome his or her body weight and generate movement of the body in an upward direction. The faster the person's body is traveling upward at the takeoff point, the higher the body will travel in the air.

Conversely, as the body falls back to the ground, the athlete wants to minimize the forces applied to the body during the landing. This is accomplished by using the muscles to control body joints as they give during landing to absorb the force. If the joints remain stiff, the landing will be more forceful, causing a larger shock to the body. Such a large landing force may cause an injury, whereas the minimized landing force results in much less trauma to the musculoskeletal system.

Optimization of effort can be characterized by the effort required to hit a golf ball a maximum distance. Generally, if a golfer uses maximum muscular effort, the resulting golf club speed is less in magnitude and accuracy than when an optimized, or near maximum, effort is used. This optimized effort enables better, smoother coordination of the complex movement, typically resulting in higher club velocities at impact with a better swing pattern and accuracy of the shot.

Instrumentation—The Key to Measuring Human Motion

Determining the best movement patterns and levels of effort for a particular sporting activity can be accomplished in two major ways: qualitatively and quantitatively. A **qualitative analysis** of an activity involves observation of the performance, not the collection of numeric data. The person performing the analysis observes the performance and, through an understanding of the ba-

---

Practical Application 13.1

THE FOSBURY FLOP

Many of the great strides made in sports performance, as evidenced by record-breaking feats, can be attributed either directly or indirectly to the science of biomechanics. For example, one of the more radical changes in the mechanical techniques associated with a sport was the Fosbury flop (see the figure on the next page). Before the 1968 Summer Olympic Games in Mexico City, Dick Fosbury introduced this biomechanically superior technique for executing a high jump. Before this, jumpers used a body-roll technique, which allowed them to attain unbelievable vertical heights, but the technique was biomechanically inefficient. After the 1968 Olympic Games, virtually every elite high jumper converted to the flop technique and improved his or her jumps as a result. Fosbury broke the world record during the 1968 Summer Games, and every record holder since has used his flop technique.

It is interesting to note that Fosbury would never have developed his technique had it not been for a change in the landing materials used in the high jump. For many years, the landing material in the pit area was either sawdust or sand. These materials allowed for the absorption of forces upon landing, but the high-tech, synthetic foam cushions introduced just before Fosbury began his career did this much better. Foam pits meant that jumpers experienced a significant reduction in the forces applied to their bodies upon landing. Furthermore the landing surface was higher above the ground. These factors provided the necessary elements to enable a radical departure from the traditional body-roll style. The mechanical modifications in jumping style would have been impossible were it not for the ingenuity leading to the development and introduction of the foam pit.

---

sic concepts of biomechanics, offers an educated opinion about what aspects of the performance need to be adjusted for improvement. The athlete, through trial and error, attempts to alter the technique to improve performance.

A **quantitative analysis** of an activity involves numeric measurement of the performance, often with high-tech instrumentation, such as high-speed video-recording systems and subsequent motion analysis performed via computerized video-digitizing and data processing designed to mathematically model the human body; computerized force-measuring platforms to measure forces produced by the body on the ground; and electromyography (EMG) for measuring the electrical activity of the muscles to determine muscle firing patterns and recruitment. These data are used to either evaluate how an elite athlete performs a skill so optimum movement patterns can be determined and/or compared to a performer with known normative values. The normative values are generated through quantitative research on large groups of athletes. These descriptive data ultimately detail how a representative group of performers, preferably elite athletes, execute the sporting skill.

As the science of biomechanics evolved alongside technologic advances used to collect biomechanical data, it is obvious that biomechanics depends strongly on sophisticated equipment to provide accurate, reliable, and quantitative measures of an athlete's performance (see Sidelight 13.1). The types of knowledge the biomechanist must have to make sense of the data will be explored next. With a knowledge of biomechanics, effective communications with the coach and

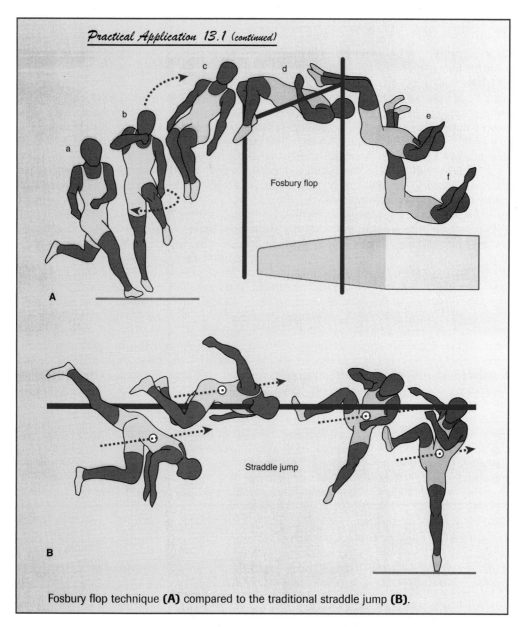

Practical Application 13.1 (continued)

Fosbury flop

Straddle jump

Fosbury flop technique **(A)** compared to the traditional straddle jump **(B)**.

athlete can take place, and scientific communication (published research articles or oral presentations at scientific meetings) can be disseminated to the exercise science community.

FOCUS ON SCIENCE

This section focuses on the biomechanical concepts needed to understand movement during sports performance. With a knowledge of these concepts, the student will begin to appreciate the tremendous mechanical complexity of human movement.

Basic Biomechanical Concepts

Sports biomechanists generally classify various forms of human motion analysis into the following categories: statics or dynamics, kinematic or kinetic, and linear or angular. Each of these is briefly discussed below. Before reading on, the student should refer to Box 12.4 to review Newton's laws of motion.

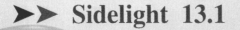

TECHNOLOGICAL ADVANCEMENT

Technology has greatly influenced the evolution of biomechanics. As instrumentation used to measure human performance improves in quality and decreases in price, the breadth and depth of biomechanics research increase. To study the movements of athletes through visual image analysis, it is necessary to use video or movie cameras that take pictures at a very fast rate. The more pictures taken per unit of time (i.e., pictures per second), the more the movement can be slowed down on the videotape or film. When cameras take pictures at high rates of speed with fast shutter openings (the time each individual picture is recorded), a superior, nonblurred still image is generated. This allows the scientist to locate important body landmarks for measurement of movement between two pictures, or points in time. When these still pictures are played back in succession with a videotape player or movie projector, the effect is one of a slow motion replay of the recorded activity.

The process of computer video digitizing, or giving numeric geometric coordinates to body landmarks over a series of moving pictures, enables the biomechanist to track and quantify the athlete's movements, including position, velocity, and acceleration of the digitized landmarks. In the 1970s and early 1980s, high-speed 16-mm film cameras were used to record the movements of athletes for more careful study in the laboratory. These expensive cameras were capable of taking up to 500 pictures per second and offered high resolution images. The problem for athletes and coaches was the delay required between recording the performance and studying the film, because it commonly took several days to develop the film. As videotape recording and playback technology came of age in the middle to late 1980s, biomechanics research began a migration toward this technology. Today, video-recording systems that take 1,000 pictures per second and provide high-quality images are affordable for many research institutions. In fact, there are video-recording systems, although quite expensive, that take up to 45,000 pictures per second.

Advances in computer hardware and software technology since the late 1970s have also made biomechanical data processing and advanced three-dimensional (3-D) human body modeling fast, accurate, and user friendly. Large volumes of biomechanical data can be processed rapidly and stored for future analysis. As computer technology improves, leading to ever more powerful, faster computer-processing systems with larger storage capacity and improved peripherals for image display, biomechanical analysis of sporting skills will soon be accomplished in real-time so that immediate, meaningful, detailed results will be available to the coach and athlete.

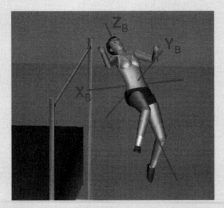

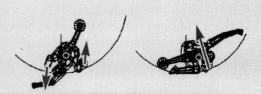

Examples of computer graphics used to study the biomechanics of sport performance. These images were made from actual performances of the high jump and discus throw. Used with permission from Dr. Jesus Dapena, Department of Kinesiology, Biomechanics Laboratory, Indiana University.

># Sidelight 13.1 (continued)

Computerized force platforms, which are firmly secured to the floor to eliminate vibrations, measure the forces generated on the ground by an athlete performing an athletic skill. As an athlete steps, lands, or stands on the platform during a performance, the interfaced computer records and stores the three-dimensional force data that are generated. These data reflect forces produced in the vertical, anteroposterior, and mediolateral directions, generating tables of numbers and/or force-time graphs. Forces are measured up to 1000 times per second for detailed analysis of forces generated even under fast movement conditions such as sprinting. Forces are measured every moment during which the body is in contact with the force platform. This enables the biomechanist to analyze force patterns generated by the athlete and to determine performance faults or potential of injury.

EMG measures the electrical activity generated by the muscle as it is stimulated by the nervous system. As the muscle's biochemical processes produce a contraction, the EMG system—through either electrodes placed on the skin (surface EMG) or fine wires placed directly into the muscle (indwelling EMG)—detects the intensity of the electrical processes of the muscle. EMG data typically are used to determine the timing of muscle contractions (onset and duration of the contraction) during a performance.

Computerized motion analysis systems, which allow multiple forms of instrumentation (video recorders, force platforms, and EMG) to be synchronized for more detailed measurement of a human's mechanical technique, use affordable, powerful computer workstations in a variety of platforms to generate synchronized data detailing an athlete's body positions, joint angles, movement speeds, accelerations, forces, torques, and muscle firing patterns. These data are output in a variety of forms, including tables of numbers, graphs, animated stick figures, and 3-D models of the body. This information is used to assess the performance level and injury potential of an athlete performing a particular sporting skill (see the figure on previous page).

Many sports activities illustrate Newton's laws of motion. First law: A barbell will remain still until a weightlifter applies an appropriate force to lift it. Second law: The greater the force used to kick a soccer ball, the greater the ball's acceleration. Third law: When a volleyball player spikes the ball, the force applied to the ball by the player's arm and hand is returned to the player's arm by the ball in the opposite direction and of equal magnitude.

Statics and Dynamics

Statics is the study of the body under conditions in which no accelerations are occurring. When acceleration of the body occurs, as happens if a person changes positions, static conditions are no longer present. *Static* means the body is either completely stationary or moving at a constant velocity. Neither of these conditions is common in sporting activities, because most involve velocity changes of various parts of the body as they move to produce the necessary body mechanics required for performing the skill. Static conditions are much more common when considering the construction of a building, bridge, or vehicle. Perhaps the closest approximations in sports are activities such as a headlock or pin hold in wrestling, a stationary flexibility position incorporated into a warmup or cooldown, and a static balance–flexibility position performed on a balance beam in gymnastics.

Dynamics is the study of a body undergoing acceleration. As a result, body segments are increasing and decreasing in velocity as the skill is performed. Varying levels of force are required to produce these accelerations. Depending on the skill and the proficiency of the athlete, the magnitudes of these forces and accelerations range from small to large. The dynamic state is the typical situation in virtually all of sports and exercise, because the nature of these activities involves the movement of various aspects of the human anatomy in a coordinated fashion. The legs in walking and running and the arm in a throw or tennis strike are examples of dynamic segments used in performing human activities.

Kinematics and Kinetics

Kinematics is the description of human motion in terms of position (displacement), velocity, and acceleration. These three variables describe motion resulting from forces produced by the muscular system or forces external to the body, such as gravity, other persons, and inanimate objects (the ground, sporting implements, etc.). However, no measures of these forces are available in the study of kinematics; therefore, it is not known exactly how much or what type of force is responsible for generating these human motions. For instance, the biomechanist may or may not know an object's mass or its **rotational inertia** or be able to make direct measures of force (as provided by a force platform system). Knowledge of at least one of these variables, however, is required if force is to be quantified.

Kinetics is the study of the forces generating the kinematic qualities described above. Quantifying the various forces applied on or by a system enables the biomechanist to determine why a body moves the way it does. This information can lead to a detailed analysis of movement mechanics and injury potential, because these forces lead directly to acceleration (increase or decrease in velocity), which, in turn, leads to changes in body position.

Linear and Angular Motion

Linear motion is the point-to-point, straight-line movement of a body in space. Depending on the complexity of the activity being monitored, the motion is generally measured in either a two-dimensional (2-D) or a three-dimensional (3-D) cartesian coordinate system (Fig. 13.1). By tracking body landmarks over time (e.g., the wrist, hip, or center of mass), the biomechanist can determine the amount of displacement, velocity, and acceleration these body points undergo during a sporting performance.

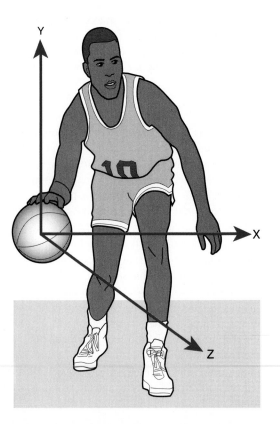

FIGURE 13.1 A three-dimensional cartesian coordinate system.

The same approach can be taken if it is desired to measure points on a golf club, tennis racquet, or ball during a sporting performance. These measures are made in the geometric planes established by the cartesian coordinate system, which are oriented to the human body and/or earth such that anteroposterior (forward and backward; z axis), vertical (up and down; y axis), and mediolateral (side to side; x axis) measures of motion are described linearly. Forces applied by or on the body in these directions lead to acceleration, or velocity changes, of these body points. Linear forces may be applied by muscles, gravity, the ground, and any number of other animate or inanimate objects.

> ☞ *Movement in a linear fashion may be along a straight line (rectilinear) or a curved line (curvilinear). An example can be found in the sport of ice skating.*

Angular motion is the measurement of how a rigid lever is rotating about an axis and is quantified through the use of a polar coordinate system. This is generally represented in the human body by body segments, e.g., the upper arm rotating about the shoulder joint (axis of rotation). By tracking over time how the lever, as established by its end points (for the upper arm: the shoulder and elbow), rotates around its proximal joint (the shoulder), the biomechanist can determine angular positional changes of the lever, rotational velocities of the lever about the joint, and increases and decreases in rotational velocity (Fig. 13.2).

These kinematic measures describe the angularly generated motion made by the athlete while performing a sports skill. This is important, because there is a direct link between the quality of angular motion of body segments, or levers, and the quality of linear motion of body landmarks located on these body levers. For example, the faster the lower leg is rotating or extending about the knee at the instant before the foot hits the soccer ball, the faster the foot is moving linearly at the moment of impact, because these points are located on the rotating lever. The faster the foot is moving linearly at impact, the greater the momentum that is imparted to the soccer ball. This impact generates the motion or flight of the ball. The rotation of the lower leg about the knee is in part the result of the contraction of muscles (quadriceps group), which causes acceleration in the direction of knee extension. The linear force of the quadriceps tendon pulling on the tibia generates a torque, or rotational force. The greater the torque produced by the mus-

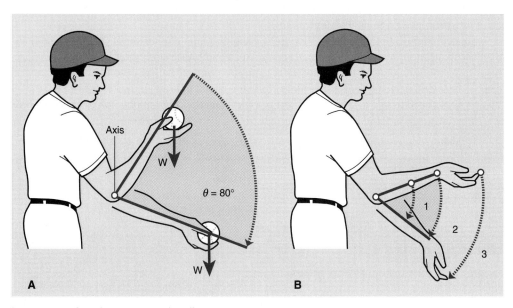

FIGURE 13.2 Angular motion at the elbow.

cles, the greater the angular accelerations generated, leading to changes in angular velocity that lead to changes in angular position.

Other points of interest in regard to measuring motion are **scalar** and vector values, displacement and distance, velocity and speed, and acceleration and deceleration. A scalar is a variable that can be described in terms of magnitude only. The numeric value associated with the scalar variable describes how much of a particular unit of measure the variable possesses. A vector, on the other hand, has a magnitude that is measured in a particular direction or along a particular axis or in a particular plane. Table 13.1 lists several variables associated with the kinematic and kinetic study of motion. Table 13.2 provides a brief description of important biomechanical variables that are basic to the study of sports biomechanics.

Advanced Biomechanical Concepts

The advanced concepts discussed in this section highlight several of the major areas that must be considered when analyzing human movement skills.

Projectiles

Any object that flies through the air free of external forces (with the exceptions of gravity and air friction) is considered a **projectile.** The object is undergoing displacement over time and is considered to be in a free-fall state, such that gravity and air friction are the only forces that affect its flight. The instant any other external force is applied to the object, and for the duration of time that it is applied, the object is no longer a projectile, because its free-fall state has been disrupted. If the external force is discontinued and the two objects separate, the original object will begin another free-fall state; but it will likely have different kinematic qualities than it had before the external force was applied.

Projectiles moving in any direction can be defined along the three axes of a cartesian coordinate system: horizontally, laterally, and vertically. If considering a thrown ball's flight between the release of the ball by the outfielder and the catch of the ball by the infielder, one must account for the displacement (straight-line measure) horizontally, laterally, and vertically as established by the initial position of the players and the release point of the ball (Fig. 13.3). A horizontal line drawn from the ball at the instant of release to the infielder establishes the horizontal axis of the cartesian coordinate system; the release point is at the origin. Vertical and lateral axes are drawn from the origin at 90° angles.

As the ball flies through the air along its path to the infielder, an arc of flight is traced, and displacements along each of the three primary axes can be measured. The horizontal displacement is measured along the horizontal axis from the point of ball release to the point of ball catch. The lateral displacement is measured along the lateral axis and indicates how much the infielder would have to move to his or her left or right from the original position to catch the ball.

Table 13.1	VARIABLES ASSOCIATED WITH THE KINEMATIC AND KINETIC STUDY OF MOTION					
			Linear		**Angular**	
Study Type	Variable	Symbol	Metric Unit	English Unit	Symbol	Unit
Kinematic	Displacement	D	m	ft	θ	rad or degree
	Velocity	v	$m \cdot sec^{-1}$	$ft \cdot sec^{-1}$	ω	$rad \cdot sec^{-1}$ or
						$degree \cdot sec^{-2}$
	Acceleration	a	$m \cdot sec^{-2}$	$ft \cdot sec^{-2}$	α	$rad \cdot sec^{-2}$ or
						$degree \cdot sec^{-2}$
Kinetic	Force	F	N	lb		
	Torque				T	$N \cdot m$ or $ft \cdot lb$

Table 13.2   **BASIC BIOMECHANICAL VARIABLES**

Variable	Description
Linear displacement	A vector describing how far an object moves in space in a particular direction along a straight line
Angular displacement	A vector quantifying how far a lever has rotated relative to a reference or baseline position over time
Linear distance	A scalar describing the total movement of a body point between two positions along the arc of its path of travel (not necessarily along a straight line); the magnitude of distance and displacement are equal when the point moves in a straight line between the two positions
Angular distance	A scalar describing the total rotational motion of a body segment about a joint between two positions; the magnitude of distance and displacement are equal when the segment is rotating in the same direction between the two positions (e.g., if a segment rotates $1\frac{1}{4}$ revolutions, the distance would be 450° (360 + 90), but the displacement would be 90° (90 + 0)
Velocity	A vector reflecting the rate of change in displacement measured in a particular direction; describes how fast an object moves along a straight line between two positions (linearly) or how fast a lever rotates about an axis in a particular direction (angularly); calculated by dividing displacement by time
Speed	A scalar accounting for how fast an object or lever is moving without regard to direction; determined by dividing distance (either linear or angular) by time
Acceleration and deceleration	A vector representing an object's increase or decrease in velocity, respectively; values are directly related to the force applied to the object or the torque applied to the lever; no related scalar
Gravitational acceleration	A force responsible for bringing an object traveling in an upward direction back to earth, because it constantly pulls against the object's motion; symbolized by g
Mass	The amount of matter an object possesses within its physical boundaries; the denser the material that makes up the object, the greater the mass
Center of mass	The theoretical point at which an object's mass, or weight, is said to be concentrated; in practice, because mass is distributed throughout the body, the point where balance is achieved
Weight	A measure representing the gravitational attraction of the earth; directly related to the object's mass
Inertia	The resistance an object offers to a change in its state of motion (velocity) or direction of motion; directly related to its mass
Force	A vector that is directly proportional to the acceleration of an object; affected by the object's mass
Torque	A vector equal to the amount of force applied to a lever multiplied by the shortest (or perpendicular) distance the force's line of action; acts from the fulcrum or axis of rotation of the lever
Angular momentum	A vector reflecting the quantity of rotational motion established around an axis; the product of rotational inertia (calculated from the mass, length, and mass distribution of a lever) and angular velocity
Linear momentum	The product of mass and velocity
Work	The product of the applied force and the distance moved by an object
Power	Work done per unit of time
Energy	The capacity to do work
Kinetic energy	Energy by virtue of an object's motion.
Potential energy	Energy generated by virtue of the position or shape of an object
Pressure	Concentration of force at any given point on the object; affected by the area over which the applied force is distributed

The vertical displacement is measured along the vertical axis and indicates how high or low the infielder must reach to catch the ball relative to the release height of the ball by the outfielder. The maximum vertical height of the ball's arc during its flight is called the apex and is measured along the vertical axis to determine how high the ball traveled in the air above the release point. By accounting for the height above the ground at release of the ball, it is possible to quantify how high in the air the ball was at its apex.

It is relatively simple to predict and quantify numerous aspects of a projectile's flight if one assumes that no air resistance affects the object while it is traveling through its arc. This is, of course, not a typical, real-world situation, but one that would occur only in a vacuum. It does, however, greatly simplify the mathematics required to describe projectile motion. Thus, for the following examples, we'll assume that there is no air resistance. Therefore, the only external force that must now be accounted for is that produced vertically by gravity.

Gravity has no effect on horizontal or lateral motions of a projectile, only vertical motion. Gravity acts as a constant accelerator or decelerator of a projectile, exerting a constant change in velocity of -9.8 m/sec/sec, or m $\cdot$ sec^{-2} (-32.2 ft /sec/sec, or ft $\cdot$ sec^{-2}). This means that a pro-

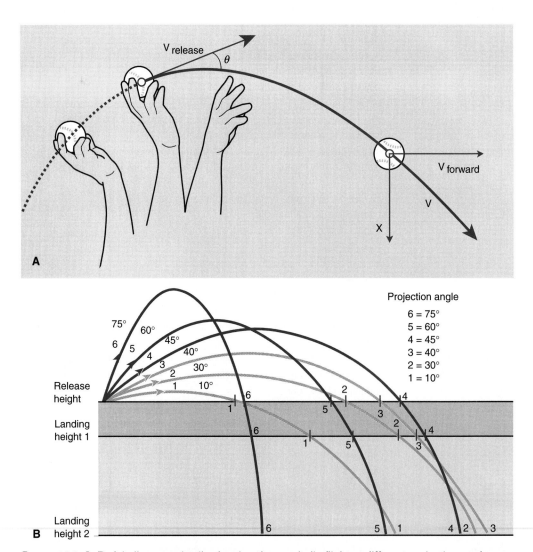

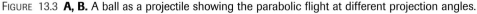

FIGURE 13.3 **A, B.** A ball as a projectile showing the parabolic flight at different projection angles.

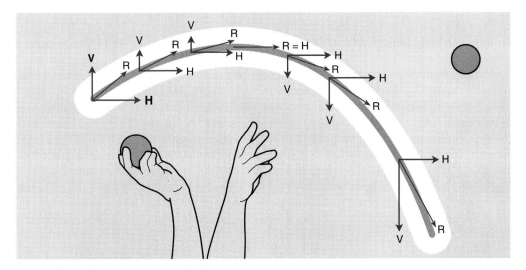

FIGURE 13.4 Changes in resultant (**R**) and vertical (**V**) velocity components during parabolic flight.

jectile's velocity is constantly changing in a vertical direction, either slowing down (if the object is ascending) or speeding up (if the object is descending). Horizontally and laterally there are no accelerations present, because air resistance has been eliminated; under these conditions, the projectile will remain at the same velocity in these directions throughout its flight.

Under the conditions set forth above, a projected object will travel along a **parabolic path** during its flight. A *parabola* is a geometric term for a curve that is symmetrical along its apex. This means the area of each side is equal; and if folded along a vertical line drawn through the apex, each side is identical in shape. Numerous predictions regarding the flight of the object can be made if one assumes parabolic flight and the symmetry of the resulting arc (Fig. 13.4).

Referring to the earlier example of the baseball players throwing and catching a ball, it would be assumed under parabolic flight conditions that the ball, once released by the outfielder at some angle to the horizon with some velocity, would travel horizontally to the infielder without any change in its horizontal velocity. Vertically, however, the ball would constantly slow down along its upward arc until reaching zero velocity at the apex of its flight, whereupon, it would immediately begin to travel along a downward arc while constantly increasing in vertical velocity.

The decrease in velocity during the ascent phase of the arc can be explained by understanding that gravity pulls downward with a constant force on the ball, which has been released with a small upward velocity. In other words, gravity acts in *opposition* to the ball's initial momentum, which was supplied by the outfielder. This force decreases the ball's velocity by -9.8 m $\cdot$ sec^{-2} for every second it is traveling upward. The faster the ball is traveling in an upward direction at release by the outfielder, the longer it will take gravity to halt the ball's upward motion to zero at the apex of the arc. As the ball passes through the apex of the arc, it immediately begins to descend back to earth. Gravity continues to exert force on the ball, causing it to reverse from ascension to descension. Now that the ball is traveling downward, gravity acts *with* the ball's motion, or momentum, causing it to increase in velocity in a downward direction over time.

The success of the throw ultimately depends on the ball's release velocity and angle of projection as provided by the outfielder during the force application of the throwing motion. If the outfielder predicts these two variables accurately and is able to generate just the right amount of effort along the correct line, the ball will arrive on time to tag out the base runner. However, if the outfielder predicts either incorrectly, the base runner's chance of advancing to the next base is improved.

Ground Reaction Forces

Ground reaction forces (GRFs) are forces applied on a person by the ground or other surface with which the person's body is in contact. These forces are applied as an equal and opposite reaction force to the force applied to the surface by the person. The more force generated by the performer onto the contact surface, as a result of body weight and musculoskeletal activity, the more force the surface returns to the performer. GRFs are typically measured in relation to a 3-D cartesian coordinate system oriented to the surface. The GRF planes are generally termed as follows: anteroposterior (AP) for forces directed forward and backward, mediolateral (ML) for forces directed left and right, and vertical for forces directed upward and downward. The GRFs are, of course, opposite to the force applied by the performer on the surface. In other words, if the person pushes downward on the surface, the surface reacts by pushing upward with equal but opposite force. If the person pushes backward on the surface, the surface pushes forward with an equal but opposite forward force. If the person pushes rightward on the surface, the surface pushes leftward with equal but opposite force.

Examples of some surfaces on which GRFs have been measured and reported in the scientific biomechanics literature are the ground, gymnasium floor surfaces, aerobic room floor surfaces, track surfaces, gymnastics bars, gymnastics landing mats, pitcher's mounds, tennis courts, and diving platforms. Forces are typically measured directly with a computerized force-measuring platform or strain gauges and indirectly through the use of accelerometers.

To explain how GRFs affect performance, consider a simple sports performance with a simple explanation focusing on force production. A standing horizontal jump is a fairly common activity in physical education settings. It requires the person to exert forces on the ground that allow the body to travel forward from the starting position through the air to a landing or finishing position. Typically, the distance from the toes at takeoff to the heels at landing are measured horizontally along the ground to determine how far the person jumped.

To maximize the horizontal displacement of the body, it is necessary for the jumper to push downward and backward with great force. The ground, in turn, pushes equally and oppositely on the performer's body. The ground, by virtue of the earth's great mass, does not move as the jumper pushes on it. Therefore, virtually all of the energy generated by the jumper's musculoskeletal system onto the ground is returned to the body as the air phase of the jump begins. The faster the jumper is traveling at takeoff in a horizontal and vertical direction, the further and higher the body will travel through the air phase to landing. The purpose of the vertical force is to generate vertical velocity, which ultimately provides the time necessary for the body to travel through a substantial air phase before landing. The horizontal force that generates horizontal velocity during the jump provides the forward momentum of the body necessary to displace it from one position to another. The combination of horizontal and vertical force applied to the ground generates an **angle of takeoff** of the body for the jump. Too much vertical effort creates a large takeoff angle, which allows the body to travel high, but not far horizontally. Too much horizontal force creates a very low angle or trajectory of the body, which does not provide a sufficient air phase to allow for horizontal travel. Obviously, the jumper must find the optimum angle of takeoff if the horizontal displacement is to be maximized.

Finally, when a jumper is attempting to propel the body vertically as in the above example or in a vertical jump, it is necessary to generate forces on the ground that exceed the body weight. When the jumper is standing perfectly still on the surface of a force-measuring platform, the platform records a force equal to the jumper's weight. However, when the jumper begins to move the body into the preparation phase of the jump by performing a dynamic partial squat, the force platform readings change. The change is a reflection of the acceleration or deceleration the body is now experiencing as a result of muscular contractions that are preparing the body for the jump (Fig. 13.5).

As the jumper first begins the preparation phase, the vertical GRF falls below the body weight. This is said to be the unweighting portion of the jump phase, which allows the body to begin moving downward in preparation for the upward movement phase. As the performer be-

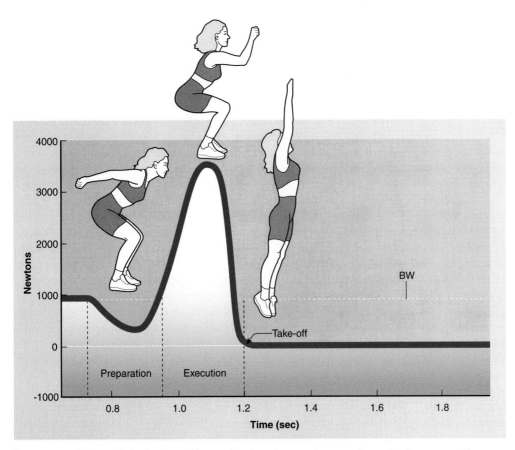

FIGURE 13.5 Phases of the horizontal jump showing changes in ground reaction forces over time generated by a force platform.

gins to push downward with great energy, the force must exceed the body weight if upward movement is to occur. The greater the ability of the jumper to produce forces above his or her body weight during this phase of the jump, the faster the jumper will be traveling vertically at takeoff and, therefore, the higher he or she will travel.

The amount of force above the body weight is generated by the musculoskeletal system. Characteristics necessary for producing these vertical GRFs are strength, muscle fiber type, coordination, and mechanical technique. Great jumpers like Michael Jordan (basketball star), Julius Erving (basketball star), Carl Lewis (Olympic track and field star), and Michael Powell (Olympic track and field star) displayed all of these characteristics: They were able to generate GRFs during their respective jumping phases that were two or more times greater than their body weight. The vertical jumpers, Jordan and Erving, would generate greater vertical forces because they needed to rise to a higher position to dunk a basketball. The horizontal jumpers, Lewis and Powell, generated lesser vertical forces during their jumping phases, because their primary goal was to travel horizontally. Of course, an additional factor that affected Lewis's and Powell's ability to generate vertical force is the fact that they were running at a world-class sprint speed when they performed their jumping phase.

Kinetic Link Principle

Coordination of body movements in sporting skills is critical for success. Many terms are used to refer to coordination: *good timing, smooth movements, effortless,* and *great skill.* Each of these terms simply means that the body's nervous system is finely tuned for stimulating the body's musculature to contract with appropriate intensity or to relax at just the right time to produce the necessary joint rotations required for a successful performance. Without this timing between the nervous and muscular systems, the skeletal system motions that result would be less effective or efficient.

Highly skilled athletes often make very complex sports skills look effortless, when, in fact, these activities can be challenging in one or more of the following requirements for success: force production (e.g., weightlifting), velocity production (e.g., sprinting, pitching, golf club swinging), specific pattern of body motions and/or positions achieved (e.g., diving, gymnastics), and conservation of energy while moving at a relatively fast velocity (e.g., distance running, cycling). Novices are often fooled by their observations of an elite athlete into believing that they, too, can perform these skills at a proficient level, because the skilled athlete does make it look effortless.

Biomechanists note that skilled athletes possess an ability to capitalize on the body's kinetic link system. This is a technical term for coordination and refers to the fact that the body segments are linked together and must create well-timed movements by virtue of muscle contractions if the performance is to be appropriate. There are two basic principles that guide the body's kinetic link system: sequential movements and simultaneous movements of the body segments.

The **sequential kinetic link principle** basically means segmental motions or joint rotations occur in a specific sequence so that time elapses between the peak rotational velocities of each involved segment (Fig. 13.6A). This coordinated effort typically leads to high velocity or momentum of the last segment involved in the performance. In sports skills in which the sequential kinetic link is employed for success, the energy or momentum flows from the core of the body (typically the trunk) to the appendages of the body (the leg segments to the foot or the arm segments to the hand). This flow is from the body's more massive segments to its least massive segments. The building of momentum in the bigger, slower segments (trunk and upper legs) of the body leads to effective transferral of momentum to the smaller, faster moving segments. In other words, failure to use the trunk appropriately adversely affects the velocity with which a ball is thrown; a club, bat or racket is swung; or a ball is kicked.

The **simultaneous kinetic link principle** dictates that major body motions occur within the same time period so that no observable difference in time exists between the contributions of the involved segments to the performance (Fig. 13.6B). This type of movement is generally employed when the athlete is challenged to move objects or his or her body, both of which offer great resistance.

Baseball pitching is a prime example of a sequential kinetic link activity. This complex skill requires the lower body to produce its actions first, followed by the lower trunk, the upper trunk, the upper arm, the lower arm, the hand, and finally, the fingers. If you can imagine attempting to throw a heavy object (such as a 16-lb shot) in the same manner as a baseball pitcher would throw a baseball, it is not hard to picture the seriousness of the injury the thrower would suffer to either the elbow or the shoulder (or both) of the throwing arm. The injury would be suffered as a result of the large torques applied to the joints by the massive object as each segment makes its individual contribution to the performance during its time phase. In the simultaneous kinetic link of shot-put activity, the athlete uses more of a pushing motion than a throwing motion to accelerate the object.

The difference between a throw and push is the timing of the involvement of the segments. During the push motion employed in the shot-put skill, virtually all major body segments are simultaneously active, so that each reaches its maximum rotational velocity at approximately the same time. This forceful movement does not allow the same magnitude of velocity to be achieved as is possible with a sound sequential application of motion, but it does allow the performer to produce the motions with much less chance for injury when accelerating a heavy object. Obviously, the stronger or more powerful the athlete, the more his or her movements can approach a sequential pattern even when moving objects of great mass. This would, of course,

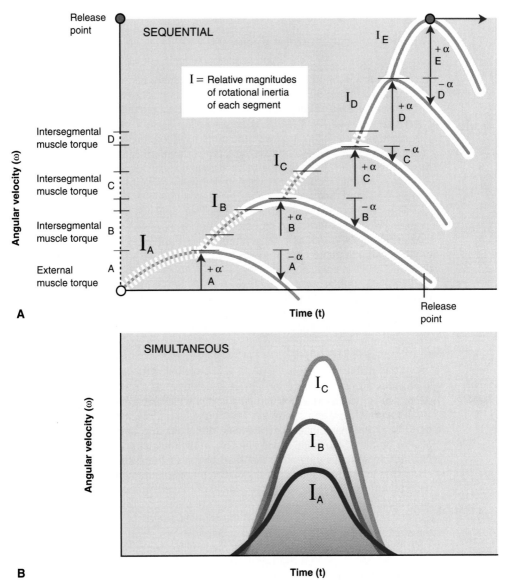

FIGURE 13.6 The (**A**) sequential and (**B**) simultaneous kinetic link principles. Notice the differences in major body motions with respect to the time axis.

be to the athlete's advantage, provided the motion can be achieved in a repeated fashion with little, if any, lasting trauma to the body.

There are activities that employ the best qualities of both the sequential and simultaneous kinetic link principles for the production of athletic performance. Some activities require both the production of great force to move a massive object (such as the body) and the production of high velocity (e.g., to propel or swing an object). The tennis serve is a great example of this.

To serve a tennis ball with great velocity and accuracy, it is necessary first to move the mass of the body forward and upward in the direction of the tossed ball and the net. This action requires a simultaneous action from the lower body in somewhat of a modified jumping activity, which also must begin the momentum transfer to the upper body. Once the jumping action has been completed, the simultaneous activities of the upper body begin, with the first contribution

A Case in Point 13.1

SQUAT LIFT: THE KING OF EXERCISES

In traditional weight training, the squat has long been considered the ultimate activity for building the body. This exercise recruits most of the major muscles of the trunk and lower body and, therefore, elicits an effective, near-total body resistance workout. The squat is generally performed with a barbell resting on the upper back/trapezius area with the arms used for collateral support. The lifter places the feet approximately shoulder width apart with the toes facing forward and slightly lateral to the body. The goal of the lift is to squat with the weights supported by the upper back to an overall lower body position (the descent phase) and then return to the starting position (the ascent phase) by standing. The depth to which the lifter descends depends on many factors, including skill, fitness level, and purpose for performing the activity as part of an overall conditioning program. Most lifters are encouraged to descend to a depth between a quarter squat (upper legs do not reach a parallel position to the floor) and a parallel squat (upper legs parallel to the floor). The muscles used in these squats are essentially the same, but the range of motion at the major joints involved in the lifts are different. In the quarter squat, the trunk forward inclination and knee angle at the bottom of the descent phase are considerably less than in the parallel squat. The parallel squat is, therefore, more challenging to the muscles and joints, causing a greater training effect to be produced but also increasing the potential for injury to the low back and knees.

From a standing position, the lift is characterized by moving the hip and knee joints through flexion, moving the ankles through dorsiflexion, and maintaining as vertical a trunk position as possible while descending. The descent should be very slow and controlled. The control is the result of eccentric contractions of the major extensor muscles of the trunk, hip, and knee, and the plantar flexors of the ankle assist primarily in the maintenance of balance. As the lifter approaches the end of the descent phase, these same muscles increase the intensity of their contractions as the momentum of the descent is halted and then reversed. With the reversal of motion, the ascent phase begins and concentric contraction of the muscles are now controlling the joints as each are extending. The extension of these joints, therefore, leads to a return to the standing posture from which the lift began.

The two most serious lifting errors made while performing this activity are descending too rapidly and allowing the trunk to flex too far forward during the descent phase. Descending too rapidly is ill-advised, because it allows an excessive amount of momentum or kinetic energy to be generated, which the muscles

---

from the lower trunk followed by the upper trunk, shoulder, elbow, wrist, and racket. Ideally, contact with the ball is made when the racket, as an extended segment of the hand, is at its maximum forward velocity. The result is a serve that, for a power server, may be in the range of 120 miles per hour (mph). A testimony to the capabilities of an elite athlete to effectively employ the kinetic link principle is the fastest serve ever recorded during a competitive tennis match: 142.5 mph, by the Australian Mark Philippoussis.

Basic Biomechanical Analysis of Movement Activities

This section discusses two skills often studied in sports biomechanics. A Case in Point 13.1 presents a biomechanical analysis of a major resistance exercise.

A Case in Point 13.1 (continued)

may not be able to overcome when challenged to halt and then reverse this motion. The faster the lifter is descending, the more muscle force is required to reverse the direction. If the athlete is lifting at a resistance close to his or her maximum or if the athlete is fatigued, it is likely that he or she will not be able to complete the ascent phase successfully or, at worst, may be injured.

When the lifter allows the trunk to flex too far forward, the forces occurring in the low back are greatly increased compared to a more upright posture. The reason for this is owing to principles of **leverage,** as discussed in Chapter 12. The trunk can be considered a lever, with a fulcrum or rotational axis formed in the lumbar (low back) area of the vertebral column. When this lever is rotated forward into flexion, the line of action of the resistive force of the barbell, not to mention the trunk weight itself, is moved from an orientation directly through the vertebral bodies to one very far forward of them.

The shifting of the line of action of the resistive forces to this extreme position causes the torque (force of the weight of the barbell and trunk–head segment times the distance from this line to the lumbar vertebrae) to increase greatly. With the increased torque, the type and magnitude of forces applied to the cartilaginous vertebral disks (in between the bony vertebral bodies) are radically different from the forces applied when the person is standing erect. Generally, the anterior portion of two adjacent vertebral bodies (e.g., L4 and L5) are forced together, a **compressive force,** while the posterior aspect of these same bones are forced apart by a tensile force.

The intervertebral disk, which acts as a buffer between these bones, is greatly affected by the condition. The compressive force applied anteriorly forces the disk's fluid core posteriorly toward the aspect of the disk that is allowed to bulge by virtue of the gap formed by the tensile force applied to the posterior aspect of the lower vertebral column. If the walls of this disk have been weakened as a result of cumulative trauma from poor biomechanics in lifting and other lumbar-intensive activities, a bulge or rupture of the disk may occur. This may lead to moderate to severe low back and leg pain, because nerves commonly are impinged owing to the disk's bulging. Surgery is often required to relieve the associated pain.

Sprinting

The elite sprinter is genetically endowed with high percentages of fast-twitch muscle fibers in the lower body muscles that are most critical for success in sprinting: the gluteal, quadriceps, and hamstring muscle groups. When combined with excellent coordination, these fast-twitch muscles enable the sprinter to move the segments of the lower body at high velocities with power and proper timing. These genetically endowed athletes fine-tune their skills with innovative training techniques that allow them to get the most from the way their body is structured.

In sprinting, angular motion is translated into linear motion by the movement of the body's limbs.

Sprinting is characterized by two major phases: the support phase, during which high muscle forces are generated to accelerate or maintain the sprinter's velocity, and the swing phase, during which the runner is airborne and the leg segments are in recovery, one preparing to strike the ground and the other beginning to swing forward from a position behind the body. A sprinter's leg spends approximately 40% of its time (~ 0.10 sec) in the support phase; the remaining time is spent in the swing phase (~ 0.13 sec). Sprinters displaying significantly greater percentages of swing time are likely to be considered overstriders. This overstriding typically results in slower running velocities. This may best be explained by considering the following simple biomechanical equation for calculating sprinting velocity of the body:

$$\text{horizontal velocity} = \text{stride rate } (SR) \times \text{stride length } (SL)$$

where **stride rate** is the number of strides taken per unit of time (typically per second) and **stride length** is the distance as measured along the ground between foot positions at takeoff and landing for the same foot. For an elite male sprinter, the typical stride length is a little greater than his height, approximately 2.5 m, and the stride rate is slightly greater than 4 strides per second (1). An elite male sprinter's maximum running velocity is $\geq 10.5 \text{ m} \cdot \text{sec}^{-1}$.

To create a high stride rate with an appropriate stride length, athletes must be able to create fast rotations of the leg segments around the joints. The upper leg must be able to rotate rapidly around the hip joint in the body's sagittal plane (the plane that divides the body into right and left halves) in both flexion and extension. The flexion motion is particularly important in the recovery of the upper leg during the swing phase, and the extension is important for moving the leg and foot to the ground. The flexion motion begins before the foot loses contact with the ground and continues until the upper leg reaches its maximum flexion position, commonly referred to by sprinters as the knee lift position. The faster this action is completed, the shorter the swing time of the leg. Provided the recovery (swing) is adequate to allow for good leg preparation for the upcoming support phase, this shortened time enhances the sprint performance.

From the point of maximum hip flexion, the upper leg rotates to the ground with the initiation of hip extension. The greater the amount of hip flexion at the end of the swing phase, the more distance the sprinter has to accelerate the upper leg into extension, which ultimately brings the foot to the ground. This fast rotation of the upper leg around the hip joint will enable better landing mechanics of the foot. If the fast rotation of the hip extension can be maintained as the support phase continues, the sprinter is able to accelerate at a higher rate or maintain running velocity while requiring a shorter time of the foot on the ground. In the latter case, the shorter time on the ground enables the runner to increase the stride rate.

Research has shown that the best sprinters in the world tend to have greater stride rates than very good sprinters, although they have fairly equal stride lengths (2). The best athletes accomplish these actions through superior coordination and a high proportion of fast-twitch muscle fibers in the primary sprinting muscle groups. Less accomplished sprinters typically demonstrate significant losses of hip extension velocity during the support phase. As a result, this class of sprinter must prolong the support phase to maintain their running velocity. In other words, less skilled sprinters lack the explosive muscle power and/or neuromuscular coordination to generate the necessary ground forces quickly; therefore, they must maintain their force production for a longer period of time. The longer they keep their foot on the ground, the lower their stride rate becomes, adversely affecting sprint performance.

In addition to the actions at the hip, the knee also plays a vital role in sprint performance. To enhance recovery of the leg from the takeoff position until foot contact, the knee joint must be flexed to an extreme angle and maintained there for a substantial portion of the swing phase. Shortly after takeoff with the hip flexing, the knee flexes, bringing the heel close to the buttocks. This action serves to shorten the leg lever, making it easier for the hip flexor muscles to swing the leg forward into a high knee lift position. If this angle is maintained for much of the middle portion of the leg swing phase and combined with near maximum muscle activity from the hip flexors, the time of leg swing is greatly diminished compared to a comparable effort with an incomplete knee flexion or a premature knee extension. Incomplete knee flexion is often associated with the mechanics of poorer sprinters or fatigue. Premature knee extension from an otherwise proper knee flexion position is also often associated with fatigue.

For an example of premature knee extension on the part of good sprinters, consider how the swing mechanics of the leg change over the course of a 400-m sprint. Early in the race, the sprinters are fresh and are better able to maintain a small knee angle, but during the last 100 m of the race, they are somewhat fatigued and the knee angle increases. Sprint velocity decreases significantly during the last portion of the race, owing in part to the poor swing mechanics of the leg, which then adversely affect many other aspects of proper sprinting mechanics.

Just before ground impact of the foot, the hamstring muscles contract forcefully to halt the knee extension that occurs at the end of the swing phase. The action of the hamstrings causes knee flexion to occur, and this continues through the early portions of the support phase. In combination with the hip extension, the knee flexion reduces the **braking force** (decelerating force) that occurs when the foot strikes the ground (Fig. 13.7).

The braking force is a result of a forward-moving foot at initial ground impact. The more successful the sprinter is at rapidly extending the hip and flexing the knee from the high knee lift position until ground impact, the less the braking force will be. Because they perform these actions effectively, the very best sprinters typically have lower braking forces than poorer sprinters. This means their foot does not kick the ground as hard in a forward direction because they are more effective at sweeping the leg in a backward direction after the maximum knee lift position. Obviously, lower braking forces mean less deceleration of the body with each foot contact. This means the better sprinter does not have to expend as much energy or as much time as the poorer sprinter to overcome this mechanical inefficiency in sprint performance.

Overhand Baseball Pitch

The primary biomechanical goal of the baseball overhand fastball pitch is to throw a ball at near maximum horizontal velocity with accuracy. Although there are numerous styles of pitching wind-ups, there is one basic style for the delivery phase of the overhand pitch (when the ball is accelerated to the release point). A fastball pitch is an example of an activity that relies more on great coordination than strength. Pitchers typically have higher proportions of fast-twitch muscle fibers, because the movement speeds required to throw a ball at greater than 90 mph are quite

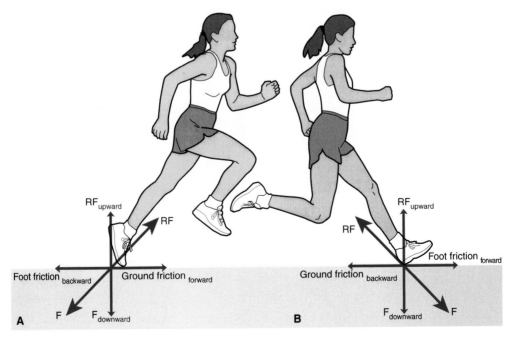

Figure 13.7 Sprinting technique.

high. However, these high speeds are built from a complex series of body movements rather than large muscular force production.

This complex series of body movements is characterized by the sequential nature in which the body segments contribute to the velocity of the ball. Basically, the lower body begins its contribution with the ground contact of the lead foot at the completion of the stride toward home plate. The forces created by the ground contact, when combined with the forward moving body, cause a rapid rotation of the lower trunk/pelvic area. This rotation is closely followed by the sequential movements of the upper trunk, upper arm, lower arm, and hand. When the hand reaches its maximum velocity, the ball is released. The velocity of each successive segment exceeds that of its preceding segment. In other words, each of these successive segment rotations accepts the momentum passed on by the preceding segment and adds its own momentum before passing it on to the next segment. As momentum builds with each successive segmental contribution, the kinetic energy of the ball increases and reaches a peak at the release point (Fig. 13.8).

The musculature in the lower and upper trunk, if used properly, is designed to produce forceful rotations of the massive trunk, which, when transferred to the shoulder, produces high rotational velocities of the upper arm. These initial actions in the body's "power core" are critical for producing a high ball velocity at release. By twisting the trunk early on away from the direction in which it will be rotating at release, the pitcher increases the distance over which this rotation can occur. The long rotational distance allows a greater rotational velocity to be achieved before passing the velocity onto the arm segments.

The rotational velocity of the trunk contributes significantly to the amount of upper arm or shoulder external rotation that occurs in the **cocking phase** of the pitch. As the trunk rotates rapidly toward the release point, the upper-arm segment is brought to a horizontal position in space with approximately 90° of abduction and the elbow is at 90° of flexion. The shoulder musculature is in somewhat of a passive state of activity at this point. As the lower and upper trunk segments accelerate toward their peak velocity, the arm segments are left behind through inertial lag. This lag causes the upper arm to externally rotate around the shoulder, thereby cocking the

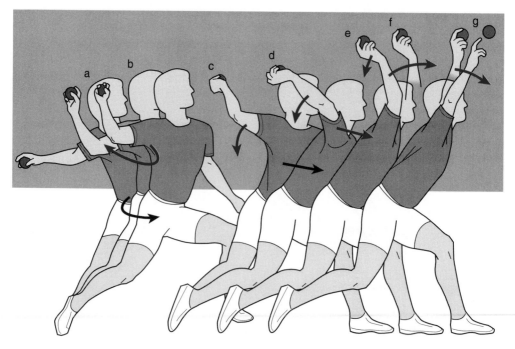

FIGURE 13.8 Overhand baseball pitch.

arm. This cocking action stimulates the anterior shoulder muscles, which fire in response to the forceful external rotation. This muscle activity is maintained as the ball begins moving toward home plate.

The ongoing muscular activity of the anterior shoulder produces a rapid internal rotation of the shoulder. Elite pitchers that throw high-speed fastballs produce peak internal shoulder rotational velocities of up to 7500°/sec. This is among the very fastest of body motions ever recorded and somewhat explains how a pitcher can achieve fastball velocities of 90 mph and more. In fact, Nolan Ryan (with the Houston Astros for many years) once threw a fastball clocked at 104 mph. These ball and arm velocities could not be achieved, however, without the important contributions of the leg and trunk segments, which lead the body in the generation of power.

The length of the body segments and the arms, in particular, are important in the generation of the pitched ball velocity. A tall pitcher with good coordination is capable of throwing a ball faster than a shorter pitcher who has an equal level of coordination. This is explained by the mechanical factors associated with a rotating lever. The end of a long lever rotating at a particular speed is moving faster linearly than the end of a shorter lever rotating at the same speed. In other words, when taller pitchers rotate their longer limbs at speeds equal to that of shorter pitchers, the ball velocity at release will be greater. It should thus not come as a surprise that taller-than-average pitchers have long dominated the ranks of Major League baseball and will likely continue to do so.

Consider how a pitcher might realistically manipulate the variables in the equation for horizontal velocity in an effort to throw the ball faster to home plate. It is necessary to keep in mind all the internal and external factors that are within the pitcher's control. Training level, technique, strength, and anthropometrics (body measures, such as height) must all be considered. Simply put, to throw the ball faster, the pitcher must be able to *(a)* apply more force to the ball, *(b)* increase the time the force is applied to the ball, *(c)* decrease the mass of the ball (against the rules), *(d)* or move the body faster as he or she strides toward the catcher. Any improvement in one or more of these areas will allow the ball to be thrown faster. The pitcher and coach would need to determine the best means by which the athlete can accomplish these performance-enhancing goals.

Finally, one must consider the biomechanical issues associated with shoulder injuries in overhand baseball pitching. Just as the pitcher must create high shoulder rotational velocities to accelerate the ball toward the catcher, he or she must create tremendously large decelerative forces to stop the internal rotation. Relatively speaking, the pitcher has a lot of time to build up the shoulder internal rotation to throw the ball with high velocity to the catcher but has little time to stop this motion so he or she can be ready to field the ball. This short time period for deceleration means the torques around the shoulder joint are quite high.

The rotator cuff is a group of relatively small muscles (supraspinatus, infraspinatus, teres major, and subscapularis) around the scapula and the rear of the shoulder that are challenged to maintain shoulder integrity and, particularly, to stop shoulder internal rotation and anterolateral separation. Because the momentum for the shoulder in regard to both the internal rotation and the anterolateral separation are high, this muscle group is challenged to the extreme with every ball thrown. As the muscles fatigue, they experience some wear and tear; injury to this muscle group occurs fairly frequently (3). If the injury is severe, it may end a pitcher's career prematurely.

ADVANCES IN SPORT BIOMECHANICS

Although numerous advancements have occurred within the science of sports biomechanics, among the most important in regard to understanding sports performance and injury prevention are the stretch–shortening cycle (elastic potential energy and contractile force of the muscles) and the kinetic link principle. These biomechanical concepts describe the interaction of muscle energy production with the movement patterns necessary to perform a sporting skill. In addition, instrumentation has played a major role in allowing this research to move forward.

Stretch–Shortening Cycle

Research into muscles' stretch–shortening cycles has allowed us to describe how the mechanics of muscle tissues affect the generation of energy and force. The stretch (eccentric) phase involves lengthening of the muscle tissues to place them on a stretch; this creates potential energy, which is released as the muscle begins the shortening phase of its action. The shortening phase is characterized by the concentric contraction of the muscles, which adds to the energy production.

The stretch–shortening cycle is a major movement component in virtually every sporting motion, particularly those that involve higher movement velocities or power production. The stretch–shortening cycle typically occurs during the transition between the preparation and execution phases of the athlete's movement. The preparation phase represents the stretching of the involved muscles, whereas the execution phase represents the shortening of the involved muscles as the body segments are accelerated. An example of this is the transition between the backswing and downswing in the golf stroke. The major hip, trunk, and arm muscles are first lengthened as the golfer prepares his or her body for the swing at the ball. As the golf club approaches a horizontal position, the golfer begins to contract the muscles in an effort to begin the shortening phase of the swing. This effort leads to the downswing, which accelerates the head of the golf club to the ball for contact.

Kinetic Link Principle

As discussed earlier, the kinetic link principle describes the mechanical coordination required for success in a movement activity. The optimum kinetic link varies from sport to sport and even among positions within a multiplayer sport. The actual movement patterns and, particularly, the movement kinematics vary from athlete to athlete performing the same skill or playing the same position. Different athletes bring different musculoskeletal and neuromuscular capabilities to the sport and, as a result, the mechanics of their techniques will differ. In some cases the differences are subtle, whereas in others they are more drastic. For example, in throwing a baseball pitch the pitcher can employ an overhand, sidearm, or submarine style delivery, all of which result in similar velocity pitches.

Research into the movement patterns required for success in sports has led to insights into the requirements for enhancing performance and has explained important aspects of injury potential. Biomechanists have explored athletes' sport techniques at all levels in an effort to discover the optimal movement patterns that lead to success. Although much has been learned about how athletes mechanically perform their skills, the challenge is to help the athletes who are performing below their potential to improve.

Instrumentation—Computer Modeling

Finally, advances in the instrumentation used to collect data in biomechanics research have allowed both the depth and the breadth of this science to expand. This instrumentation was discussed earlier; however, the role of computer software and mathematical modeling of the body was not emphasized. In recent years, tremendous advances have been made in the sophistication of 3-D computer graphics models of the body, computer-animation software, and the ability to synchronize the instrumentation used to measure performance so that in-depth measures of performance are possible. Today, biomechanists can generate humanlike, 3-D computer animations of the athlete that can be viewed from any position desired. This allows the scientist, coach, and athlete to see and measure sports performance. As these measures continue to improve and, particularly, the time to generate them decreases, sports biomechanics will play an even greater role in training the athlete.

SUMMARY POINTS

- Sports biomechanics, the combination of the sciences of applied anatomy and mechanical physics, focuses on the forces and movement techniques associated with performance enhancement and injury prevention in sports, exercise, and other motion activities.
- For a particular movement skill, the performer must determine whether the physical effort should be maximized, minimized, or optimized to afford the greatest success.
- Use of high-tech instrumentation is necessary for quantitative analysis.
- Performance of movement skills combines linear and angular motions of the body and its segments.
- Important kinematic variables in the study of human motion are linear and angular displacement, velocity, acceleration, and linear and angular momentum.
- Important kinetic variables in the study of human motion are force, torque, work, power, and pressure.
- Projectiles are airborne objects or bodies that are affected by only gravity and air resistance.
- Parabolic flight is a special category of projectile motion in which air resistance is negligible, thereby allowing the projectile to travel on a parabolic path while airborne.
- Ground reaction forces are the equal and opposite forces applied on a body by virtue of that body's interaction with a surface, such as the ground, the floor, an object, or some apparatus.
- Leverage in the human body is a combination of segmental lengths; force applications on the segments by muscles, gravity, and objects; and the length of the lever arms to the axis of rotation (joints) for each of the respective forces applied to the lever.
- Muscle contractions affect joint motions, causing body segments either to begin or to stop rotating, which, in turn, affects the linear motion of points situated along these levers.
- The sequential and simultaneous kinetic link motions of the body joints or segments generate movement of the body as a whole or objects under the control of the performer. The weight of the body or object to be propelled determines which principle is used.

REVIEW QUESTIONS

1. Define sport biomechanics.
2. Discuss the biomechanical concepts and variables of kinematics and kinetics.
3. List several sports activities for each of the following variables. In each case, the variable is the most important biomechanical principle for the production of a successful performance.
   Horizontal velocity of the body
   Vertical velocity of the body
   Horizontal velocity of an object
   Resultant velocity (combination of horizontal and vertical) of a body or object when angle of takeoff is important
   Horizontal force application involving an impact

4. For the following activities indicate which form of kinetic link is used in performing the skill and briefly discuss why.

Golf swing

Standing vertical jump

Javelin throw

Free throw (arm actions)

Overhead (military) press (arm actions)

References

1. Mann RV, Herman JA, Johnson BF, et al. The elite athlete project: sprints and hurdles. USOC technical reports 1–11, Colorado Springs, U.S. Olympic Training Center, 1982–83.
2. Mann R, Herman J. Kinematic analysis of Olympic sprint performance: men's 200 meters. Int J Sport Biomech 1985;1:151–162.
3. Dillman CJ, Fleisig GS, Andrews JR. Biomechanics of pitching with emphasis upon shoulder kinematics. J Orthop Sports Phys Ther 1993;18:402–408.

Suggested Readings

Biomechanics research at the Olympic Games, 1984–1994. Champaign, IL: Human Kinetics, 1994.

Hall SJ. Basic biomechanics. St. Louis: Mosby-Year Book, 1995.

Hay JG. The biomechanics of sports techniques. Englewood Cliffs, NJ: Prentice-Hall, 1978.

Kreighbaum E, Barthels KM. Biomechanics: a qualitative approach for studying human movement. New York: Macmillan, 1996.

14

Athletic Training

James M. Rankin

Objectives

1. Describe how athletic training is integrated into the healthcare delivery system in the United States.
2. Cite the basic principles related to the domains of athletic training.
3. Describe the principles of injury evaluation, emergency care, and treatment of athletic injuries.
4. Explain the integration of rehabilitative exercise and therapeutic modalities to return an athlete to competition.
5. Describe the education process for becoming an athletic trainer.

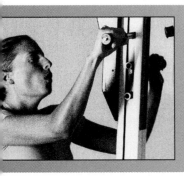

Athletic training is the allied health profession dealing with the prevention, care, and **rehabilitation** of injuries to physically active individuals. Athletic training is an interdisciplinary profession drawing on medicine, anatomy, physiology, biomechanics, exercise physiology, nutrition, pharmacology, psychology, physics, and management. Athletic training is closely aligned within its scope of practice with sports medicine, which is narrowly defined as pertaining to the assessment, emergency care, treatment, and rehabilitation of sports-related neuromuscular injuries.

> ⚷ *The American College of Sports Medicine defines sports medicine as the physiologic, pathologic, psychological, and biomechanical phenomena associated with exercise and sports.*

Athletic training began between 1900 and 1925 in the United States as a service to athletes on men's sports teams. The first athletic training text published was by a physician (1). From these origins, athletic training has evolved into a profession that practices in different clinical environments: individual and team sports in educational and professional settings, sports medicine and orthopedic clinics, and industrial settings. As a profession, athletic training is still evolving and redefining its scope of patient coverage and education standards. Athletic trainers have a limited scope of medical practice, falling under the auspices of medical (M.D.) and osteopathic (D.O.) physicians. In many jurisdictions, athletic training is defined by state practice acts within state law.

DEFINITION, DESCRIPTION, AND SCOPE

The term *athletic trainer* can be confusing. In other areas of sports, the word *trainer* has vastly different meanings. A trainer could be a boxer's coach, a racing horse's coach, a designer of individual workouts for Hollywood celebrities, or an individual instructor at the local gym. In Europe and other parts of the world, a trainer coaches team and individual sports. Athletic training is separate from training and defines an allied health profession. Figure 14.1 shows how athletic training fits within the scope of exercise science and gives the general content organization of athletic training education programs.

Athletic Medicine

Physicians and athletic trainers make up the primary athletic medicine team. The physician may be a team physician hired by the agency to supervise all aspects of medical care to the athletes at that agency or the athlete's primary care physician (family physician). The medical team approach uses a number of specialists who can provide immediate support services. Types of specialists include orthopedic surgeons, dentists, physical therapists, optometrists, podiatrists, and equipment managers (2). Related support specialists include exercise physiologists, nutritionists, sport psychologists, and substance abuse counselors. In addition, the team must work in conjunction with position coaches, athletic directors, administrators, and strength coaches

> ⚷ *The sports medicine team is headed by the physician. The athletic trainer is the on-site representative of the physician; he or she evaluates injuries, providing the physician with the information necessary to make a definitive diagnosis.*

Job Sites

Athletic trainers practice at a variety of job sites. The largest job placement area is currently in sports medicine clinics. In this clinic setting, athletic trainers are involved in the treatment and rehabilitation of injuries sustained by physically active individuals who may or may not be part

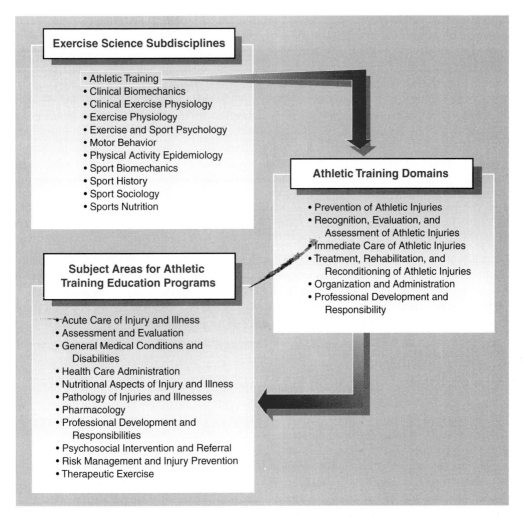

Exercise Science Subdisciplines

• Athletic Training
• Clinical Biomechanics
• Clinical Exercise Physiology
• Exercise Physiology
• Exercise and Sport Psychology
• Motor Behavior
• Physical Activity Epidemiology
• Sport Biomechanics
• Sport History
• Sport Sociology
• Sports Nutrition

Athletic Training Domains

• Prevention of Athletic Injuries
• Recognition, Evaluation, and
  Assessment of Athletic Injuries
• Immediate Care of Athletic Injuries
• Treatment, Rehabilitation, and
  Reconditioning of Athletic Injuries
• Organization and Administration
• Professional Development and
  Responsibility

Subject Areas for Athletic Training Education Programs

• Acute Care of Injury and Illness
• Assessment and Evaluation
• General Medical Conditions and
  Disabilities
• Health Care Administration
• Nutritional Aspects of Injury and Illness
• Pathology of Injuries and Illnesses
• Pharmacology
• Professional Development and
  Responsibilities
• Psychosocial Intervention and Referral
• Risk Management and Injury Prevention
• Therapeutic Exercise

FIGURE 14.1 General content organization of athletic training educational programs.

of organized sports. Many athletic trainers in clinics work in conjunction with physical or occupational therapists, orthopedic surgeons, and other medical personnel. Approximately half of clinic-based staff athletic trainers will have outreach placements in high schools that contract for athletic training services. Additional roles for clinical athletic trainers include marketing, administration, and owning a clinic.

The second largest placement area is in a secondary school as a teacher and athletic trainer. The advantage to this combination is continuity of care during the day. The athletic trainer gets to know the athlete and can work with him or her at other times during the day than practice. The disadvantage is the athletic trainer is working two full-time jobs.

The third largest site is at colleges and universities, which employ slightly less than 10% of trainers. There are many practical reasons why entry-level athletic trainers prefer this setting, including shared interests with the athletes, the chance to work with fast-healing bodies in excellent physical condition, and the high level of athletes' compliance with physician's orders and rehabilitation programs. The job market in colleges is stagnant at this time; few or no new jobs are being created. However, there is a greatly expanding market for athletic trainers with doctoral degrees who can become members of the teaching faculty and direct athletic training education programs.

The job market is limited in professional sports; only 1% of all athletic trainers are hired by professional teams. Unfortunately, until the women's professional basketball leagues were formed, few women worked at any level of professional sports, and none was employed in the principal organizations of men's professional team sports in the United States. There have been women in minor league ice hockey and the Continental Basketball Association (in which half the teams once had female athletic trainers).

Finally, job placement is expanding in the industrial setting; the athletic trainer practices on employees who are physically active at their job sites. The athletic trainer in the corporate setting is the go-between for employees (athletes), supervisors (coaches), and plant physicians (team physicians). Businesses and corporations are adding athletic trainers to their work sites, because it is cost effective to treat and rehabilitate workers within the facility; this setup decreases both lost time and lost productivity.

Domains of the Body of Knowledge

The body of knowledge making up the core of athletic training has been divided into six domains by the National Athletic Trainers' Association (NATA) Board of Certification, Inc.: prevention of athletic injuries; recognition, **evaluation,** and assessment of athletic injuries; immediate care of athletic injuries; treatment, rehabilitation, and reconditioning of athletic injuries; organization and administration; and professional development and responsibility (3).

Prevention of Athletic Injuries

Exercise and sports activities carry the inherent danger of injury at any time. One of the main duties of an athletic trainer is to ensure that the competitive environment is as safe as it is humanly possible to make it. The single most important part of **injury prevention** is for the participant to be fit before engaging in the sports or activity. Preparticipation physical examinations given by physicians qualify individuals for the physical demands of the activity. These examinations may even uncover old injuries from participation in another environment.

Athletic trainers need to take the time to inform physically active people that injury can happen at any time and in any place. Prevention is as much the responsibility of the athlete (or worker), as it is the coach's, supervisor's, and athletic training staff's. Once an injury has occurred, it is necessary that the person and those around him or her know what **signs** and **symptoms** signify an increase in the severity of the injury and which indicate that the healing process is proceeding as expected.

Minimizing the risk of injury owing to unsafe conditions reduces the incidence of injury. Extraneous pieces of equipment laying on a playing surface or in a work area and broken safety and competitive equipment are inherently dangerous. Simply having two separate groups of athletes work in opposite directions on the field instead of approaching directions decreases unintended collisions. Requiring that active people wear mandated safety equipment will significantly minimize injury.

In the industrial setting, athletic trainers may spend significant time with the worker on job-specific training before a worker becomes part of the production community. Workers are instructed in proper body movements that minimize the risk of injury. Athletic trainers may also devote significant time to running work-site fitness centers, assessing body mechanics, and implementing lifetime fitness programming.

Exercising caution in adverse environmental conditions is an extremely important way to reduce risk. Heat illness, cold injury, air pollution, and **circadian dysrhythmia** are real problems. Every year, between 5 and 10 U.S. high school football players die from **heat stroke** during August practices in a hot environment. Heat stroke is a preventable situation when reasonable care is shown. Those most at risk are overfat, underconditioned young males in areas of the country where both high temperature and high humidity are a problem.

Recognition, Evaluation, and Assessment of Athletic Injuries

In collegiate, high school, and professional settings, athletic trainers are the eyes and ears of physicians at practice and competition sites. It would not be practical to employ a physician to attend practices and competitions for all sports. When an injury occurs, the athletic trainer is most likely the first person to intervene. A systematic approach to injury evaluation is critical, including creating a comprehensive written record for communication with physicians and other sports medicine team personnel. The athletic trainer then communicates the results of the evaluation to the supervising physician who incorporates this information into a definitive diagnosis. Athletic trainers act as the bridge between physicians and athletes (or workers), coaches (or supervisors), and families and often between the athletic program and the media concerning the extent of injury to a particular athlete. Athletic trainers must possess current certification in cardiopulmonary resuscitation (CPR) from the American Red Cross, the American Heart Association, or the National Safety Council (4). In addition, first aid certification is strongly encouraged.

There are a number of injury evaluation systems in use that all have certain elements in common. A **primary survey,** either formal or informal, is completed first. This is followed by a **secondary survey,** which evaluates the specific complaint of the athlete (Fig. 14.2). Care must be taken at all times to avoid exposure to **bloodborne pathogens** from contact with blood and other bodily fluids when performing an evaluation or first aid procedure (5). Occupational Safety and Health Administration (OSHA) guidelines require that athletic trainers use latex gloves and proper disposal and cleanup procedures any time blood or other fluids are present. Athletic trainers are considered category I for risk of exposure to hepatitis B and HIV. This means trainers are required to have been immunized against hepatitis B or must have signed a waiver declining the protection.

When an athlete is unconscious, a primary survey is required, which includes assessing the ABCs (airway, breathing, and circulation). The emergency medical service (EMS) needs to be activated and notified of the level of emergency. CPR, rescue breathing, or careful monitoring of an unconscious individual is initiated, depending on the circumstances. Practical Application 14.1 points out the importance of proper assessment of the unconscious athlete.

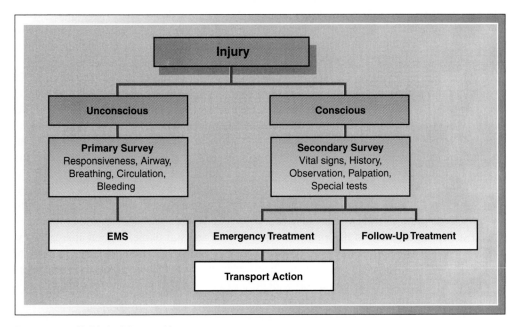

FIGURE 14.2 Field decision-making process.

Practical Application 14.1

CATASTROPHIC INJURY AND UNQUALIFIED PERSONNEL

During a high school football game, a wide receiver made top-of-the-head to top-of-the-head contact with the defensive player tackling him. When the pile cleared, the player was face down and not moving. A teammate lifted the unconscious player's arm and dropped it. The teammate then used the arm to roll the player over. The coach came over to the player, and without any evaluation of the injury, removed the player's helmet. The player is now quadriplegic.

What would an athletic trainer have done differently? Were the teammate and coach negligent in their actions? Would an athletic trainer have made a difference in the final outcome?

Athletic trainers have been trained to deal with catastrophic situations. First an athletic trainer would conduct a formal primary survey—assessing the ABCs—and then check for possible severe bleeding. If the athletic trainer ascertained that the athlete was in a life-threatening situation, he or she would have immediately contacted emergency medical service. If the athlete regained consciousness during the wait for transportation, the athletic trainer would have calmed the athlete and kept him in the same position until the emergency medical technicians could put an extraction collar on him.

Would the athlete be quadriplegic today if the athletic trainer had taken these steps? Obviously, that cannot be established; however, it is certain that the athlete had no chance of escaping quadriplegia because of the way his injury was handled.

If the injured athlete is conscious, a primary survey is still a necessary part of an athletic trainer's thought process. The survey can be as simple as noting that owing to talking or screaming, for example, there is obviously an open airway and the athlete is breathing. Depending on the injury, careful monitoring of the athlete's level of consciousness may still be an important consideration in overall management.

Once the primary survey is completed, the secondary survey is conducted. This begins with taking an **injury history.** What happened, when, and how are important for obtaining an accurate diagnosis from the physician later. The athletic trainer must determine if the athlete had ever injured that body part before and learn the outcome of any previous injury. This information has a bearing on any structural and functional testing done on the new injury site. If at any point the results indicate an unfavorable outcome from further testing, the evaluation should be terminated, and transportation of the athlete to an appropriate medical facility should be initiated.

After the history (or perhaps during the history), the athlete's body language is observed. This is followed by a more formal **observation** of the injured area; the athletic trainer is looking for obvious deformities and any change in skin color and/or shape and size of various structures. The next step is **palpation** of the injured area, both bone and soft tissue. A good approach is to first ask the athlete to point to the most painful area. Then the athletic trainer begins to touch the body part away from the most painful area, finally arriving last at the site of greatest discomfort. The touch sensation establishes a rapport with the person and suggests to the athlete that the athletic trainer is not attempting to hurt him or her.

Special testing is often done to establish the structural and functional integrity of an injured body area. Initially, circulation beyond the injury site, response to touch, and ability to activate muscle are assessed. When all of these have been found normal, the **range of motion** (ROM) of the injured area is tested in three successive stages: active range of motion, passive range of motion, and resistive range of motion. In active range of motion testing, the athlete moves the body part in response to the athletic trainer's commands. Next, the athletic trainer moves the body part, comparing what the person will do willingly and what the athletic trainer can do when antagonistic muscles are relaxed (passive ROM). Finally, the athlete again moves the injured body part through the normal range of motion, but this time against manual resistance supplied by the athletic trainer (resistive ROM).

The examination proceeds to special tests, usually specific structure tests designed to identify the presence of injury. The tests chosen will be based on all previous information obtained during the evaluation. Should these be normal, the injured person is subjected to functional testing, i.e., activity-specific movements to determine if the person may safely return to full activity. For these (and all other tests) bilateral comparisons are made to take into account the variability found in individual people.

When an injury evaluation is complete, the athletic trainer must either release the person to return to activity (mild injuries), remove the athlete and refer him or her to a physician (moderate to severe injuries), or activate EMS for transportation of the athlete to the nearest appropriate facility (some severe and all potentially catastrophic injuries).

At the conclusion of the injury evaluation, the athletic trainer completes a written record. All test results should be recorded for use by the physician and other personnel for diagnosis and treatment of the injury. With a properly executed injury evaluation and therapy record, other athletic trainers can supervise rehabilitation, continuing with the rehabilitation plans developed by the original athletic trainer and physician.

When constructing a written record, it is of paramount importance that everyone who will use the record has the same understanding of the terminology used. To this end, a number of record-keeping formats have been created. Perhaps the most accepted format is known as SOAP, which stands for subjective, objective, assessment, and plan (6). Subjective information is what the athlete tells you. Much of history taking is subjective. Objective information is quantifiable. Signs, observation, palpation, and special tests all give objective information. Assessment is the professional opinion of the athletic trainer or other healthcare professional about the nature and extent of the injury. Plan includes all treatments rendered and disposition of the injury, whether referral or continued local intervention and rehabilitation.

Immediate Care of Athletic Injuries

Acute injuries are most often seen by the athletic trainer before any other healthcare professional (Fig. 14.3). The most common first aid treatment for acute musculoskeletal injuries is rest, ice, compression, and elevation, or the RICE method (see A Case in Point 14.1). Rest may mean removal from physical activity for a time or resting a particular body part by using crutches and slings. In extreme cases, physicians will enforce rest by placing the joint or bones in a cast. Ice is the most common form of cold applied to injury sites. Wrapping ice packs onto the body using elastic wraps adds the dimension of compression and helps limit swelling. After the application of cold, the person should be sent home in a compression wrap and given instructions to repeat the cold application regularly. The extremities should be elevated to allow gravity to assist in lymphatic drainage. Between 4 and 6 in. of elevation is usually enough; for example, place a bed pillow under a sprained ankle.

When a primary survey is performed it may be necessary to initiate rescue breathing or CPR. Athletic trainers must be certified in CPR (and all coaches should be as well), because there have been many reported incidents of high school, college, and professional athletes suffering undiagnosed cardiovascular defects that lead to death. Any athletic training setting must have an **emergency care plan.** Such a plan will not prevent injuries; however, a well thought out and executed plan will greatly limit secondary injury caused by inappropriate movement, treatment, or

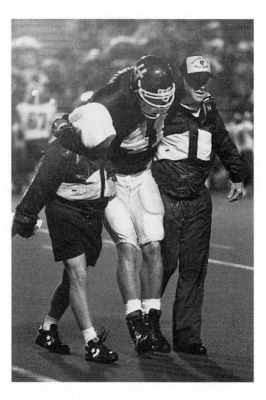

FIGURE 14.3 Acute injury.

time spent activating EMS. The emergency care plan should be a written document that emphasizes the roles, personnel, and equipment that are required to triage an injury and begin emergency first aid.

Emergency medical system personnel are not always at sporting events in a "stand-by
mode" to take over life-threatening injuries. Usually, the athletic trainer is the first qualified person to respond. In situations in which there is an on-field injury and the athletic trainer responds,
the evaluation is made immediately by the athletic trainer even if EMS personnel are at the site.
Once the athletic trainer makes the decision to involve them, EMS personnel take charge of the
care of the injured athlete.

Former NATA president Barton once stated that if an athletic trainer practices at the college
or university setting for more than 5 years, he or she will see at least one catastrophic, potentially
life-threatening situation (8). When such an injury happens, the emergency plan must be activated. The senior-ranking athletic trainer or designate should take charge and assess the patient.
Other persons will be assigned roles as needed. These roles should be practiced at least monthly,
and personnel should be able to function comfortably in more than one role, because all of the
personnel will not always be available. It is a good idea to consult with an EMS professional
while creating the plan to find out the best traffic flow plan for each area and for overall advice
on the emergency procedures.

Treatment, Rehabilitation, and Reconditioning of Athletic Injuries

The immediate effects of injury include pain, swelling, decreased range of motion, and loss of
function. These cause a period of inactivity that can lead to disuse atrophy and decreased
strength, endurance, and neuromuscular coordination. The old phrase that you "use it or lose it"
certainly applies to muscle. One NATA study looked at the effectiveness of athletic trainers in
various settings. Athletes rated their readiness to return to activity on a 1 (low) to 4 (high) scale
before and after they had seen an athletic trainer and gone through a prescribed treatment pro-

gram (7). Results indicated the average readiness to return to activity before treatment in a sports medicine clinic was 2.35; average readiness increased to 3.40 after treatment. Average readiness in high schools was 2.50 before seeing an athletic trainer and 3.72 after. Similar results were seen in college settings (2.66 before and 3.73 after) and industrial settings (2.64 before and 3.59 after).

Joints, ligaments, and bone all need intermittently applied stresses to maintain or expand their tissue content and the efficiency of their function. Cardiovascular impairments due to disuse include a decrease in heart rate of 0.5 beat per minute per day immobilized, and concurrent decreases in stroke volume, cardiac output, and respiratory function (5). To combat these problems, systematic rehabilitation involving various forms of active, passive, and resistive exercise are used. To maintain cardiorespiratory function, exercises incorporating upper body ergometers, cycling, or a swimming pool are excellent. These should be chosen to minimize stress on the injured body part while providing a total body workout.

Restoration of the normal range of motion incorporates both physiologic movements and accessory movements about a joint. Physiologic movements are those normally ascribed to a joint. Accessory movements are small movements that reposition the bones for maximum efficiency of physiologic movement. For example, flexion and extension are the physiologic movements at the knee, and anterior or posterior tibial translation and tibial rotation are accessory movements.

A Case in Point 14.1

THE ANKLE SPRAIN

A female high school basketball comes into the sports-care center in a private clinic with a 2-hr-old sprain to her right ankle; it's rated grade 2 by the on-site physician. There is a moderate amount of swelling, pain, and dysfunction. Her team is playing again the following Wednesday and against the team's biggest rival on Saturday. There is one week until the next game.

What can be done to minimize time lost and allow the athlete to play on Saturday? What must be done to safeguard the health of this athlete?

The RICE method is immediately employed after the injury. The athlete is treated for 20 min per session until that evening. She is sent home with a compression wrap and on crutches with instructions to use partial weight bearing and continue the cold every 2 hr at home until bedtime. She is instructed to sleep with her foot on a standard bed pillow.

The next day, cold treatments are resumed with the addition of mild closed kinetic chain multiaxial ankle platform. The activity is repeated once during the day, the RICE treatments continue; the physician prescribes an anti-inflammatory/analgesic medication. The level of activity on the ankle platform is increased or decreased, depending on the athlete's pain. The ankle is always treated with cold after any exercise session.

The basketball player's ankle is initially placed in an rigid air-cell-padded brace; when she can walk without a limp, the crutches are removed. At a later stage, the brace is replaced by an functional brace in conjunction with tape. Although there is great variation in the speed of healing among individuals, college-age athletes, on average, heal faster than the general population because they are young and in excellent physical condition, have good nutritional status, are goal motivated and adhere to prescribed rehabilitation programs.

Care must be exercised not to push the athlete back into participation too soon. This could delay healing or even cause further injury, such as a **stress fracture** or injury to another body part in the closed kinetic chain.

Athletic trainers assess whether range of motion is adversely affected by forces or pathology altering physiologic or accessory movements. The two are intimately related and must be properly integrated for normal function about a joint. To increase physiologic movements, large muscle activity through active, passive, and resistive range of motion is performed throughout the range of motion, stressing the end points of the range to increase the function. Accessory movements are more often restored with joint mobilization techniques.

Exercise comes in a variety of forms. Isometric exercise involves tightening a muscle, but not moving the joint through a range of motion. Strength is increased, but only for about a 15° angle around the joint position angle. Thus to get a complete workout at the shoulder for flexion (normal range 0 to 180), 12 separate exercises would need to be performed, one in each 15° arc. For some joints and activities, this is sufficient, but for many others this is extremely inefficient.

Isotonic exercise moves a joint through a range of motion and has two components: concentric and eccentric. Concentric contraction involves shortening the muscle against the force of gravity. A typical bench press or arm curl with the arm down at the side is a concentric activity. Eccentric contractions attempt to shorten the muscle, but the contractile elements are lengthened by the superior force of gravity, so the body simply controls the rate of gravity moving the mass. In a bench press, with the arm fully extended the weight is then returned toward the body in an eccentric contraction. The same muscles that pushed the weight up concentrically now lengthen to control gravity's effect and return the weight to the starting position.

Both concentric and eccentric contractions can be performed using free weights or machines. Often in rehabilitation, a weight will be moved to a position by contracting muscles in both limbs. The weight is controlled back to the starting position by eccentric contraction. In this way, greater weights can be moved eccentrically than concentrically. However, there is greater residual muscle soreness from eccentric contractions.

One type of isotonic exercise is isokinetic exercise. This allows movements at functional speeds owing to the principle of accommodating resistance. The speed of the contraction is preset and the force generated is variable at the preset speed. An advantage of isokinetic exercise is the capability to complete a full range of motion.

Closed kinetic chain activities are those that deal with the terminal segment, such as the hand or foot of a limb, in contact with an external surface. Forces are transmitted up the chain of joints to the trunk. An example of a closed chain activity is using a slide board to simulate speed skating motions during the rehabilitation of anterior cruciate ligament injuries. Proprioceptive input from the foot helps sequence motor units at appropriate forces and times. Closed chain activities have gained great popularity in physical therapy and athletic training rehabilitation programming in recent years.

In open kinetic chain activity, the terminal segments are not in contact with external surfaces. This decreases or eliminates the effect of proprioception in the terminal segment from the sensory input side of restoring function. An example of an open chain activity is using a knee extension bench where the arm is fixed to the tibia above the ankle. Proprioceptive input from the foot does not affect contraction sequences.

The recovery of proprioception, normal range of motion, and neuromuscular coordination are primary goals of the rehabilitation process. **Functional progression** is the movement from the acute **inflammation** phase to the **repair** phase to the remodeling phase and may take days to months to complete, depending on the extent and severity of an injury. The restoration of normal range of motion controlled by normal strength–power relationships is facilitated by a proper mixture of **therapeutic modalities** and therapeutic exercise. Athletic trainers need to first develop a written plan with both short- and long-term goals of the rehabilitation process, the methodology that will be used to reach the goals, and the outcomes that signify passage to the next stage of the process (see Sidelight 14.1). An athlete may be returned to competition before the completion of the rehabilitation program. This does not release the athlete from further exercise to finish the progression to full recovery.

➤➤ Sidelight 14.1

TREATMENT PLAN FOR A SPRAINED ANKLE

The following is a well-devised plan an injured athlete will follow to return to competition-level play.

SHORT-TERM GOALS
- Minimize swelling, discomfort, pain, and loss of function.
- Restore full ROM, strength, power, and endurance.
- Maintain cardiovascular and respiratory function.
- Proceed through functional progressions

LONG-TERM GOAL
- Return to competition-level of play.

TREATMENT
- Acute

   Ice bags surrounding ankle held in place with compression wrap, leg elevated for 20 min.

   Ice, compression, and elevation for 20 min every 2 hr for the following 24 hr, excluding sleep.

   Compression elastic wrap when patient leaves facility, remove to ice ankle, and replace.

   Crutches if the patient cannot walk without a limp.

- Postacute

   Tilt board, smallest ball setting, circles, and begin alphabet movements; continue cold treatments after activity.

   ROM activity; continue cold treatments after activity.

      Using towel, rubber tubing, or rubber sheeting, perform dorsiflexion, inversion, eversion, and plantar flexion.

      Stretch the gastrocnemius and soleus.

   Tilt board, increase ball settings when the activity does not induce pain; continue cold treatments after activity.

   Strengthening exercises; continue cold treatments after activity until 10 postinjury and there is no residual soreness from the rehabilitation activity.

      Tilt board with counterweights, continuing to increase ball size as indicated by pain.

      Walk in a straight line, then in large S, then in sharp-cornered Z; decrease the diameter of the S and the Z as indicated by pain.

      Jog in a straight line, then in a large S, then in a sharp-cornered Z; decrease the diameter of the S and then the Z as indicated by pain.

      Run in a straight line at half speed, then three-quarter speed, then at full speed.

      Run in a large S, then in a sharp-cornered Z at half speed, then three-quarter speed, then at full speed; decrease the diameter of the S and then the Z as indicated by pain.

      Sports-specific activity at half speed, then three-quarter speed, then full speed.

Organization and Administration

The area of organization and administration encompasses **personnel management,** facility management and design, budgeting, preparticipation physical examinations, medical record keeping, insurance, and public relations (8). Personnel management functions include the hiring and use of personnel. Decisions must first be made on the scope of coverage for a particular athletic training setting, hours of operation, and patient load before deciding how to equip and staff the facility. Managing the activity at a particular site includes decisions on who is treated and the hours of operation. Basic policies and procedures at a site may or may not be the same at all other sites in a system. Working with a budget to purchase expendable supplies and permanent equipment sometimes requires advanced imagination to cover an athletic trainer's needs.

Concern for and control of exposure to the legal system is an extremely important **health-care administration** function. Negligence is certainly a consideration in any healthcare setting. Negligence is a branch of tort law that excludes contracts but recognizes legal responsibility for harm done to others. Juries usually award damages to the injured party, most often in the form of money.

Elements of negligence: duty, breach of duty, causation, and damage.

All four elements of negligence must exist for a negligence claim to be successful. Most often breach of duty is defined as an act of commission in which the accused does something that a reasonable and careful person would not do or an act of omission in which the accused fails to do something that a reasonable and careful person would do. An example of doing something that should not be done would be moving a seriously injured athlete off the playing field at the request of the officials who wish to restart the competition while EMS is en route. An example of failing to do what is required would be allowing an athlete to return to play with only a superficial examination, missing a potentially life-threatening closed-head injury such as a severe concussion.

Defenses against negligence include the assumption of risk by the athlete for common injuries that occur within a sport; statutes of limitation, which specify a time limit to the filing of negligence actions; and waivers, which are contracts between the athlete and the administration whereby the athlete receives the right to participate in return for agreeing to hold the athletic administration blameless for injury incurred during practice and competition. Unfortunately, waivers are only as binding as the court agrees that they are. They can be found to be not in the best public interest and, therefore, declared null and void.

A large portion of legal energies in athletic training programs are directed toward risk management through prevention of athletic injuries, especially owing to unsafe conditions. Any danger that is considered foreseeable can lead to a negligence action. Knowingly allowing the use of faulty or broken equipment, allowing coaches or supervisors to teach illegal, unethical, or unsafe techniques can have similar consequences.

Medical record keeping is a critical area in any healthcare setting. Complete, accurate, and legible records inform others about the initial impression of the injury, decisions regarding referral and emergency treatment, follow-up care, and rehabilitation programs implemented. The information is used to communicate with physicians, other athletic trainers and allied medical personnel, lawyers, and insurance companies. The information is confidential without the express permission of the athlete.

Professional Development and Responsibility

The athletic trainer has a duty to maintain his or her knowledge and skills at the current standard of practice. Because this standard may change, it is important that athletic trainers continue to upgrade their skills through continuing education programs offered through a variety of outlets. In addition, athletic trainers have a duty to help educate the student athletic trainers who work with them, acting as mentors and clinical instructors. Athletic training is a profession in which classroom knowledge must be placed into practice frequently during the learning process to implant it firmly in long-term memory.

FOCUS ON SCIENCE

Once an injury takes place, the athletic trainer can have a major influence on the course of the injury through the use of therapeutic modalities. Correctly used, modalities help limit the inflammatory response to the injury and increase the rate of repair and remodeling, minimizing the time lost by the athlete. Incorrectly used, modalities may lengthen healing time or lead to further medical complications.

Common Athletic Injuries

Athletic injuries are usually either from direct trauma or from overuse. To classify injuries, the symptoms, signs, and functional significance of the trauma are evaluated. A symptom is subjective information described by the athlete. Pain is a symptom, as are nausea, lightheadedness, and dizziness. A sign is information gathered through objective assessment, such as heart rate, blood pressure, and body temperature.

Injuries lead to a loss of function or the inability to move a body part throughout a normal range of motion and against normal resistance. When someone **sprains** an ankle, swelling inhibits the range of motion. Signs, symptoms, and loss of function increase as the severity of the injury increases. Box 14.1 lists items found in a typical field kit used by athletic trainers.

Contusions (bruises) are compression injuries that range from superficial damage to deep muscle or bone bruising with significant hematoma. They are caused by a direct blow to a body part and result in pain and swelling. Skin discoloration (ecchymosis) may follow the contusion and is often characterized by a dark purple color which turns greenish yellow as healing progresses.

Strains stretch a muscle, a tendon, or muscle–tendon unit beyond normal physiologic limits. The cause of muscle strains is debatable. Certainly absorbing the outside forces generated by a collision or inappropriate placement of body parts causes some strains, but most strains are attributed to abnormal muscle contraction (5). Also, muscle fatigue before injury may be a contributing factor (9). Strains result in pain on movement, pain on stretch, and loss of function.

Strains are graded according to severity. First-degree strains involve minimal stretching or microtrauma, minimal pain, and loss of function. Second-degree strains are more extensive, with partial tearing of some tissue, moderate pain, loss of function, hematoma formation, muscle spasm, and inflammation. Third-degree strains are severe injuries, with a complete tearing of a muscle, tendon, or musculotendinous interface accompanied by a severe loss of function, significant pain, severe loss of strength, hematoma formation, possible calcium formation during the healing process, and a possible palpable defect in the muscle (9).

Overuse injuries are common in athletics and are caused by repetitive microtrauma. Before an original injury has been allowed to heal, the mechanism of injury is repeated again and again. Without visible or palpable defects, there is pain on movement and passive stretch, some swelling, loss of function, and inflammation (9). Tendinitis, an inflamed tendon, is a common overuse injury.

Sprains are a stretch beyond normal physiologic limits of a ligament in the same way that strains involve muscle or tendon. It should be noted that a person cannot strain ligaments, just as a person cannot sprain tendons. Sprains are characterized by pain, point tenderness, and mild loss of function to complete joint instability, swelling, hemorrhage, and inflammation.

Strains are injury to muscles, tendons, or musculotendinous interfaces. Sprains are injury to ligaments and joint capsules.

Sprains are graded in a similar fashion to strains. A first-degree sprain stretches a ligament without tearing fibers and without deformity. It is accompanied by mild pain, minimal swelling, point tenderness, inflammation, and loss of function. First-degree sprains respond readily to treatment, and athletes usually may return to competition in a few days. Second-degree sprains are more significant, with partial tearing of the ligament, moderate to strong pain, moderate swelling, inflammation, and loss of function. They may result in substantial lost time and rehabilitation. Third-degree sprains involve a severe loss of joint function, often with complete tearing of the ligament. There is severe pain, swelling, joint instability, and in-

Box **14.1**
Suggested Supplies for a Field Kit

Students should realize that this type of list quickly becomes obsolete and requires constant updating with new technology. Also note that there are no over-the-counter medications in this list. There is legal risk if these are given without the direct supervision of a physician.

Adhesive bandages (plastic or flexible cloth)
  1" × 3"
  2" × 2"
  Knuckle covers
Athletic tape (linen with zinc oxide base)
  3–5 rolls 1 1/2 inch
  2–3 rolls 1 inch
  3–5 rolls 2 inch elastic
  2–3 rolls 3 inch elastic
Heel and lace pads (2" × 4" foam)
Tape underwrap
Tape cutters
Bandage scissors
Latex gloves
Biohazard disposal bags
Surface cleanup kit
CPR mask
Antiseptic hand cleaner
Petroleum jelly
Eye irrigating solution (sterile)
Eye patch
Roller gauze
Gauze pads
  2" × 2" nonsterile
  3" × 3" or 4" × 4" sterile
Sling
Contact lens solution
Pocket mirror
Alcohol
Hydrogen peroxide
Analgesic balm
Triple antibiotic ointment
Penlight
Tweezers
Dental cotton
Injury report forms
Pens
Sticky notes
Access to a cell phone or regular phone, and money to use it if necessary
Photocopy of parent information card giving permission to treat

flammation (9). This injury often requires surgical intervention or extensive rehabilitation and time away from sports activity. Many of the special tests that athletic trainers use assess joint laxity and ligament stability. When moving a joint through its full ROM, a sharply defined end point (called the end feel) to this range is good, whereas a soft mushy ending usually indicates a third-degree injury.

Dislocations (luxations) involve the joints of the extremities. This is a complete disruption of articulating joint surfaces with tearing of most, if not all, ligaments surrounding a joint. Common sites for dislocations include the interphalangeal joints of the fingers, wrist, elbow, glenohumeral (shoulder) joint, and the patella. A dislocated acromioclavicular joint is termed a shoulder separation rather than a dislocation. Dislocations should be treated as **fractures,** splinted in the position they are found, and referred to a physician or emergency room for treatment. In a **subluxation** (partial dislocation) the joint surfaces have become disassociated, but spontaneous reduction (moving back into the normal position) of the deformity has taken place.

Fractures are a disruption in the continuity of a bone caused by stress. Stress is consolidated at points where bones change their shape or direction (5). The forces adversely affecting bone can operate independently or in conjunction with each other. Spiral fractures are caused by twisting forces, and oblique fractures are caused by compression, bending, and twisting. Transverse fractures are caused by bending forces.

Open fractures present more of a challenge to the athletic trainer for immediate management, because outside pathogens enter the open wound and fracture. Closed fractures remain under the skin. Any fracture that is displaced does collateral damage to surrounding tissues. Fractures should be splinted in the position that they are found, and the patient transported to a physician or emergency room.

Neurologic injuries are also a part of sports participation. When body parts are injured, the displacement of body elements can stretch or tear peripheral nerves. Closed-head injuries include concussions and vascular damage (see A Case in Point 14.2). Fragments from a fractured cervical vertebra can penetrate the spinal cord, damaging nervous transmission below the level

A Case in Point 14.2

CONCUSSION

Two opposing soccer players attempted to head a ball during a game. The first player hit the ball, the second player hit the first player in the forehead causing a grade 3 concussion. When the athletic trainer got to the athlete, he was on his hands and knees staring at the ground and unresponsive for approximately 5 min. Finally, he began to answer questions. He remembered nothing from warming up for the game until he heard the athletic trainer talking to him. He had no radiating pain through any body segment, but he did have a large headache. His pupils were equal and reactive to light. When EMS arrived, the athlete was transported to the local hospital where he was held overnight for observation and then released.

When can this athlete return to his sport? What are the possible consequences of returning too early?

This athlete can return when cleared by the team physician, most likely 7 days after all symptoms have been resolved, including headaches, body pain, balance, or other irregularities. As much as possible, the amnesia should also be resolved. Should the athlete return too early, he risks second-impact syndrome, a potentially fatal complication that comes in response to a relatively minor second brain injury before the first injury has healed.

of the injury. A bulging lumbar disk can put pressure on spinal nerve roots, leading to atrophy of musculature, abnormal pain sensations, and gait problems.

An athletic trainer's worst nightmare is to come across an athlete who is unconscious and face-down. All unconscious athletes should be assumed to have a closed-head injury and severe cervical trauma until proven otherwise. With the individual face-down, it is paramount to assess the ABCs. Should it be necessary to begin CPR the athlete must be properly positioned using the correct technique.

Inflammatory Response

Inflammation is a process whereby the body seeks to control the deleterious effects of trauma, bacterial and viral invasion, and decreased blood supply. The classic signs and symptoms include pain, redness, temperature, swelling, and loss of function.

The early phase of inflammation begins immediately after injury and lasts as long as 3 days. The late phase overlaps the early phase and continues for about a week longer (10). For the first few seconds the arteries constrict, which allows white blood cells in the capillaries to line the walls. Following this, there is a more general dilation of blood vessels with increased blood flow. The capillaries then begin to leak (increased vascular permeability). White blood cells and proteins move outside into the tissues. This attracts water from plasma and swelling occurs. In later stages of inflammation, a protein system in the blood becomes activated, which increases the development of the inflammatory process; attracts more white blood cells; and increases phagocytosis, vascular permeability, and attraction of white blood cells.

Along the edge of the traumatic damage, cells do not function normally. Each cell has enzymes that destroy that cell when it becomes damaged beyond repair. These enzymes digest cell membranes and then attach to structures on the cell membranes of uninjured cells, causing additional cell death. This is a secondary injury owing to enzymes.

In addition, swelling decreases blood flow through an area. The swelling is compounded by the shutting down of the lymphatic system. The additional pressure on the vascular system leads to a decrease in the availability of oxygen and glucose to normal cells on the periphery of the injury site, leading to a secondary injury owing to hypoxia (lack of oxygen).

Factors that limit the amount of damage include blood clotting and accumulation of blood into a hematoma. Blood clotting is a complex process that begins with the exposure of platelets to molecules that are not normally found in the vascular system. The platelets begin to get sticky and clump together, which is sometimes enough to seal capillaries. For larger vascular injuries, the process continues. Chemicals from the platelets travel through the blood to the liver, leading to the production of a chemical that helps the clot to form. With this chemical at the injury site, one of the proteins in the blood binds to the platelet plug. If the bleeding is in a local internal area, a hematoma forms, which limits range of motion.

Tissue Repair

The process of repair begins on the 3rd day after the injury and continues for about 3 weeks. The 1st week involves scar formation, especially synthesis of collagen, a protein molecule. With collagen formation, developing capillaries bud from intact capillaries on the outer edge of the wound and a scar takes on a reddish granular appearance. Then the scar begins to contract. Some individuals will scar more than others, a process that can limit function and requires therapeutic intervention. Muscle and nerve tissue have little or no ability to reform the original tissue, hence collagen scar repairs these tissues.

Remodeling begins on day 9. Collagen is initially laid down in random directions. During remodeling, the collagen molecules are reordered along stress lines through an injury site. When this is complete, the scar is still only 70% of the strength of the original tissue and has fewer blood vessels. Furthermore, as the collagen is replaced, capillaries will be removed. The final scar has few blood vessels and a white appearance. Remodeling can go on for a year or more.

Several factors modify the inflammatory and repair process. Physicians use drugs to inhibit the process. Nonsteroidal anti-inflammatory drugs (NSAIDs), such as aspirin and ibuprofen, and corticosteroids, such as prednisone, inhibit the development of inflammation. Placing an injured body part in a cast or immobilizer is clearly beneficial during the early inflammation phases; but if used for prolonged periods of time, immobilization leads to atrophy and the development of adhesions. Some therapeutic agents, including electrical stimulation, hyperbaric oxygen, and therapeutic ultrasound, have positive effects on repair and remodeling (11).

Therapeutic Modalities

Therapeutic modalities are a combination of physical agents, machines, massage, and manual exercise used to modify an inflammatory response, restore tissue, or increase strength and range of motion. For acute inflammation, cold has been the treatment of choice in athletic medicine for more than 40 years. Cold minimizes the accumulation of edema and decreases hemorrhage, possibly by decreasing the metabolic demands of the injured tissue. Cold also provides a strong analgesic effect. It is important to realize that cold will not decrease edema that is already present.

There is some confusion in the scientific literature as to when it is permissible to switch from cold to heat. Some studies suggest that after 48 to 72 hr heat should replace cold (12). This appears to be beneficial for tissue that is at rest for a few days during early rehabilitation. In an athletic population, however, switching to heat too early may cause problems. Most athletes continue to perform some form of activity when injured, which may lead to increased edema formation. Knight (12) suggested that for an active population it is not safe to switch to heat until about day 14, and then only when rehabilitative exercise does not induce any further pain.

Cold treatments average 20 min (with variation for relative body fat under the skin). Methods of application include crushed ice packs (bags), ice cups in a massaging action, slush buckets, cold whirlpools, chemical gel packs, and single-use chemical packs. For acute musculoskeletal trauma where RICE is the treatment of choice, ice packs wrapped against the body with a compression wrap appears to work the best.

The exact mechanism by which cold works is poorly understood. At one point it was thought that cold could induce a vasodilation allowing increased blood flow (13), but preventing swelling. Later research established that cold in fact decreased blood flow through an area, although the mechanism is still unclear (14). What is known is that cold has a positive effect in preventing edema and in decreasing pain. Cold has also been shown to have a positive influence on muscle spasm, possibly by decreasing pain and breaking the pain–spasm cycle.

A major effect of cold was thought to be a decrease in the secondary injury caused by decreased blood flow as a result of swelling (12). This theory remained unsubstantiated until a 1997 study by Merrick and co-workers (15) investigated cellular destruction and the influence of cold. The authors conclusively demonstrated that cold works by decreasing blood flow to the injury.

Heating modalities have been used most successfully on postacute and chronic inflammation. Superficial heat is produced by moist heat packs, paraffin baths, warm whirlpools, and fluidotherapy. The penetrating level of these forms of heat is usually not into skeletal muscle. Their actions then, to relieve pain and muscle spasm, must be mediated through the nervous system to some degree. Deep heat comes in the form of ultrasound and diathermy. These modalities heat tissues within the body, targeting especially muscle. They will increase blood flow, increase metabolic rate, decrease pain and muscle spasm, and assist in the resolution of posttraumatic edema.

ADVANCES IN ATHLETIC TRAINING

Athletic training is still a developing profession. Originally, a student in athletic training would obtain a degree in physical education and then work in an apprenticeship arrangement with an athletic trainer. In 1959 a list of formal course work in athletic training was proposed. The apprenticeship evolved into an internship, with some additional course work and fine tuning of the clinical requirements.

In 1970, Certified Athletic Trainer (ATC) became the entry-level credential. Formal education programs were developed at a number of universities under guidelines from the NATA Professional Education Committee. Completion of an approved program was one route to certification, as was completion of an apprenticeship program, completion of a physical therapy program, or being actively engaged in the practice of athletic training for a minimum of 5 years. Over the years, the latter two were abandoned, leaving approved programs and the internship route as avenues to certification.

The 1983 *Guidelines for Development and Implementation of NATA-approved Undergraduate Athletic Training Education Programs* (16) introduced competency-based education. The competencies were divided into six domains identified by the NATA Board of Certification in *Role Delineation Study* (3). The NATA Education Council is in the process of finalizing a new draft of the competencies that will divide the athletic core body of knowledge into approximately 11 areas. There will be a corresponding addition of clinical proficiencies demonstrating application skills for the knowledge base from the competencies.

In the 1980s, athletic trainers could see the profession evolving in a similar process to physical therapy. It became apparent that state credentialing of athletic trainers would become a necessity. To accomplish this goal, accreditation of athletic training education programs was necessary. A major step toward accreditation came in 1990 when the profession of athletic training was formally recognized as an allied health profession by the American Medical Association.

In 1994, the first accredited athletic training education programs were endorsed by the Committee on Allied Health and Accreditation (CAHEA) which was shortly thereafter replaced by the Commission on Accreditation of Allied Health Education Programs (CAAHEP) to accredit entry-level athletic trainer education programs. The guidelines have been replaced by the current *Standards and Guidelines for an Accredited Education Program for the Athletic Trainer* (17).

NATA created the Education Task Force in June 1994 to look at all aspects of athletic training education and propose reforms leading to standardization of education programming. In 1996, the NATA board of directors adopted 18 reforms for educating athletic trainers. Among these was the recommendation that NATA and the NATA Board of Certification work to initiate regulations, to take effect in 2004, that only graduates of accredited athletic training education programs would be eligible to take the certification examination (18).

During the 1990s, there was an explosive growth in the credentialing of athletic trainers by state governments. Much of the reform movement within NATA was prompted by the interaction of state credentialing bodies with other allied health professions and state legislatures. Athletic trainers are now credentialed in about 38 states, either by licensure, registration, certification, or exemption from another regulated profession's practice act. Credentialing by state governments has led to a tightening of educational standards, and state practice acts control who can be served by athletic trainers and what those services may be.

SUMMARY POINTS

- Athletic training is an allied health profession that works cooperatively with physicians and other medical and allied health professions in all aspects of healthcare delivery to athletes.
- Athletic training is the allied health profession dealing with the prevention, care, and rehabilitation of injuries to active individuals.
- The domains identified by the NATA Board of Certification describe the body of knowledge required to practice athletic training.

- Prevention of athletic injuries is a vastly underrated area, encompassing preparticipation physical examinations, physical conditioning for specific sport activities, and ensuring a safe competitive site from both physical and environmental aspects.
- Recognition, evaluation, and emergency care of athletic injuries is the area most people associate with athletic trainers. Having a specific plan for evaluation is stressed, including the necessity of keeping complete and accurate records.
- The primary survey covers life-threatening situations, assessing the ABCs, and serious bleeding.
- The secondary survey covers the injury at hand, evaluating the history of the injury, observing the body for obvious indications of injury, palpating involved structures, and conducting special tests to determine the exact nature of the injury.
- Common types of injuries include contusions, strains, sprains, luxations, fractures, epiphyseal injuries, neurologic injuries, and skin conditions.
- Rehabilitation of athletic injuries involves preparing and executing a plan for the return of an individual to competitive levels of play.
- Rehabilitation combines the use of therapeutic modalities and therapeutic exercise.
- Healthcare administration involves day-to-day management of the site and resources to deliver athletic training services, planning and executing emergency care plans to deal with serious injury, setting up preparticipation physical examinations, and legal considerations.
- Professional development and responsibility involves keeping abreast of the profession through continuing education activities.

REVIEW QUESTIONS

1. Define athletic training.
2. List each domain of athletic training and identify the principal activities associated with that domain.
3. In what settings are athletic trainers employed?
4. Explain the difference between a sign and a symptom.
5. Explain the differences between a strain and a sprain.
6. List common therapeutic modalities used in athletic training.

References

1. Bilik SE. The trainer's bible. New York: Reed, 1956.
2. Anderson MK, Hall SJ. Sports injury management. Baltimore: Williams & Wilkins, 1995.
3. National Athletic Trainers' Association. Role delineation study. Greenville, NC: NATA, 1999.
4. National Athletic Trainers' Association. Credentialing information. Greenville, NC: NATA, 1996.
5. Arnheim DD, Prentice WE. Principles of athletic training. Madison, WI: Brown & Benchmark, 1997.
6. Kettenbach G. Writing SOAP notes. 2nd ed. Philadelphia: Davis, 1995.
7. The results are in: athletic training outcomes study. NATA News 1997;(May):22–23.
8. Rankin JM, Ingersoll CD. Athletic training management: concepts and applications. St. Louis: Mosby, 1995.
9. Gallaspy JB, May JD. Signs and symptoms of athletic injuries. St. Louis: Mosby, 1996.
10. Clark RAF. Overview and general considerations of wound repair. In: RAF Clark, PM Henson, eds. The molecular and cellular biology of wound repair. New York: Plenum, 1988:4–17.
11. Michlovitz SL. Thermal agents in rehabilitation. 3rd ed. Philadelphia: Davis, 1996.
12. Knight KL. Cryotherapy in sports injury management. Champaign, IL: Human Kinetics, 1995.
13. Moore RJ, Nicollette RL, Behnke RS. The therapeutic use of cold (cryotherapy) in the care of athletic injuries. Athletic Training 1967;2:6–13.
14. Knight KL, Aquino J, Johannes SM, Urban CD. A re-examination of Lewis' cold-induced vasodilation in the finger and ankle. Athletic Training 1980;15:238–250.

15. Merrick MA, Rankin JM, Andres FA, Hinman CL. A preliminary examination of cryotherapy and secondary injury in skeletal muscle. Med Sci Sports Exer 1999;31:1516–1521.
16. National Athletic Trainers' Association. Guidelines for development and implementation of NATA-approved undergraduate athletic training education programs. Greenville, NC: NATA, 1983.
17. Committee for the Accreditation of Allied Health Education Programs. Standards and guidelines for an accredited education program for the athletic trainer. Chicago: CAAHEP, 1998.
18. Delforge GD, Behnke RS. The history and evolution of athletic training education in the United States. J Athletic Training 1999;34:53–61.

Suggested Readings

Kisner C, Colby LA. Therapeutic exercise. 3rd ed. Philadelphia: Davis, 1996.

Konin J, ed. Clinical athletic training. Thorofare, NJ: Slack, 1997.

Magee DJ. Orthopedic physical assessment. 3rd ed. Philadelphia: Saunders, 1997.

Pfeiffer RP, Mangus BC. Concepts of athletic training. 2nd ed. Boston: Jones & Bartlett, 1997.

Prentice WD. Rehabilitation techniques in sports medicine. 3rd ed. St. Louis: McGraw-Hill, 1999.

Rankin JM, Ingersoll CD. Athletic training management: concepts and applications. St. Louis: Mosby, 1995.

Starkey C. Therapeutic modalities for athletic trainers. 2nd ed. Philadelphia: Davis, 1999.

BEHAVIORAL KNOWLEDGE BASE

Our understanding of human movement would be incomplete without delving into the mental and emotional processes that are part of our basic nature. Thus two important subdisciplines of exercise science, exercise and sports psychology (Chapter 15) and motor behavior (Chapter 16), seek to understand human movement in behavioral terms.

Science can ascertain many factors that lead to world-record sports performances, including nutritional, physiologic, and biomechanical factors. However, unless we understand what motivates top athletes to pursue and achieve top performances or why certain individuals continue to exercise while others do not, our understanding of human movement would be lacking. The psychological makeup of individuals, then, is an important realm of study within exercise science. These and other topics are covered in Chapter 15.

Likewise, exercise science is concerned with understanding the processes that lead to movement, both skilled and unskilled. These processes involve both the central and peripheral nervous systems and the neural circuits that innervate muscle groups. This, coupled with how developmental factors across the lifespan changes human movement, is the topic of Chapter 16.

15

Exercise and Sports Psychology

STEVEN J. PETRUZZELLO

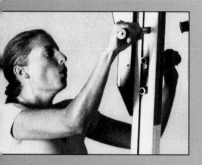

Objectives

1. Explain how the subdiscipline of exercise and sports psychology fits within the discipline of exercise science.
2. Distinguish among the various areas of study that usually fall under exercise and sports psychology.
3. Describe the prominent approaches for studying personality, including some of the major issues and findings from the area.
4. Explain arousal and its effects on performance.
5. Describe the prominent motivational theories in exercise and sports, including representative findings from motivational research.
6. Describe how exercise influences thoughts and emotions.

Although exercise and sports psychology has enjoyed a tremendous surge of interest since the 1980s, the importance of the relationship between bodily movement and the mind has been known for centuries. The ancient Greeks espoused exercise as an important component of both physical and mental health. This philosophy carried over into the sixteenth century, when Mendez (1) wrote *Book of Bodily Exercise,* which included the effects of exercise on the mind. Noted psychologist and philosopher James (2) spoke of the importance of physical activity when he addressed the American Association for the Advancement of Physical Education, saying,

> Everyone knows the effect of physical exercise on the mood: how much more cheerful and courageous one feels when the body has been toned up, than when it is "run down." . . . Those feelings are sometimes of worry, breathlessness, anxiety, tension; sometimes of peace and repose. It is certain that physical exercise will tend to train the body toward the latter feelings. The latter feelings are certainly an essential ingredient in all perfect human character.

Thus at its most basic core, exercise and sports psychology is concerned with the psychology of human movement as it is reflected in the behavior, thoughts, and feelings of the individual(s) engaging in that movement. As such, exercise and sports psychology has borrowed many of the theories and methodologies from its parent discipline of psychology.

Although our ancestors recognized the intimate link between body and mind, it wasn't until the late 1960s to early 1970s that any systematic investigation of issues relevant to the psychology of exercise and sports began to emerge. Since its revival at that time, exercise and sports psychology has had two primary research objectives: determination of the psychological antecedents of participation in sports and physical activity and determination of the psychological consequences of participation in sports and physical activity.

Examples of the first objective include research that attempts to determine what personality factors might lead someone to participate in sports and/or physical activity, and research that examines the effects of precompetition anxiety or confidence on performance. The second objective is represented by research that examines how an exercise training program might influence anxiety, depression, or well-being and research in how sports performance might influence feelings of **self-confidence** or **self-efficacy.**

DEFINITION, DESCRIPTION, AND SCOPE

Exercise and sports psychology has grown to encompass a vast array of issues relevant to the psychology of physical activity. Boxes 15.1 and 15.2 list important research questions in each major area.

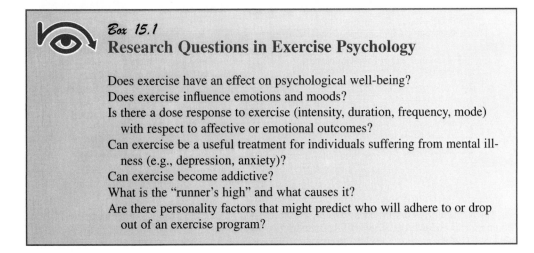

Box 15.1
Research Questions in Exercise Psychology

Does exercise have an effect on psychological well-being?
Does exercise influence emotions and moods?
Is there a dose response to exercise (intensity, duration, frequency, mode) with respect to affective or emotional outcomes?
Can exercise be a useful treatment for individuals suffering from mental illness (e.g., depression, anxiety)?
Can exercise become addictive?
What is the "runner's high" and what causes it?
Are there personality factors that might predict who will adhere to or drop out of an exercise program?

> ### Box 15.2
> ## Research Questions in Sport Psychology
>
> Is there an athletic personality?
> What is the relationship between anxiety and performance?
> How does attention influence performance?
> Are there psychological predictors of athletic injury?
> Does relaxation have a role in improving sports performance?
> Is self-confidence an important predictor of sports performance?
> Is there an optimal balance between the amount of mental practice relative
> to the amount of physical practice to produce the best performance?

The Framework of Exercise and Sports Psychology

In attempting to define the boundaries of the field, Rejeski and Brawley (3) proposed a framework similar to that shown in Figure 15.1. In their conceptualization, exercise and sports psychology is composed of four distinct yet related areas: health psychology, exercise psychology, sports psychology, and rehabilitation psychology. They further clarify their model with the following assumptions: *(a)* Content in each of the areas is linked to the discipline of psychology, *(b)* examination of relevant issues involves the use of a wide range of models and techniques from various aspects of psychology (e.g., experimental, social, personality, psychophysiology, clinical), and *(c)* each of the four areas is distinct and yet has important relationships with each

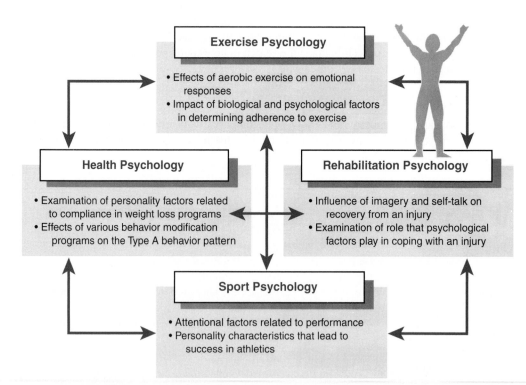

FIGURE 15.1 General content organization of exercise and sports psychology courses and texts. Modified from Rejeski WJ, Brawley LR. Defining the boundaries of sport psychology. Sport Psychol 1988;2:231–242.

of the other areas. Rejeski and Brawley (3) define exercise psychology as "the application of the educational, scientific, and professional contributions of psychology to the promotion, explanation, maintenance, and enhancement of behaviors related to physical work capacity." Sports psychology is defined as "educational, scientific, and professional contributions of psychology to the promotion, maintenance, and enhancement of sport-related behavior."

Because there is a great deal of overlap between health psychology (educational, scientific, and professional contributions of psychology to the promotion and maintenance of health and the prevention and treatment of illness) and exercise psychology, these two areas are combined in this chapter, with the emphasis on exercise. In addition, because of the scope of this chapter, rehabilitation psychology (application of psychological knowledge to physical disability) is not discussed in any detail, and certain aspects of sports psychology will not be mentioned. Even restricting the scope of this chapter to exercise and sports psychology, the breadth of these areas is still rather wide. As such, a number of sports psychology issues are not covered. Group processes, which includes issues such as group and team dynamics, group cohesion, leadership, and communication, are not discussed, nor are performance enhancement issues.

Analysis in Exercise and Sports Psychology

Exercise and sports psychology lends itself well to a variety of analytical methods in an attempt to examine psychological phenomena. The most popular approach historically has been constructionist, which has its roots in the tradition of cognitive psychology. From this perspective, a great deal of weight is given to the individual's subjective experience. The predominant analytic strategy used in this perspective is the self-report, which typically involves the use of standardized questionnaires or psychological inventories. Some examples include Spielberger's State–Trait Anxiety Inventory, the Profile of Mood States (POMS), the Beck Depression Inventory in the exercise domain, the Sport Competition Anxiety Test (SCAT), Competitive State Anxiety Inventory 2 (CSAI-2), and the Test of Attentional and Interpersonal Style (TAIS) in the sports domain.

To a much lesser extent, observational approaches have also been used. This level of analysis involves watching individuals and recording what they do. There are some well-developed procedures for performing observational analyses, most notably the Coaching Behavior Assessment System (CBAS). The use of such a system requires extensive training for the observers so that all observers are recording behaviors in the same fashion. This particular constraint is likely part of the reason that the observational approach has been relatively unpopular.

Another approach has grown from the notion that individuals' experiences before, during, and after sports or exercise and their behaviors and physiologic processes all reveal important information about human nature. This psychophysiologic approach consists of examining phenomena from both a psychological and physiologic perspective (i.e., a multilevel approach). The underlying belief is that insight into psychological phenomena can be gained by examining physiologic events. It is important to mention that much of what is currently known in exercise and sports psychology has been derived from research using only a single level of analysis approach. Unfortunately, despite its potential, the psychophysiologic approach has not been used much in exercise and sports psychology.

FOCUS ON SCIENCE

Many issues have been studied in exercise and sports psychology. Some have been popular and hence have received a great deal of research attention; other issues have been less popular and have not been examined as thoroughly. In this section, the areas and issues that have been historically popular within exercise and sports psychology are presented, and the major findings are reviewed. By necessity these are only overviews. More comprehensive accounts can be found in Suggested Reading.

Personality

Consider the following statements:

Sports build character.

There is a personality type that is more likely to be successful in sports.

A long-term program of exercise can lead to a more stable, less anxious personality.

Statements such as these are derived from the belief that personality plays an important role in both sports performance and exercise and health behaviors. However, there is no overwhelming scientific support for any of these statements, but not for lack of trying. Personality research in exercise and sports psychology has been popular. Some authors have stated that personality research underlies much of what exercise and sports psychologist study (4).

Overview and Definition

Little consensus exists about how personality is defined. One way to understand personality is to examine how it is conceptualized. A particularly useful model for such a conceptualization comes from Hollander (5), who views personality as multilayered, in some ways like the layers of an onion; the innermost layers are relatively stable and the outermost layers are more readily changeable based on the individual's interactions with his or her surroundings (Fig. 15.2).

At the center is what is referred to as the psychological core, thought to be the most stable and least changeable aspect of personality. This is developed from early interactions with the environment (e.g., parents, objects) and includes such aspects of personality as perceptions of the external world; perceptions of the self; and basic attitudes, values, interests, and motives. In other words, our **self-concept** is at the center of our personality.

Emanating from the core are typical responses, behaviors that are consistent with our core and are usually fairly consistent over time. Finally, the buffer zone from the social environment is the layer referred to as role-related behaviors. This layer represents the most changeable aspect of the personality, because it includes behaviors that vary based on the situation or surroundings the person might be in. It is important to note, however, that these behaviors remain consistent with the psychological core and typical responses.

It is through such models that the consistent yet dynamic nature of personality can be illustrated. Personality is relatively stable over time (e.g., months, years) and yet is capable of change and modification. This point has had important implications for research examining sports performance and exercise and health behavior.

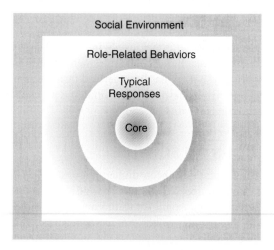

Figure 15.2 Hollander's conceptual model of the structure of personality.

Approaches to Studying Personality

Numerous approaches have been used to study personality in exercise and sports psychology. The two most prominent approaches are dispositional and learning; the emphasis of the former is on the person, whereas the emphasis of the latter is on the environment. Both approaches essentially endorse what has been termed an *interactionist approach* to studying personality (see Sidelight 15.1). Dispositional approaches include biologic theories and the trait theories. Learning approaches include conditioning or behaviorist theories and social learning theories. Social learning theories will be revisited in the section on **motivation.**

Personality has been most often studied from either a dispositional or social learning perspective. Dispositional approaches focus on the individual, with extreme versions discounting the effect of environmental factors. Such theories typically emphasize some aspect of biology as being important in determining personality. Social learning approaches also focus on the individual, but place much more emphasis on the influence that environmental factors have in shaping personality.

One of the classic dispositional theories comes from the ancient Greeks. It was their belief that personality was intimately linked to the body's "humors" (e.g., fluids). More or less of one type of humor resulted in distinct personality profiles. As such, it was thought that a preponderance of blood resulted in a sanguine, or cheerful, disposition. A greater proportion of black bile, on the other hand, led to melancholy or a depressed personality. Yellow bile was associated with irritability, and phlegm was related to indifference and apathy. The solution to problematic personalities was the alteration of these bodily fluids. One can imagine some fairly gruesome scenes resulting from such practices!

Trait theory has been a popular approach to studying personality. **Traits** are relatively enduring, highly consistent internal attributes that an individual possesses. Examples include moody, anxious, touchy, restless, optimistic, active, sociable, outgoing, lively, carefree, calm, and even tempered. Cattell (6) proposed that personality consisted of 16 factors that were derived through complex statistical procedures. He developed the popular 16 Personality Factor (16PF) Questionnaire to measure them. This was a widely used approach to studying personality, particularly in the sports domain, in the 1960s and 1970s.

Eysenck (7) favored an approach that examined the relationships among traits, particularly what he termed the *superordinate dimensions* that derived from these relationships. Unlike Cattell, Eysenck believed personality could be captured most effectively with only three dimensions: **extroversion–introversion** (outgoing, sociable vs. shy, inhibited), **neuroticism–stability** (anxious, excitable vs. even tempered, easygoing), and **psychoticism–superego** (egocentric, impulsive vs. cooperative, caring). Another important aspect of Eysenck's model is that each dimension is proposed to have a biologic basis, highlighting the notion that personality is not some ephemeral construction but is intimately linked with biologic processing. Eysenck's work has shown that Cattell's 16 factors essentially boil down to the three superordinate dimensions.

One major problem with research in the personality area is that so many of the studies are conducted out of convenience; for example, a sample of athletes is available, so an investigator has them complete one or multiple personality inventories, the data are analyzed, and findings are then presented. Based on the results of many such studies, numerous reviewers have concluded that there is no relationship between personality and athletic performance. A more useful approach involves using a theoretical framework, deriving testable hypotheses from that framework, and then using a measurement tool and a subject sample that will allow testing of the hypotheses. Results from studies that have adopted such an approach have shown some consistent relationships between personality and performance.

INTERACTIONIST APPROACH TO STUDYING PERSONALITY

A point of great contention and vigorous debate in the study of personality has centered on whether focusing on the person or the situation is the more effective way to study personality. This has been termed the *person–situation debate* and dates to the late 1960s. The person perspective, usually referred to as the trait approach, emphasizes that personality is derived from stable, enduring attributes of the individual, which lead to consistent responses over time and across situations. The situation perspective, on the other hand, emphasizes that behavior is best explained by examining the environment and the individual's reaction to that environment. Extreme positions from both perspectives basically give no credence to the other position. Currently, it appears that a more moderate position, one that espouses both the person and the situation and, more important, the interaction between the two, offers the best understanding of the influence of personality on behavior.

Another related and important issue in the personality area involves the distinction between states and traits. As noted, traits are seen as relatively enduring dispositions that exert a consistent influence on behavior in a variety of situations. States, on the other hand, are viewed as the psychological reactions to the situation in which the individual finds himself or herself and are consistent with the individual's traits. For example, a highly trait anxious person would tend to be a worrisome, nervous individual regardless of the situation. When placed in a stressful situation such as standing at the free-throw line in the closing seconds of a close basketball game, this individual would be expected to respond with a high amount of state anxiety. This typically manifests itself cognitively as extreme nervousness or tension and somatically with sweaty palms, tense muscles, and an unsettled stomach. Carron[a] noted that skeptics called for abandoning the trait approach altogether, because of its failure to account for physical activity behavior. This prompted some scientists to argue that instead of abandoning the trait approach, the approach should be more adequately used. Coupling such traits with situational factors such as psychological states should serve to enhance predictive power.

[a]*Carron AV. Social psychology of sport. Ithaca, NY: Mouvement Publications, 1980.*

Eysenck's model provides meaningful and testable predictions for the sports and exercise domains. For example, because extroverts seek out sensory stimulation and are well able to tolerate pain, it is hypothesized that this personality would be more likely to take up sports and would be more successful in sports than introverts. Eysenck et al. (8) present numerous pieces of evidence that support such predictions. It has also been found that physical activity is often inversely related with neuroticism. Although the search for an athletic personality has not provided any breakthrough answers whereby we can definitively state that personality factors X, Y, and Z will guarantee athletic success, the evidence points to the factors of independence and extroversion as being most related to success in sports.

Another popular question in the personality area has been whether sports and exercise can change personality. Scientists have asked whether independent, extroverted individuals are developed through sports participation or if independent, extroverted people gravitate toward sports. Although the issue hasn't been definitively resolved, the majority of the evidence points to the gravitational explanation.

Does this mean that sports can't influence personality? On the contrary, more recent studies have shown that engaging in structured sports programs (e.g., midnight basketball leagues in inner cities) can lead to positive changes, such as less deviant behavior, which could be considered aspects of personality. In the exercise domain, a great deal of work has shown that long-term exercise programs often result in reductions in the traits, such as anxiety and neuroticism (9). This work clearly demonstrates the fact that personality can change. It is possible, over a period of weeks, months, or years, for personality to change as a result of regular physical activity. This change is usually in the direction of reduced negative factors (neuroticism) and enhanced positive factors (extroversion), changes that are quite consistent with Eysenck's theoretical formulations.

Motivation

What drives an individual to stick to an exercise program with a fervent regularity, while another drops out within 3 months of beginning? What leads an individual to continue in a sport even though he or she has experienced a series of failures and disappointments? What leads one individual to become involved in sports or physical activity, while another actively avoids such pursuits? These questions relate to the concept of motivation in exercise and sports psychology. What is motivation? What pushes some people to do things others would not do? How is motivation most often studied? How can it be assessed? These and other issues are the focus of this section.

> *Motivation itself is made up of three components. First, motivation is involved in the choices we make to participate in some activities and/or avoid participating in others. Second, motivation refers to how much an individual invests in an activity. Two different people may choose to invest widely differing amounts of time in an exercise program. Third, motivation is persistence, which is what keeps an individual engaged in a behavior, often in the face of obstacles or setbacks.*

Approaches to Studying Motivation

Motivation in the exercise and sports psychology domain has most often been studied from an achievement framework. Achievement motivation was initially studied within the McClelland-Atkinson model, one of the earliest and most influential models. In fact, many of the current motivational models are derivatives of this model. The model itself proposes a complex mathematical approach to predict and explain the need for achievement, a concept developed within the model, using both personality (i.e., individual) and situational (i.e., environmental) factors.

Numerous social-psychological theories of motivation have grown out of the initial McClelland-Atkinson model. Most of these have adopted a cognitive approach to achievement motivation, wherein strivings for achievement are assumed to be caused by cognitive mechanisms. One of the most important of these cognitive constructs is self-confidence, or the perception an individual has of her or his own ability. Self-confidence is the belief an individual has that he or she can successfully execute an activity or a plan. Perhaps not surprisingly, self-confidence and its situationally specific derivative self-efficacy, have been shown to be significantly related to successful sports performance. So strong is this finding that some believe it is the most important cognitive factor in sports.

Two social psychological theories have been prominent in the exercise and sports psychology motivation literature. The first is Bandura's (10) social cognitive theory, of which self-perception of ability is paramount, and the second is Weiner's (11) attribution theory. Both have had application in sports and the exercise literature.

Social Cognitive Theory

Social cognitive theory is the most recent version of Bandura's social learning theory (12). A major component of this theoretical framework is the notion of self-efficacy, which is proposed to be the cognitive mechanism mediating motivation and thus behavior. Self-efficacy represents the convictions or beliefs an individual has that he or she can carry out a course of action to achieve a particular outcome. An important point is that this belief is not concerned with the skills that individuals actually possess but is instead centered on their own judgment of what they can do with those skills. As it has often been referred to in the literature, self-efficacy is essentially self-confidence that is specific to a particular situation. It is a key factor in determining behavior, but only when the proper incentives and requisite skills are present. Self-efficacy has been shown to

typically has its greatest effects on attention through its effect on the breadth of attention. Essentially, the hypothesis is that, as arousal increases, the attentional field narrows. This is effective to some extent. Returning to the notion of the inverted U hypothesis, as arousal increases from low to moderate levels, the attentional field is narrowed. This facilitates performance, because the narrowing of attention eliminates unnecessary, irrelevant stimuli from the attentional field.

For example, as an athlete begins to get aroused before a game, he or she is no longer concerned about what friends in the stands might be doing or what the public address announcer is saying. Attention is focused on the task at hand. However, as arousal continues to increase, attention is narrowed even further, potentially allowing the athlete to miss important, relevant environmental and situational cues. The result is that performance suffers. Imagine the football quarterback who has become overly aroused. As he drops back to pass, because of a narrowed attentional field he is unable to spot an open secondary receiver after the primary receiver is covered. That important environmental information has been lost to the attentional field because of the heightened arousal. Also, in the case of the weightlifter who forgets to chalk his hands, too much arousal can lead him to forget important aspects of his normal pretask routine, which could be disastrous for performance. Obviously, numerous factors can impinge on or facilitate attention. Both internal (e.g., personality) and external (e.g., task demands, crowd noise, weather) factors interact with arousal to influence the kind of attentional processing that occurs during performance. The stage of attention that the individual is operating in (e.g., automatic, effortful) is also an important consideration. What follows is a sampling of some of the ways in which attention can be inferred from a variety of responses (e.g., self-report, performance, physiologic responses).

BEHAVIORAL MEASURES OF ATTENTION   Attention can be assessed in a variety of ways, often depending on the perspective within which it is examined. Experimental psychologists working within the tradition of cognitive psychology have used a paradigm that involves a behavioral assessment of attention. This paradigm is referred to as a dual-task paradigm. As the name implies, two tasks compete for the subject's attention.

The underlying assumption of this approach is that the individual has a fixed attentional capacity. In other words, there is only so much attention to go around; and when it is used up, there is no more. The rationale for the dual-task paradigm is that, if the primary task requires a sizable amount of the total attentional capacity, only a minimal amount can be allocated to a secondary task. As such, if attention is maintained on the primary task, there should be a performance decrement on the secondary task.

Imagine the point guard on a basketball team. Bringing the ball up court requires that attention be directed to a number of things: dribbling the ball, calling a play, determining the location of teammates and opponents, etc. Now imagine the attentional demands placed on a novice compared to a professional National Basketball Association (NBA) point guard. The novice has to devote most, if not all, of his attention to simply dribbling the ball. All of the other aspects of the situation are either ignored or are attended to minimally. Dribbling suffers as attention is diverted away from the task. The NBA point guard, on the other hand, needs to devote little attention to the task of dribbling the ball; therefore, he can devote more attention to the other tasks.

An example of the dual-task paradigm from the sports domain is to ask the subject to perform a primary task, e.g., in rifle shooting, the subject tries to shoot each shot as close to the center of the target as possible. The secondary task may involve the performance of a reaction time task. While the subject is performing the primary task, he or she is given a stimulus to which the he or she must respond as quickly and accurately as possible. If attention is fully directed to the primary task, performance on the reaction time task suffers (i.e., response times are slow). To the extent that attention is diverted from the primary task whenever the secondary task must be performed, shooting performance deteriorates.

The dual-task technique has been used in sports, but the question arises: Is it a good technique to use? The manipulation required for the dual-task paradigm to work essentially disrupts performance. The technique can reveal a good deal about information processing, but it does little to tell us about attentional processes in real sports situations. It is also debatable whether there is actually a limit to attentional capacity, the assumption of which underlies the dual-task technique.

SELF-REPORT MEASURES OF ATTENTION   Another way to think about attention draws from an individual difference approach. This has also been referred to as attentional style. Different people are affected in different ways by task demands and situational factors. As is the case with much of exercise and sports psychology, the major assessment strategy in this context is self-report, usually via questionnaire.

The most prevalent attention scale used in sports is Nideffer's (18) TAIS. The TAIS was developed out of the conceptual framing of attention as two-dimensional. Nideffer believed that attention could have a width dimension (broad vs. narrow) and a direction dimension (internal vs. external). These dimensions make intuitive sense and have been generally accepted. The problem, however, lies in the assessment of these dimensions, which is what the TAIS purports to do. The TAIS has been roundly criticized for not being a good predictor of sports performance, a quality it should have if it is to be a useful instrument. The TAIS also appears to fail in its ability to assess both dimensions of attention. It seems to measure width of attention but not direction.

Besides these shortcomings, the TAIS and other self-report measures of attention suffer from at least two other limitations. First, it is questionable whether athletes (or any individuals, for that matter) can actually access the cognitive operations that occur during attentionally demanding activities and then put those operations into words. More often than not, what individuals report when asked what they were attending to is based on prior assumptions regarding the causes of behavior rather than what was actually occurring. One need only recall the typical response to the often-asked question that asks athletes what were they thinking about when they performed the game-winning move. More often than not, their response is simply, "I don't know." The second major problem with using self-report assessments of attention is that athletes will not complete questionnaires when it's perhaps most important, i.e., immediately before performance. If they do consent to do so, performance is likely to be adversely affected.

PSYCHOPHYSIOLOGIC MEASURES OF ATTENTION   A third assessment strategy involves the psychophysiologic approach. The idea is that the psychological construct of attention can be determined based on physiologic responses of the body immediately before performance. Assessments of bodily responses during this **preparatory period** is also potentially less disruptive to performance. A growing amount of information has been, and is being, gathered regarding attention using such an approach. These findings will be discussed later in this chapter.

Exercise and Mental Health

Exercise has long been recognized as having the potential to influence our moods and emotions. In essence, mental health is thought to be intimately linked to physical health. A great deal of research has examined how exercise affects aspects of mental health like anxiety and depression (9,19,20). More recently, the ability of exercise to enhance positive aspects of mental health has also been examined.

Anxiety and Depression

Based on the large number of studies to date, it is safe to say that exercise is associated with reductions in anxiety and depression. Both single bouts of activity (acute exercise) and long-term programs of regular exercise (chronic exercise) have been shown to reduce state and trait levels, respectively, of anxiety and depression. These effects hold for those suffering from mild to moderate levels of anxiety and depression and for those who have normal levels of anxiety and depression. Both aerobic and anaerobic (e.g., resistance training) forms of exercise reduce depression, but only aerobic exercise works to alleviate anxiety. Little research to date has examined anaerobic exercise effects on anxiety, however, so this should be considered a tentative finding.

Even though there has been ample research on anxiety and depression, there is little that has examined the **dose-response** nature of the exercise effects. This would entail examining how varying doses of exercise, in terms of intensity, duration, and frequency, affect psychological status. One report indicates that to reduce anxiety or depression, an exerciser must workout for at least 20 min at not less than 60% of maximum heart rate or oxygen capacity (21).

Unfortunately, no solid evidence exists to support such assertions. Some evidence suggests that durations of as little as 5 min may result in favorable psychological changes (9). The main problem with making any conclusive statements about minimal durations and intensities is the overall failure of the research to systematically examine these variables. Fortunately, it does seem that as the length of chronic exercise training increases, reductions in anxiety and depression occur. Obviously, this suggests that making exercise a regular lifestyle habit is healthful in terms of mental health (although carrying this healthy habit to the extreme can be problematic; see A Case In Point 15.1). When reading the exercise and mental health literature, be aware of these limitations in making conclusions about exercise effects.

Psychological Well-Being

The vast majority of research examining psychological changes associated with exercise and physical activity has focused on reductions in negative emotions. There is growing evidence, however, that exercise can also be effective in enhancing and improving positive psychological

---

A Case in Point 15.1

TAKING EXERCISE TO THE EXTREME

Although a regular regimen of exercise is generally thought to be healthy, taking it to the extreme can lead to problems. Most of us tend to think of athletes as healthy individuals. However, athletes involved in heavy training can sometimes experience significant mental health disturbances. Athletes in sports like swimming and distance running often overtrain. Such physical training involves high mileage as a way of conditioning the cardiovascular system so that when the athlete tapers (i.e., reduces the training load) before important competitions, the body responds with fast times.

Research has shown that such intensive training changes the psychological state of the athlete. Essentially, the individual experiences increased tension and depression and decreased feelings of vigor and energy. Although this is not unexpected given such intensive training, some athletes may become clinically depressed. If this occurs, the only thing the athlete can do is to stop training completely; reducing the training load doesn't help at this point.

Research with swimmers has shown that such negative psychological changes are actually fairly tightly linked with the training load. The athlete's mental health is negatively affected when the training load increases, but it is positively affected when the training load decreases. It has been proposed that psychological monitoring of the athletes during the course of their season could help prevent some cases of more severe psychological disturbances.

states. One of the most consistently reported effects from exercise of even mild intensities has been an increase in feelings of energy. For example, Thayer (13) has consistently shown that a 10-min walk is more effective—not only at reducing tension but also at increasing energy—than eating a candy bar or smoking cigarettes.

Another aspect of mental health that has recently gained more attention is the concept of **psychological well-being.** Simply put, psychological well-being is a preponderance of positive emotion over negative emotion along with favorable thoughts, such as satisfaction with life. It should be relatively easy to see that if exercise reduces negative emotions like anxiety and depression and increases positive emotions like energy and vigor, then it should also result in better psychological well-being. Exercise and physical activity has also been shown to increase self-confidence, self-esteem, and cognitive function.

How Does Exercise Produce Psychological Changes?

Although it is clear that exercise has positive effects, how and why this happens remain to be determined. Numerous explanations have been proposed for the mental health effects of exercise, but four have become classic explanations, not because they are necessarily any better explanations but because they have been so frequently mentioned (22). These include the distraction hypothesis, endorphin hypothesis, thermogenic hypothesis, and monoamine hypothesis.

Of the four hypotheses most often mentioned as the cause for the affective changes that occur with exercise, the distraction hypothesis is the lone strictly psychological explanation. Its basic premise is that the reason for the improved emotional profile after exercise is because the act of exercising provides a distraction from the normal cares and worries that often lead to stress and negative emotions. In essence, exercise provides a time-out from these usual concerns, a chance to leave them behind for a while. Although there is some evidence to support this hypothesis, there is equally solid evidence that refutes it. As such, it remains a potential explanation.

The hypothesis that has created the biggest stir has been the endorphin hypothesis. The popular press has parlayed this explanation into the mainstream so that it is nearly impossible to read an article about exercise from a popular magazine without seeing reference made to the body's own natural painkillers as the reason for why exercise makes us feel better. It is true that **endorphins,** a class of stress hormones, are released in response to a stressor. Exercise, of course, is a stressor to the body; and as such, endorphin concentrations are elevated in response to exercise of even mild intensities and remain elevated for some time after the exercise is over. Because it is during the same time that people typically report feeling better (i.e., less anxious, less depressed), it has become popular to claim that the endorphins are responsible for this improved mood.

Some research has supported this assertion, showing that elevated levels of endorphins are related to such feelings. More sophisticated studies have blocked endorphins from exerting their influence and shown that the psychological changes do not occur, i.e., anxiety reduction and other mood changes do not take place. On the other hand, studies with just as much methodological sophistication have blocked endorphins in the same manner and still shown psychological changes consistent with the feel-better phenomenon.

As it stands today, it is difficult to conclude that endorphins are indeed the reason for the enhanced mood states typically reported after exercise. Solid evidence refutes such a notion; yet equally solid evidence supports it. Although it would be foolish to make claims either way, the popular media has done just that; but because of their presentation of the research, endorphins have been touted as the reason for feeling better when we exercise. Much more research needs to be done before any such claims can be made.

The thermogenic hypothesis has also been cited as a reason for the emotional changes occurring with exercise. The basic premise is that with exercise of sufficient intensity and/or duration body temperature is elevated. In fact, it may be somewhat surprising to realize that the ele-

Practical Application 15.1

EXERCISE, BODY TEMPERATURE INCREASES, AND REDUCED ANXIETY LEVEL

Here is one way that exercise is thought to lead to feelings of reduced anxiety. During exercise, body temperature is elevated and remains elevated for some period of time after exercise is terminated; this state is detected by the hypothalamus in the brain. This information is relayed from the hypothalamus to the thalamus, which initiates a series of events. Skeletal muscles receive a reduction of neural stimulation from the motor cortex and thus relax. This further results in a reduction of sensory stimulation back to the brain, which may promote a feeling of arousal reduction or relaxation. In this manner, the elevated temperature caused by exercise is hypothesized to lead to a more relaxed state after the exercise ends (thermogenic hypothesis). This relaxed state is often interpreted as a reduction in anxiety.

vations that occur with exercise are often of the same magnitude as when the body develops a fever, for example, when suffering from the flu. Body temperatures greater than 40°C have been reported after distance running (e.g., 10 km, marathons). Such elevations in body temperatures are also seen with sauna bathing, an activity often used as therapy for various maladies.

It is thought that with elevated temperature, whether from exercise or other activities, a variety of positive effects are set into motion (see Practical Application 15.1). Studies have shown reductions in muscle tension after exercise, and others have documented psychological changes. At present, studies that have directly tested the thermogenic hypothesis have essentially failed to support it. It is possible that temperature changes may still have a place in explaining exercise effects, but it may require the measurement of more relevant sites (e.g., brain temperature) or it may be that the changes in temperature simply set in motion other psychophysiologic changes that lead to the exercise-induced emotional changes.

Finally, the monoamine hypothesis places emphasis on changes in brain chemistry (i.e., neurotransmitters) as the causal mechanism for exercise-induced emotional changes. These emotion influencing neurotransmitters include norepinephrine, dopamine, and serotonin; and their effects are often localized to brain structures known to have an important role in emotion (e.g., frontal lobes, amygdala). Initial work with animals has shown that exercise alters levels of these neurotransmitters in the brain (i.e., release into or uptake from synapses is changed). Some initial work in exercising humans has shown promise in delineating whether these, and other, neurotransmitters could explain the altered emotional states associated with exercise.

The above hypotheses for explaining the exercise-related psychological changes so often seen are not the only ones; and obviously there is still a long way to go before any definitive answers are determined. In all likelihood, one single explanation will probably not provide a sufficient answer to the question. Instead, a combination of factors, both psychological and physiologic, will likely be the best solution. Regardless of the actual cause for why exercise is associated with psychological change, it is important to realize that the changes take place. The available evidence is strong enough for psychological benefits to be included in the 1996 surgeon general's report (23) as some of the many benefits that accrue from a physically active lifestyle.

ADVANCES IN EXERCISE AND SPORTS PSYCHOLOGY

Exercise and sports psychology is a growing and exciting subdiscipline of exercise science. All of the areas discussed in this overview have many unanswered questions, yet there has been much progress through the systematic efforts of researchers. Sophisticated theories have been developed, some specific to physical activity, that should prove helpful in the quest to more fully understand why we exercise (or don't) and how the experience of physical activity can be made more meaningful. The following are a few of the advances that have been made in this effort.

Sports Personality Research

Schurr et al. (24) have examined higher-order factors from the 16PF in a sample of nearly 2000 male collegiate athletes and nonathletes. They further subdivided the athletes based on level of success (letter winners vs. nonletter winners) and sports type. Sports type was divided into sports in which aggression was focused against an opponent in a direct (e.g., football) or parallel (e.g., golf) manner, into team or individual sports, and into individual parallel aggressive sports of long (e.g., golf) or short (e.g., gymnastics) duration.

Another unique feature of this work was the use of complex statistical analyses. Schurr and co-workers (24) found that no single personality profile could differentiate athletes from nonathletes, but numerous differences were found when the various categorizations based on sports type were examined (Table 15.2). The fact that they were able to find the expected relationships indicates how important classification can be in the sports domain. It also illustrates the need to use sophisticated analyses that can simultaneously account for multiple variables, which increases the chance of uncovering relationships among highly complex human behaviors.

Psychophysiologic Approaches to Studying Attention

Psychophysiologic approaches have been adopted as a way of avoiding some of the problems inherent in self-report and behavioral paradigms for studying attention (e.g., disruption of performance, inaccurate verbal reports of what happened, inability to measure attention when it is most important). To reiterate, physiologic responses during attentionally demanding situations are thought to reflect attention. The two most common classes of measurement are cardiac responses and electrocortical, or brain, responses.

An interesting phenomenon occurs when an individual directs attention to either environmental cues or internal factors. As attention is directed toward the environment, heart rate slows down (cardiac deceleration) in an attempt to capture relevant cues from the situation. When that attention is directed internally, heart rate speeds up (cardiac acceleration) in an effort to reject these situational cues.

Table 15.2	MAJOR DIFFERENCES IN PERSONALITY BETWEEN ATHLETES AND NONATHLETES AND AMONG ATHLETES FROM DIFFERENT SPORTS[a]	
Reference Group	**Compared To**	**Personality Profile**
Team sport athletes	Nonathletes	Less abstract reasoning; more extroverted; more dependent; less ego strength
Individual sport athletes	Nonathletes	Less abstract reasoning; less anxious; more dependent; more objective
Direct sport athletes	Nonathletes	Less abstract reasoning; more extroverted; more independent; more objective
Parallel sport athletes	Nonathletes	Less abstract reasoning; less anxious; less independent; more ego strength
Individual sport athletes	Team sport athletes	Less dependent; less anxious; less extroverted; less emotional; more objective
Direct sport athletes	Parallel sport athletes	More aggressive

[a]Reprinted by permission from Schurr KT, Ashley MA, Joy KL. A multivariate analysis of male athlete characteristics: sport type and success. Multivariate Exper Clin Res 1977;3:53–68.

For example, as an athlete focuses his or her attention on an environmental stimulus, like listening for the starter's pistol or looking at the bull's eye, his or her heart rate slows. This is not the same sort of large physiologic change that would be seen when an individual goes from running a 100-m dash to slowing down to a jog. Rather, the heart rate change is smaller, on the order of 5 to 10 beats per minute. As such, the response is examined on a beat-by-beat basis.

It has been suggested that these changes in cardiac function facilitate attentional processes by regulating the amount of information sent to the central nervous system, which results in increased or decreased sensorimotor performance. The fact that the direction and magnitude of the cardiac response have been related to performance has led to the suggestion that they are good indicators of individual's attentional state. It has been hypothesized that experienced athletes would have better attentional skills and would show a pattern of cardiac deceleration during the preparatory period before response execution.

In addition to controlled laboratory studies in which these response patterns have been shown, cardiac responses have been examined in sports situations such as simulated races, rifle shooting, archery, and golf. Like the laboratory studies, the more real-world sports studies have shown predictable heart rate responses before the athlete initiates the sport skill and relationships between the cardiac changes and performance. For instance, it has been shown that novice athletes show little slowing of heart rate before task performance; but after a period of training, the same athletes show cardiac deceleration patterns similar to more experienced athletes. Other research has shown that the degree of the deceleration response is associated with performance. In much of the sports research that has used this measure of attention, the athlete's normal performance routine is unimpaired. This is important. because it shows that the psychophysiologic approach can be used to examine attention in real sports situations without disrupting performance.

In addition to using cardiac responses as indices of attention, changes in brain activity have also proven useful in understanding attentional processes. The most common measure of brain activity is the electroencephalogram (EEG), which is a recording, from the scalp, of electrical potentials occurring in the brain. EEG has been used, because it has been shown to successfully differentiate varying states of attentional focus and it is known to be a stable and reliable measure. The vast majority of research in sports that has examined EEG responses during response execution has examined patterns from the same brain regions (e.g., temporal or occipital lobes) in both the left and right hemispheres. It has been thought that the two hemispheres are involved in different kinds of information processing. For example, the left hemisphere has traditionally been thought of as the site of logical, analytical, sequential thought processing, whereas the right hemisphere has been thought of as the site of creative, free-flowing, parallel thought processing.

The evidence has shown that, as the time to perform a skill approaches, there is a general shift in brain activity across the two hemispheres. Left hemisphere activity is progressively reduced before response execution, whereas right hemisphere activity increases. These findings have been interpreted as indicating that highly skilled athletes have the ability to focus attention in a way that reduces the mental activity of the left hemisphere, thereby making the right hemisphere more dominant. Such a change in mental functioning reduces distracting thoughts that could negatively affect performance. There is limited evidence showing that athletes can be trained to develop the appropriate kind of thought processing; when this occurs, performance is significantly affected.

Both coaches and scientists believe that excessive self-talk and thinking disrupt performance. The more appropriate mind-set for optimal performance is one that is free of self-analysis and conscious concern with details of the skill. Keeping in mind the criticism of self-reports with respect to attention, there is anecdotal evidence that individuals who have less left hemisphere activity feel as if they are in an appropriate mental state for effective performance. In some ways, the research evidence seems to support Nike's "just do it" slogan, i.e., instead of thinking too much and overanalyzing what to do, it is better to get into a mind-set that is free of a focus on details and strategy, at least immediately before performing the skill. There is still much work left to do before we have a complete understanding of attentional processes and how these processes affect performance.

Exercise and Brain Function

Another exciting area of research in exercise psychology is the examination of brain function as it is affected by exercise and in terms of how it influences our thoughts and feelings. Some of this work has incorporated animal models to examine changes in brain neurotransmitters thought to be involved in such processes. Interesting work is also being carried out with humans to determine how factors like brain blood flow, brain electrical activity, and by-products of brain neurotransmitters are linked with emotions and thoughts.

Research is beginning to demonstrate that blood flow to the brain changes as a function of exercise. In and of itself, this should be no great surprise. There do appear to be differential changes in blood flow, however, depending on the region of the brain being examined. For example, the temporal, parietal, and frontal regions of the brain have been shown to have fairly sizable increases in blood flow as exercise intensity increases from low to moderate levels. Related work in animals has shown that such changes also occur at deeper levels of the brain and may be localized to brain structures involved in processing certain types of information (e.g., emotions).

Studies examining electrical activity of the brain before, during, and after exercise have also revealed interesting findings. For example, electrical activity recorded from the scalp before exercise has been shown to predict how an individual will feel after that exercise. This electrical activity seems to be lateralized; greater activity in the left anterior hemisphere is related to more positive feelings after exercise. This work has provided interesting links between exercise, brain activity, and emotions (25).

Others have examined how regular exercise training might influence brain function. One classic study demonstrated that the brain function of older, physically active adults was much more similar to a group of younger adults than to a group of older sedentary adults (26). Their central nervous systems were more efficient in performing the cognitive tasks they were given. They were able to process information more quickly and more accurately, at least in part because of their regular level of physical activity. In essence, exercise seems to be able to slow the changes that are typically associated with aging.

Even with the advances that have been made regarding how the brain itself functions as a result of acute and chronic exercise, relatively little is known about how such functions relate to an individual's thoughts, emotions, and behaviors. This is, however, an exciting area of current research in exercise and sports psychology.

SUMMARY POINTS

- Exercise psychology is the science of how psychological principles can be used in the promotion, explanation, maintenance, and enhancement of physical activity behaviors.
- Sports psychology is the science of how psychological principles can be used in the promotion, explanation, maintenance, and enhancement of sports-related behaviors.
- Phenomena in exercise and sports psychology can be analyzed from multiple levels, including self-report, observation, and psychophysiology.
- Personality dimensions of extroversion–introversion and neuroticism–stability have been shown to be related to both exercise and sports behaviors. Extroverts typically do better in sports; regular exercise can lead to less neuroticism and greater emotional stability.

- The evidence supports the notion that independent, extroverted individuals gravitate toward sports as opposed to sports participation leading to independent, extroverted personalities.
- Motivation is composed of choice, intensity, and persistence.
- Self-efficacy, a person's belief that he or she can perform some activity to achieve a goal, has been consistently shown to be related to performance.
- Causal attributions are reasons people give for why things happen. The classic categories include ability, effort, luck, and task difficulty.
- The most consistent relationship between arousal and performance has been explained according to the inverted U hypothesis. This states that as arousal increases from low to moderate levels, performance increases; as arousal continues to more extreme levels, performance deteriorates.
- Attention research in sports psychology typically involves either a self-report or behavioral approach, both of which have limitations. Psychophysiologic approaches to attention have revealed consistent changes in heart rate and brain activity immediately before task performance. Such physiologic changes have been related to actual performance.
- Exercise has been shown to reduce negative mental health and to enhance psychological well-being. The explanation for such changes is currently unknown.
- One of the most promising areas of current research in exercise and sports psychology involves the study of brain function at multiple levels (e.g., neurochemical, metabolic, electrical), how such function is influenced by exercise, and how it relates to psychological events.

REVIEW QUESTIONS

1. What are the primary research objectives in the exercise and sports psychology area?
2. What has been the most commonly used measurement strategy in exercise and sports psychology?
3. What is the primary difference between exercise psychology and sports psychology?
4. Which dispositional theory of personality has been used to study personality in the physical activity domain?
5. How are personality states and traits distinguished?
6. What is meant by the term *self-serving bias*?
7. What are the two most prominent models for studying arousal–performance relationships? Briefly describe each model.
8. What are the ways in which attention can be studied?
9. Of the various hypotheses for explaining why exercise might lead to improved mental health, which is focused on brain neurotransmitters?
10. Are endorphins responsible for the feel-better phenomenon associated with exercise? Why or why not?

References

1. Mendez C. Book of bodily exercise. F. Guerra, trans. New Haven, CT: Licht, 1960 (1553).
2. James W. Physical training in the educational curriculum. Am Phys Educ Rev 1899;4:220–221.
3. Rejeski WJ, Brawley LR. Defining the boundaries of sport psychology. Sport Psychol 1988;2:231–242.
4. Vealey RS. Personality and sport: a comprehensive view. In: TS Horn, ed. Advances in sport psychology. Champaign, IL: Human Kinetics, 1992:25–59.
5. Hollander EP, Principles and methods of social psychology. New York, NY: Oxford University Press, 1967.

6. Cattell RB. The scientific analysis of personality. Baltimore: Penguin, 1965.
7. Eysenck HJ. A model for personality. Berlin: Springer-Verlag, 1981.
8. Eysenck HJ, Nias DK, Cox DN. Sport and personality. Adv Behav Res Ther 1982;4:1–56.
9. Petruzzello SJ, Landers DM, Hatfield BD, et al. A meta- analysis on the anxiety reducing effects of acute and chronic exercise: outcomes and mechanisms. Sports Med 1991;11:143–182.
10. Bandura A. Social foundations of thought and action. Englewood Cliffs, NJ: Prentice-Hall, 1986.
11. Weiner B. An attributional theory of motivation and emotion. New York: Springer, 1986.
12. Feltz, D.L. Self-confidence and sports performance. Exer Sport Sci Rev 1988;16:423–457.
13. Thayer RE. The biopsychology of mood and arousal. New York: Oxford University Press, 1989.
14. Dienstbier RA. Arousal and physiological toughness: implications for mental and physical health. Psychol Rev 1989;96:84–100.
15. Spence JT, Spence KW. The motivational components of manifest anxiety: drive and drive stimuli. In: CD Spielberger, ed. Anxiety and behavior. New York: Academic, 1966.
16. Landers DM, Boutcher SH. Arousal-performance relationships. In: JM Williams, ed. Applied sport psychology: personal growth to peak performance. Mountain View, CA: Mayfield, 1993:197–218.
17. Oxendine JB. Psychology of motor learning. Englewood Cliffs, NJ: Prentice Hall, 1984.
18. Nideffer RM. Predicting human behavior: a theory and test of attention and interpersonal style. San Diego: Enhanced Performance Associates, 1978.
19. Landers DM, Petruzzello SJ. Physical activity, fitness, and anxiety. In: C Bouchard, RJ Shephard, T Stephens, eds. Physical activity, fitness, and health. Champaign, IL: Human Kinetics, 1994:868–882.
20. Morgan WP. Physical activity, fitness, and depression. In: C Bouchard, RJ Shephard, T Stephens, eds. Physical activity, fitness, and health. Champaign, IL: Human Kinetics, 1994:851–867.
21. Dishman RK. Mental health. In: V Seefeldt, ed. Physical activity and well-being. Reston, VA: American Alliance for Health, Physical Education, Recreation and Dance, 1986:303–341.
22. Morgan WP, O'Connor PJ. Exercise and mental health. In: RK Dishman, ed. Exercise adherence: its impact on public health. Champaign, IL: Human Kinetics, 1988:91–121.
23. U.S. Department of Health and Human Services. The surgeon general's report on physical activity and health. Washington, DC: GPO, 1996.
24. Schurr KT, Ashley MA, Joy KL. A multivariate analysis of male athlete characteristics: sport type and success. Multivariate Exper Clin Res 1977;3:53–68.
25. Petruzzello SJ, Tate AK. Brain activation, affect, and aerobic exercise: an examination of both state-independent and state-dependent relationships. Psychophysiology 1997;34:527–533.
26. Dustman RE, Emmerson RY, Ruhling RO, et al. Age and fitness effects on EEG, ERPs, visual sensitivity, and cognition. Neurobiol Aging 1990;11:193–200.

Suggested Readings

Horn TS, ed. Advances in sport psychology. Champaign, IL: Human Kinetics, 1992.

Morgan WP, ed. Physical activity and mental health. Washington, DC: Taylor & Francis, 1996.

Singer RN, Murphy M, Tennant LK, eds. Handbook of research on sport psychology. New York: Macmillan, 1993.

Weinberg RS, Gould D. Foundations of sport and exercise psychology. Champaign, IL: Human Kinetics, 1995.

16

Motor Behavior

MARK A. GUADAGNOL

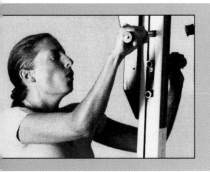

Objectives

1. Explain how motor behavior is integrated into the greater discipline of exercise science.
2. Identify the subcategories of motor behavior.
3. Describe how movement patterns and skills are learned.
4. Describe the way in which movement is controlled.
5. Identify the factors that influence control of movement.
6. Describe the changes in motor development across the life span.

This chapter continues the exploration of the behavioral knowledge base of exercise science by introducing the subdiscipline of motor behavior, which represents a marriage between the study of psychological and physiological processes. The word *motor,* defined as producing movement, has obvious significance within the discipline of exercise science. Important concepts, such as motor fitness, perceptual motor activity, and motor skills, are examined by exercise science students at many points in their academic preparation. It is within the context of motor behavior that these and many other such terms take on the special meaning regarding how motor skill is produced.

The concept of movement is too multidimensional to consider all its many aspects within this chapter. For instance, movement includes activities as diverse as painting, driving a car, and speaking, all aspects of movement that go well beyond exercise. Movement also has important biologic functions. At a basic level, movement is necessary for the survival of an organism and its species. For instance, eating, procreating, and locomotion all require movement. If we were unable to move, locomotion would be impossible, as would reaching, communicating, and seeing. Therefore, the study of motor behavior has many applications across a wide spectrum of movement activities.

In addition, this chapter focuses on movements that can be thought of as learned movements. These types of movements are often called **skills,** which generally take long periods of time to master. Perhaps Guthrie (1) defined skills best: "Skills consist of the ability to bring about some end result with maximum certainty and minimum outlay of energy, or time and energy." Movement skills can be wonderfully elegant forms of expression, as anyone who has watched Mikhail Baryshnikov leap or Michael Jordan dunking a basketball will attest. The study of movement, and hence the study of motor behavior, gives us insight into the skill of which Guthrie spoke. The purpose of this chapter is to describe briefly the three divisions of motor behavior and how movement skills develop and are learned.

DEFINITION, DESCRIPTION, AND SCOPE

Motor behavior includes three cognate disciplines: motor learning, motor control, and motor development (Fig. 16.1). Motor learning is concerned with understanding how people learn movements, i.e., how a relatively permanent change in behavior results from practice or experience. This relatively permanent change manifests itself in a more efficient orchestration of movements.

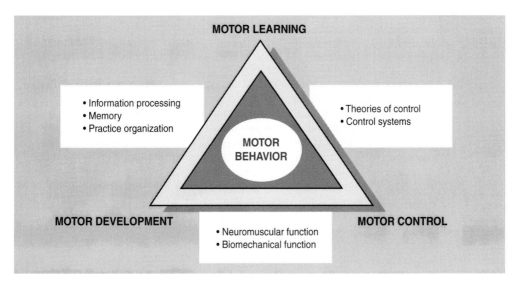

FIGURE 16.1 General content organization of motor behavior.

Issues such as how memory works, how to organize practice for efficient **learning,** and how we learn to process information fall under the domain of motor learning. Motor learning has its roots in psychology and education, yet the application of its principles is found in physical and occupational therapy, coaching, teaching, and human factors engineering.

Motor control is concerned with understanding the mechanisms by which the neuromuscular system orchestrates the myriad movements made by the organism and the manner in which these mechanisms are constrained. In other words, motor control is concerned with how our **central nervous system** (CNS; brain and spinal cord) plans and executes movements. Issues such as stabilizing the body before movement and carrying out rapid tasks are addressed through motor control.

Finally, motor development is concerned with understanding the change in movement orchestration that results from system maturation, rather than practice or experience. With motor development we are concerned with how our learning and control of movements change as we mature both physically and mentally. The field of motor development formerly dealt largely with development from infancy to adulthood. Now, it includes work with older adults. Therefore, motor development focuses not only on how we change as we grow to adulthood but, more generally, on how we change as we age.

There are two important things to note about the divisions of motor behavior. First, these divisions, although obviously related, are generally studied separately. This is partially because of the history of each division and the fact that the individuals studying them come from different areas of science. Second, the study of motor behavior is not just a study of sports skills or exercise. It can also be applied to a variety of other skills such as driving a car, drawing and writing, typing, and playing a musical instrument.

FOCUS ON SCIENCE

This section presents an overview of the subdiscipline of motor behavior, including a nonexhaustive review of the research associated with each area. Many of the studies cited use non-

A Case in Point 16.1

MAKING PRACTICE PAY OFF FOR YOU

Have you ever wondered the best way to practice something to learn it quickly? There are numerous ways practice can be organized, but one recent example comes from work done by Guadagnoli and co-workers.[a] The main research question in this study was, How should practice be organized to teach the skill of putting in golf? The conclusion was that practice should be stable for novice players and variable for experienced players. In general terms, this means that novice players should attempt several similar putts, for instance, from 4 ft away, before varying the putt distance. As the learner progresses he or she should change targets more frequently. For example, the novice player may putt 10 balls to the same hole before changing targets, whereas the more experienced player may want to change targets after putting only 3 balls to a single hole. In short, the experienced player, while performing in competition, will find that stable practices won't help much.

[a]Guadagnoli MA, Holcomb WR, Weber T. The relationship between contextual interference effects and performer experience on the learning of a putting task. J Hum Movement Stud 1999;37:19–36.

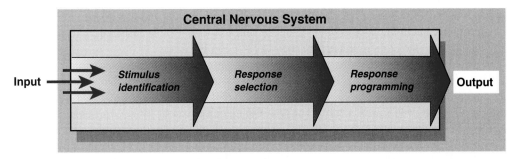

FIGURE 16.2 Information processing model demonstrating how humans process information. The model flows from left to right

sports-related tasks; in these cases take a moment to think about the results of the studies and how they can be applied to some motor skill you are trying to learn.

Motor Learning

How would you like to learn five times faster? Have you ever been curious about how memory works? Do you ever wonder why you seem to understand something in class, or during practice, but not on a test or during a game? Why does it take us so long to react to an external stimulus some times but not other times? If you have ever thought about these questions, you share some interests with motor learning researchers. As mentioned, motor learning is the study of how we learn motor skills, but there is a lot more to it than that. In general, one can think of it as understanding how we learn, how we process information, how we best organize practice to make for efficient learning, and how memory works (see A Case in Point 16.1).

Do we learn motor skills the same way we learn verbal skills, that is, how to read or how to do mathematics? Franklin Henry, generally regarded as the father of motor behavior, argued that motor learning and **verbal learning** are different. Verbal learning is learning what to do, whereas motor learning is learning how to do. Although it is not obvious from a scientific perspective that there are fundamental differences between the two, we know that there are many findings in the verbal literature that correlate with findings in the motor literature. In general, it seems that some of the findings in motor learning research can be applied to verbal learning, and visa versa. Therefore, many of the same strategies from motor learning can help with verbal learning. Important categories of motor learning research are presented next.

Information Processing

The study of information processing comes from cognitive psychology, and relates to how we process information. Because we are constantly bombarded by information, we must decide what is important and what is not and then organize the commands so the muscles can respond. Information processing is generally broken down into three stages (Fig. 16.2): taking information in from our environment (stimulus identification), deciding what to do with the information (response selection), and organizing and executing the response (response programming).

The challenge in studying human information processing is that it cannot be directly observed. Remember, information processing takes place in the brain; and even if we could directly examine the brain, we would not know exactly what each stage of information processing looks like. Therefore, indirect methods are used to hypothesize the activity of the brain during information processing. One indirect method is to analyze how quickly one responds. That is, we can measure the time from when a stimulus (any external cue in the environment) is presented until the person makes a response. This time is generally referred to as **reaction time,** which indicates how long it takes a person to process the information involved in making a decision and to respond. The method of using reaction time to analyze a person's mental processing is termed the **chronometric method.** Factors that influence reaction time enable researchers to determine what happens in the brain to initiate this response.

Researchers have generally regarded information processing as happening one stage at a time, a view that has continued to define the field in more recent research and reviews. This approach to information processing employs the manipulation of one stage at a time to see how it affects overall reaction time. Through the manipulation of processes in one stage, researchers speculate on the role of that particular stage in processing information. For example, two distinct stimulus–response arrangements are shown in Figure 16.3. On the left there is one stimulus (light) and one response (key). The job of the subject is to push the response button with the right index finger as soon as the light comes on (150 msec is a typical response time). On the right side of the figure there are two stimulus lights and two response alternatives, left and right. The job of the subject is to push the response button that is directly below the stimulus light that is illuminated. In this arrangement, it may take 250 msec to respond. In both cases, the subject is responding to a light; therefore, the stimulus identification is the same for the two conditions. In both cases, the subject is responding by pressing a response key, so the response programming is the same for the two conditions. However, in the first condition the subject has no choice to make, whereas in the second situation there is a choice. Therefore, the response selection is different for the two conditions. The difference in reaction time between the two conditions is the result of response selection. In fact, a finding known as Hick's law predicts that as the number of response choices increases so does reaction time (2), i.e., when we have more choices it takes more time to chose, and we are more likely to make the wrong choice.

Any batter who has faced a pitcher who has an arsenal of multiple pitches has personally experienced Hick's law. If the pitcher has only one pitch (an 80 mile per hour fastball, for example), the batter will have no decision about which pitch is coming and is, therefore, likely to be successful. However, if the pitcher has several pitches (e.g., fastball, curveball, change-up, and slider), the batter has a much more difficult task. Because most pitchers have more than one pitch, the batter's job is difficult. This is one of the reasons that a batter who gets a hit 3 out of 10 (30%) tries is considered a very good batter.

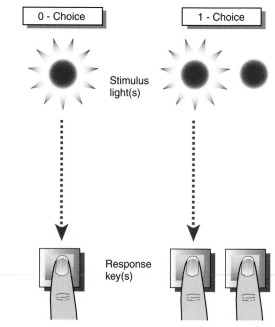

FIGURE 16.3 Zero- and one-choice stimulus–response arrangements. The subject is told to press the button under the light that turns on.

What is involved in responding to some external stimulus like a baseball? First, the person must recognize that something is changing in the environment, that some stimulus has appeared, such as a baseball being thrown. The person must then choose the appropriate response to that stimulus, such as swinging at the ball or not. Finally, the brain must organize a specific set of commands to send out to the muscles. These commands give specific directions about how to stabilize the body and where and when to swing the bat.

Stimulus identification, the detection and identification of a stimulus (such as a baseball), is affected by the intensity and clarity of the stimulus. In women's softball, a neon yellow ball is usually used to increase the intensity and clarity of the ball so the batter can identify it more easily. An important aspect to stimulus identification is that the brain must be aroused to the point at which it contacts memory. Memory is important to make an association between the stimulus and something meaningful. Once an appropriate meaning is attached, the stimulus can be passed on to the response selection stage.

In the response selection stage of processing, the subject decides on an appropriate response. The variables of greatest interest to the response selection stage are the number of stimulus–response alternatives and stimulus–response compatibility. Practice may affect both of these variables. The compatibility between a stimulus and a response has been extensively explored; generally, the more closely related (compatible) the stimulus is to the response relationship, the faster the response (3).

In the response programming stage, the commands to the muscles are organized and initiated. The most prevalent variable to be manipulated in this stage is that of the complexity of the response. The **duration** of the response has also been addressed. Evidence has indicated that as the complexity of the response to be made increases, the reaction time increases (4). In addition, the amount of time one has to prepare muscular commands seems to affect response programming (4,5).

Information processing can be used in a practical way to speed up or slow down an individual's reaction time. To begin with, certain strategies allow for a particular amount of anticipation or preparation for a movement. Other strategies can specifically affect each of the three stages previously mentioned. In a sports setting, one can gain an advantage, for example, by making plays look alike (stimulus identification), increasing the opponents options (response selection), or making the opponent perform a more complicated task (response programming).

Each of these manipulations and their referenced studies have demonstrated effects on the three major stages of information processing. The challenges to each individual stage have been shown to increase the overall reaction time. By employing these methods, some researchers have claimed that the stages are discrete and distinct, whereas others indicate that there are alternatives to the idea that information processing is serial, asserting that we are able to perform the processes of more than one stage concurrently (6,7).

Memory

Perhaps the most widely used model to explain memory, proposed by Atkinson and Shiffrin (8), is called the multistore memory model because it has more than two stores or memory divisions. In fact, the model has three stores: short-term sensory store (STSS), short-term memory (STM), and long-term memory (LTM). In Figure 16.4, the arrow going from STM to LTM signifies information going into the LTM store. This process is known as encoding. The arrow going from LTM to STM signifies information moving from the permanent storehouse (LTM) to the working memory (STM). This process is called decoding.

Each memory store has a specific duty and a defined **capacity** and limitation. The **capacity** of a memory store is the amount of information it can hold. The duration is the length of time that information can be held. The STSS takes information in from the environment through the senses (e.g., vision, audition). It has an unlimited capacity but a duration of less than 1 sec. This means that we can hold a lot of information for a very short period of time. The STSS holds in-

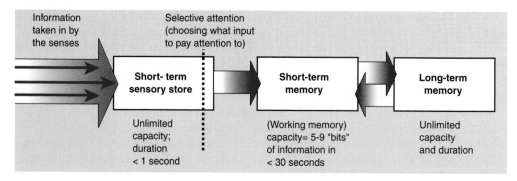

FIGURE 16.4 How information flows *(arrows)* through the multistore memory model.

formation while we decide if it is important enough to attend to. This decision is made by a process called **selective attention,** whereby we actively choose one unit of information to pay attention to at a time. The information that is attended to is sent to the next memory store, STM.

STM, was originally at the heart of memory, because it is our conscious memory, also known as working memory (9). The capacity of STM is considered to be five to nine bits, or units, of information (10). What exactly constitutes a bit depends on how the information is organized. For example, the letters *m, p, i, r, e, c, a,* and *f* constitute eight bits of information to be remembered. However, when the letters are reorganized to *campfire,* there is only one bit of information to remember. Recently, there has been a great deal of interest in how the presentation of information and the organization of practice can affect how one organizes information. You can see how grouping information, known as *chunking,* could be helpful to learning.

The duration of STM is considered to be less than 30 sec if uninterrupted. However, this may not be particularly important. A simple experiment that demonstrates this phenomenon is to empty your mind and think of nothing for the next 30 sec. You quickly realize that it is difficult, if not impossible, to not let anything into your consciousness for even 30 sec. If you were successful, this means that you did not see, hear, or think anything. If this were true, you could not have noticed when 30 sec had passed because you could not have noticed your watch.

If information is deemed important enough to store it permanently, it is sent from STM to LTM. LTM has an unlimited capacity and duration. A question that may arise is that if the capacity and duration are unlimited, why do we sometimes forget things that we used to know? The answer (barring an accident or illness that affected the brain) is that we haven't lost the information from LTM, but have failed to retrieve it. This means that we still have the information, but we don't know how to access it. This is similar to working on a word processor. Sometimes we have saved a file on a disk or the hard drive and we cannot remember where it is. It is still where we saved it, but we can't access it.

It is important to note that memory can be thought of as retaining information, which, by definition, is learning. Therefore, to understand learning, an understanding of memory is important. Motor learning theorists have gone to great lengths to understand memory and ways that practice can be organized to optimize the efficiency with which we learn (11).

Practice Organization and Learning

Inherent in the discussion of learning is the **practice–learning distinction.** Typically, **performance** is defined as observable behavior. Learning is defined as a relatively permanent change in behavior that results from practice or experience. Because learning results from a change in one's internal state, i.e., a change in memory, it cannot be directly observed and must be inferred from performance, typically via a retention test.

The practice–learning distinction is critical, because one's performance during practice is not necessarily an index of learning (11). In fact, many studies have demonstrated a practice–learning paradox in which variables affect practice performance and retention performance (learning) in an opposite manner. For example, practicing variations of a task, instead of practicing the same task over and over again, has been shown to hinder practice performance but enhance learning (12,13). For example, putting a golf ball to several targets (rather than repeatedly to the same target) may hinder practice performance but enhance learning (12). It appears that a practice organization that does not sufficiently challenge the performer (such as low practice variability or too much feedback) enhances practice performance, but hinders learning. This information is important, because instructors commonly provide frequent feedback to students, noting that students perform better than when feedback is infrequently given. The students' performance during practice is generally taken as an index of learning. However, in a test situation (a measure of learning), when the frequent feedback is not available, performance is likely to be poor. In this example, instructors help students resolve motor problems instead of challenging the students to learn.

The organization of the practice is critically important to learning. For example, if a student must learn a variety of tasks, is it better to present all the tasks in each practice session or to present just one task per session? This question and others will be addressed next.

CONTEXTUAL INTERFERENCE   The term **contextual interference** was introduced by Battig (14) to describe the interference that results from practicing a variety of tasks within the context of a single practice situation. A high degree of contextual interference can be established by having the performer practice several skills during the same practice session. Shooting a basketball from a variety of locations to learn a jump shot is an example of high contextual interference. A low degree of contextual interference can be established by having the performer practice only one task during a practice session. Shooting a basketball repeatedly from the same location is an example of low contextual interference. It has been demonstrated that low contextual interference practice (relative to high contextual interference) leads to superior practice performance, but much poorer learning (15). This is an example of the practice–retention paradox. This paradox may be performer dependent. It appears that for inexperienced individuals, high levels of contextual interference during practice is not more beneficial for learning than low levels. In fact, it has been demonstrated that until the performer is experienced at a task, high levels of contextual interference may be detrimental to efficient learning, but after some degree of competency is reached, high contextual interference is beneficial. Therefore, early in practice, decreasing extraneous interference is desired, but as the performer becomes more proficient, more interference is desired.

VARIABILITY OF PRACTICE   A concept similar to contextual interference, practicing variations of a task compared to practicing the same task over and over again, has been shown to hinder practice performance but enhance learning (13). Like contextual interference, variability appears to be performer dependent. For example, it has been demonstrated that practice variability affects children differently from the way it affects adults, suggesting that one's ability and previous knowledge, relative to the practice organization, influences learning (16,17).

Knowledge of Results

Feedback describing a successful performance after a practice session is a critically important factor in performance and learning. Understandably then, the relationship between feedback and the learning of motor skills has for some time been a source of interest for practitioners and theorists alike. Experimentally, this relationship has been studied chiefly via **knowledge of results** (KR), usually defined as error information in addition to what the performer can get on his or her own. In other words, KR is information given to the performer by a therapist, teacher, or coach about the performer's success on an attempted response. An example of KR is telling a pitcher that he or she threw a strike. Currently, scheduling of KR is being investigated under a variety of conditions. One such variation that has drawn recent attention is known as summary KR.

SUMMARY KNOWLEDGE OF RESULTS   The **summary knowledge of results** method requires a subject to complete several (e.g., five) trials of a simple motor task without receiving KR. After the trials have been completed, KR about those trials is given to the subject. This procedure is similar to a coach waiting for a quarterback to complete a series of downs before giving KR about the series. In a laboratory setting, summary KR has been shown to be strongly detrimental to practice performance compared to when KR is given immediately after each trial (11). The fact that summary KR hinders practice performance but facilitates learning was first introduced into motor learning research by Lavery (18). Lavery's findings contradict both intuition and the traditional view of learning, which suggests that any variation of KR that provides more precise, frequent, and/or accurate information on movement outcome has a positive effect on learning (19,20). However, it may be that if KR is given to the performer immediately after a response, the performer is not motivated to process other information (e.g., internal feedback). Rather, the performer uses the KR to guide trial-to-trial performance instead of actually learning to solve the motor problem.

Although Lavery established that immediate KR may be detrimental to learning, he also confirmed that some degree of KR is beneficial for learning. Other researchers built on these results to find the optimal length of summary KR. Optimal length is task dependent (21), i.e., a task of great complexity requires more help to solve the motor problem than does a simple task. From an applied standpoint, this suggests that if an individual is to learn a complex task (e.g., a double-twist back-flip dive), more immediate KR should be given than if the same athlete were learning a simple task (e.g., a front dive). It has also been suggested that optimal feedback may be performer dependent (11). It was found that as a learner practices, the optimal summary length increases. That is, inexperienced individuals perform better during both practice and competition if the summary length is short; as the athlete becomes more skilled, a short summary may lead to better performance during practice but produces less learning. Therefore, keeping the task constant, the expert may need less immediate KR than the novice.

FADING KNOWLEDGE OF RESULTS   **Fading knowledge of results** is systematically reducing the amount of KR throughout the practice period. For example, KR may be given after each trial early in practice, after every 3rd trial toward the middle of practice, and only after every 10th trial late in practice. This fading technique has been shown to be beneficial for learning. Once again, it appears that helping the performer solve the motor problem early in practice and reducing the help as skill proficiency increases is a highly effective practice schedule.

Part–Whole Practice

When riding a bike with training wheels, the child learns some of the skills of riding a bicycle (steering and braking) before learning all the skills (including balance). As most practitioners are aware, part–whole practice is common in the teaching of many complex skills (e.g., learning the breaststroke). A question that arises is whether or not part–whole practice makes for more efficient learning than practicing a whole task. To answer this question, researchers have used a dichotomy in which skills are classified by complexity (number of parts) and organization (dependency relationship between parts).

Researchers have suggested that skills high in complexity and low in organization (e.g., shooting a jump shot in basketball) benefit from part–whole practice. Skills that are low in complexity and high in organization (e.g., running a pass pattern) benefit from practicing the skill as a whole. Unfortunately, all skills do not fall into such a simple dichotomy. Therefore, a progressive-part method of practice has been suggested. Using this method, separate parts of a skill are practiced independently but ordered according to the order in which each part occurs in the skill. As parts are learned, they are progressively linked together until the skill is practiced as a whole. The progressive-part practice organization provides strong constraints early in practice, when parts are practiced independently, but provides fewer constraints as the task becomes more well learned.

Using the example of riding a bicycle, first we start with peddling. Because there are training wheels on the bike, balance is not part of the equation; and if we go only in a straight direction, steering is not a factor either. That is, balance and steering are constrained in the task. Eventually, we start changing direction by steering, and it becomes part of the equation. Finally, the training wheels are taken off and balance becomes part of the equation. Essentially, the efficiency of a progressive–part practice organization suggests that the cognitive training wheels of the task should strongly constrain skills early in practice and the constraints should lessen skill proficiency increases.

The literature suggests two important points: practice performance does not necessarily indicate learning, as shown through the practice–retention paradox; and as the level of the performer increases, the extent to which that performer is helped should decrease. From this information, a principle of the relationship between practice and learning has been developed.

PARADOX PRINCIPLE   There are several paradoxes in learning that can be better understood through motor learning. For example, have you ever wondered why you do well during practice but poorly in a game? Maybe you have had an experience where during a study session, you think you know the information but still perform poorly on a test. Yet there are other situations where you may not perform well during practice or you may struggle in studying for a test, but in fact you perform quite well when you are tested on the field or in the classroom. These are all examples of the practice–learning paradox. That is, practice performance does not necessarily indicate how much one is learning. This paradox involves all the motor learning discussed thus far in this chapter.

LEARNING AND TASK DIFFICULTY   Figure 16.5 shows the hypothetical relationship between practice performance and **task difficulty,** which is defined as the difficulty of the motor problem one must resolve to successfully complete a task. For example, trying to make a 20-ft. sloping putt is more difficult than trying to make a 2-ft. straight putt. Task difficulty has been manipulated through changes in task complexity, as in the putting example. Task difficulty can also be manipulated by changing the quality and/or quantity of feedback, practice organization, and/or experience level.

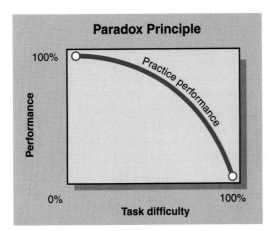

FIGURE 16.5 Task difficulty and practice performance. As task difficulty increases, performance decreases.

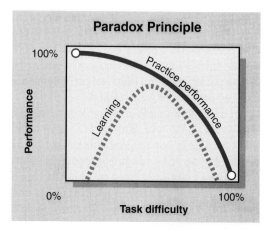

FIGURE 16.6 Task difficulty, practice, and learning performance. As task difficulty increases, learning increases until the point at which the performer is optimally challenged.

As shown in Figure 16.5, as task difficulty increases, practice performance decreases. That is, as the motor problem becomes more difficult, performance deteriorates. This is a fairly straightforward and obvious prediction. However, learners are generally not as concerned with practice performance as they are with what happens during a test or competition (i.e., learning).

Figure 16.6 shows the hypothetical relationship between learning and task difficulty. As you can see, learning increases with increasing task difficulty, to a point. At that point, known as the **challenge point,** the student is being optimally challenged to enhance learning. Notice that at the challenge point, practice performance is not optimal, but learning is optimal. Increasing the task difficulty beyond this point further hinders practice performance and begins to hinder learning.

Previous findings are consistent with the notion that to a point, a more difficult practice organization leads to poorer practice performance, but superior retention performance (11,15). These findings have shown that practice performance does not necessarily indicate learning, and too much or too little relative difficulty hinders learning. For example, in the summary KR experiments cited earlier, it was found that increasing summary length enhanced learning to a point. Beyond that point, learning was hindered by an excessively long summary length.

What amount of difficulty is optimal for learning? Optimal difficulty depends on the level of the performer and the complexity of the task. Within a task, difficulty may be manipulated by some type of cognitive training wheel. That is, if the task is too simple (e.g., the teacher constantly gives feedback to the performer) the cognitive training wheels could be adjusted to increase the task difficulty (less feedback may encourage the student to solve the motor problem). On the other hand, if the task is too difficult, the difficulty could be decreased by adjusting the cognitive training wheels.

Completing the picture of learning and task difficulty is **relative task difficulty,** which is defined as the difficulty of the motor problem one must resolve to successfully complete a task relative to the performer completing the task. As discussed, when keeping the task constant, the relative task difficulty depends on the level of the performer. For example, the task of trying to hit a golf ball provides little difficulty to a professional golfer but tremendous difficulty to a novice golfer. In the same sense, the task of tying one's shoe laces is much more difficult for a five-year-old than for a teenager. Accordingly, practice organization should be adjusted as the performer's level changes. That is, the difficulty of the task should increase as the performer becomes more proficient. The specifics of the extent to which one should be challenged during practice to optimize learning has not been well documented.

Motor learning seems to be most efficient when the learner is challenged most efficiently. This does not mean the learner is challenged to optimize practice performance but that he or she is challenged to optimize learning.

Motor Control

Motor control is concerned with understanding the mechanisms by which the neural and muscular systems coordinate the myriad movements we make.

Neuroanatomy

Neuroanatomy is the study of the functions of the brain, spinal cord, and peripheral nervous system (Fig. 16.7). The brain and spinal cord taken together are known as the central nervous system. The CNS is made up of **neurons,** defined as nerve cells that send and receive messages throughout the CNS. Some of the neurons associated with the CNS carry messages to and from the brain. Motor (efferent) neurons send commands to the motor system (i.e., the muscles). **Sensory (afferent) neurons** send signals from the senses to the CNS.

The neurons in the brain carry messages among areas in the brain that are specialized for specific purposes. Much of what we know about the function of the brain was learned by study-

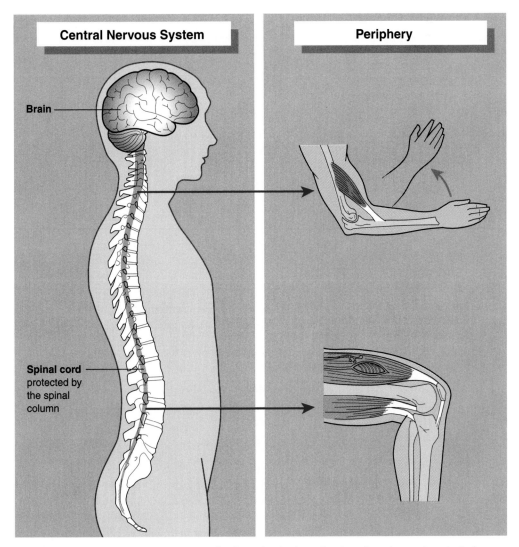

FIGURE 16.7 The central nervous system (brain and spinal cord), where learning and control of movements take place.

ing people who were victims of injury to different areas of the brain. Sometimes these injuries are very serious and with drastic outcomes. Medical science has been able to elucidate brain function in each area, but this remains one of the least understood fields of physiology. Generally, the brain can be divided into five areas: cerebellum, basal ganglia, supplementary motor cortex, premotor cortex, and motor cortex.

CEREBELLUM   The cerebellum is the area of the brain that receives afferent signals. When the cerebellum is damaged, different animals are affected in different ways. Cats demonstrate decerebrate (elimination of cerebral function) rigidity, a syndrome in which the limbs become extremely rigid. Humans and other primates demonstrate hypotonia, a state of low muscle tone. In humans, cerebellar damage affects coordination. For example, balance suffers, walking heel to toe becomes almost impossible, eye movements are affected, the ability to point to a target is impaired to the extent that the individual performs a homing-in maneuver. Simple sequential movements, like turning the palm up and down, is very difficult. Individuals with cerebellar damage are often misunderstood, because their motor functions may mimic those of an intoxicated person. In fact, individuals who suffer from cerebellar damage have often been accused of being alcoholics based solely on their behavior.

BASAL GANGLIA   The basal ganglia are a set of interconnected structures in the forebrain. One of the diseases associated with damage to the basal ganglia is Huntington disease (HD). The disease starts as occasional clumsiness and forgetfulness; but eventually the afflicted person falls prey to uncontrollable ballistic (i.e., fast) movements, an inability to reason, and finally death. HD is hereditary and has been traced to seventeenth-century Salem, Massachusetts, the period known for the Salem Witch trials in which some of those individuals accused of being witches undoubtedly manifested the uncontrollable behavior typical of HD.

Another disease resulting from basal ganglia damage is Parkinson disease, which manifests as shuffled walking, a shaking motion known as resting tremors, slowness to initiate and complete movements, and strong rigidity. Parkinson disease results from a deficit in the neurotransmitter dopamine. L-Dopa and deprenyl are used to lessen the symptoms of the disease.

Based on injury or illness, it is hypothesized that the basal ganglia serve three main functions: movement organization, scale and amplitude of movement, and perceptual–motor integration. The basal ganglia are believed to help in choosing and organizing how we are to move. A second role is scale amplitude of the movement. Such decisions as how much force to put into picking up a milk jug are partially the role of the basal ganglia (if we apply too much force, we may hit the top of the refrigerator with the jug). Related to scaling movements is perceptual–motor integration. This means coordinating our environment with our goal. Hitting a ball requires us to perceive the flight of the ball and estimate how long it will take for us to swing a bat to meet the ball. This is an example of how we perceive our environment and coordinate it with our motor (muscular) activity.

SUPPLEMENTARY MOTOR CORTEX   The supplementary motor cortex is important for planning movements. It takes information from other areas of the brain, such as the basal ganglia and cerebellum, and starts to organize a movement. Information from the supplementary motor cortex is sent to the premotor cortex for further processing.

PREMOTOR CORTEX   The premotor cortex sends efferent signals to the proximal musculature, like the trunk and shoulders. What would happen if information was sent to the distal musculature without first stabilizing the proximal musculature? If you tried to hurriedly raise your hand in class without your trunk being stabilized by the premotor cortex, you would likely fall forward on your desk. The premotor cortex also receives signals that help with spatial orientation. The premotor cortex first evaluates its initial conditions and then starts the plan of action, stabilizing the system before movement. Once the premotor cortex has stabilized the system, movement plans are sent to the motor cortex.

MOTOR CORTEX   The motor cortex was the first place localized brain function was found. Interestingly, the motor cortex was mapped primarily by neurosurgeons poking parts of the cortex to see what they do. This was not done just for the doctor's amusement, rather it was a practice commonly done for victims of epilepsy. An epileptic seizure that started in one part of the motor cortex may spread to another area and cause a deadly seizure. To keep this from happening, the doctor would find out where the seizure started (in the hand, for instance), open the skull and poke in different parts until the area associated with the hand was found, and that area would be removed, in the hope of stopping the seizures. The motor cortex appears to be a trigger for movement, because it is one of the last areas to be active before movement begins. Besides being a trigger, the motor cortex also receives feedback and sends signals to distal musculature.

PERIPHERAL MOTOR SYSTEM   The peripheral motor system consists of the nerves and muscles those nerves innervate. A motor unit is the fundamental functional unit of the peripheral motor system and is made up of a motor neuron and all the muscle fibers it innervates. What this means is that we don't have a single neuron for each muscle fiber or each muscle. In some cases, like in the eyes and tongue, we need fine control, so we have a motor neuron that controls just a few muscle fibers. In this way, control is precise but not powerful. Other areas, like the quadriceps muscles of the anterior thigh, have one motor neuron for many muscle fibers. In this way, control is powerful but not precise.

General Motor Control Theories

The fact that motor neurons innervate a muscle is only half the story. The sensory information coming back from the periphery is important. In fact, the first theory of motor learning was based on the interaction between motor and sensory neurons. In 1971 Adams (19) presented the **closed-loop** theory of motor learning. *Closed loop* means that feedback (e.g., vision, audition, proprioception) in the form of sensory information necessary to control the movement is received during the movement. Early experimental evidence for the closed-loop system came from Keele and Posner (22), but it may be intuitively perceived when we notice that we can correct movements midstream. Correction can occur because the movements are being performed with feedback. The advantage of this type of system is accuracy, because movements can be controlled as they are happening. Evaluating the feedback to control movements takes time; therefore, one disadvantage to a closed-loop system is lack of speed. An example of this system is the automatic pilot mechanisms on airplanes that receive feedback from navigation instruments to make course corrections.

In 1975 Schmidt (20) introduced a theory of motor learning that incorporated an **open-loop** mechanism. *Open loop* means that we do not receive feedback on-line (i.e., during the movement). Instead, movements are completely preplanned. That is, movements are controlled by a motor program made up of a predefined set of commands that, once sent out, complete a movement without the intervention of feedback. Early evidence for the open-loop system came from Henry and Rogers (23). The advantage of this type of system is speed, because the time it takes to provide feedback is eliminated. An example of this system is the traffic turn signal that is preset to change colors at fixed time intervals regardless of the traffic needs. Figure 16.8 illustrates both closed- and open-loop control systems.

Whether humans can be viewed completely as servomechanisms (control systems operating by positive and negative feedback) and the extent to which open-loop systems are operative are still concerns of active research.

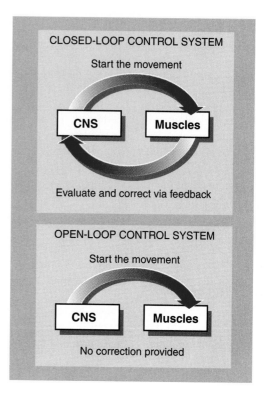

FIGURE 16.8 Closed-loop control systems involve the use of feedback, the determination of error, and correction of the error for better performance.

Motor Development

Motor development, sometimes called life-span development, is concerned with the study of motor performance throughout life. Motor development differs from motor learning and control in at least three ways. First, motor development is arguably more wedded to physiology than control and learning. Physical maturation and growth play such a great role in one's motor development that these factors must be central in most studies of the area.

Second, the methods of study in motor development often differ from motor learning and control. Longitudinal and cross-sectional studies are much more prevalent in developmental studies than in studies of learning and control. Furthermore, the findings we will discuss in motor development, particularly with infants and children, are descriptive rather than experimental. Descriptive studies describe what happens, whereas experimental studies attempt to explain why something happened. Descriptive results generally come from observation, whereas experimental results come from manipulating variables within a study. Finally, the origins of the field of motor development come primarily from education, although the areas of physiology and educational psychology also play a role in the study of motor development.

Methods of Study

Descriptive research is generally defined as describing the current state of the problem. With this type of research, experimental variables are not manipulated and conclusions about why an effect occurs are not justified. For example, consider a study that concluded that a strong relationship exists between alcohol consumption and longevity (how long one lives). This finding is the result of charting how much alcohol one consumes on a weekly basis and then recording the individual's age at death. To say that there is a strong relationship between alcohol consumption and longevity is simply describing the state of the problem. From this description, one cannot say why alcohol and longevity are related. The study only allows a description, not an explanation, of what happens.

Experimental research is generally defined as manipulating a variable or variables to investigate the effect on some outcome. In this case conclusions about why an effect occurs are justified. For example, we could perform an experimental study to see if alcohol consumption affects longevity. One way to do this would be to get several individuals who do not consume alcohol and give them a prescribed number of alcoholic beverages, per week, for the rest of their lives. If individuals who drink two to three glasses of alcohol a week live longer, as the descriptive study suggests, we can conclude that alcohol affects longevity. Three types of experimental research are longitudinal, cross-sectional, and sequential.

Longitudinal Studies   The **longitudinal method** is the study of motor development over time. For example, studying changes in an individual's throwing pattern from age 4 to 14 is longitudinal research. Studying the intelligence of an individual, or group of individuals, from age 20 to 80 is a longitudinal study. This method is probably the most reliable of the three types of experimental research, because societal and technological factors do not play large parts in the results. In the example of assessing intelligence over the life span, the method of assessing intelligence can affect the results. If a computer test was used to assess intelligence, for example, it may give an undue advantage to individuals familiar with computers. Their intelligence, as tested on a computer, may be artificially inflated or deflated based on the method of assessment.

Learning over the course of the study is a problem often seen in longitudinal studies. Repeated testing may affect the data just because the subjects learn how to take the test. If you were given the same test year after year, it would likely affect your results. Perhaps the most prohibitive aspects of longitudinal studies is time. To examine intelligence for an individual from age 20 until 80 takes 60 years!

Cross-Sectional Studies   The **cross-sectional method** resolves some of the problems of the longitudinal method. Whereas the longitudinal method requires one to collect data on the same individuals over a part of the life span, the cross-sectional method requires one to collect data on individuals of different ages who represent different parts of the life span. Thus all the data can be collected at once; therefore, handling the problem of the time length of the study. Furthermore, because each individual is tested once, the problem of repeated testing is handled.

Unfortunately, cross-sectional research is not without its problems. The biggest problem, as mentioned earlier, is that different age groups might differ in performance for reasons other than age (e.g., societal and technological factors).

Sequential Studies   The **sequential method** combines the longitudinal and cross-sectional methods. The method involves studying several different samples (cross-sectional) over a number of years (longitudinal). This method allows individuals differing in age or education, for example, to be compared at the same time to identify current behavioral differences.

Life Span Stages

Generally the life span is divided into five stages: infancy, childhood, adolescence, adulthood, and older adulthood. Each of these stages is marked by either developmental markers or age, but there is not always agreement between motor development scientists. Some researchers suggest seven stages: prenatal, infancy, early childhood, later childhood, adolescence, adulthood, and older adulthood (25). Even within stages, scientists are not in complete agreement. For example, Haywood (24) describes the childhood period as extending from 1 to 10 years; but Gabbard (25) states that the childhood stage extends from 2 to 12 years of age. He identified particular phases of movement that might be expected to emerge during each of the life span stages.

Infancy   A large part of the information about infancy comes from descriptive research. Descriptive research simply describes what infants do, not why they do it. A lot of this description involves **primitive reflexes,** which are associated with infants' basic needs, such as nourishment and security (see Box 16.1).

One of the interesting questions regarding these reflexes is what happens to them as we age. For example, the tonic neck reflex is elicited when the infant's head is turned to the side. The response to the head turning is an extension of the arm and leg on that side. Obviously such reflexive actions aren't noticeable in adults; rather, they are present to only about the first year of life. Therefore, it appears that these reflexes are integrated into our normal movements and/or suppressed as the nervous system matures (see Practical Application 16.1). Not all movements displayed by infants are reflexive. One of the most significant contributions of the work conducted by maturational theorists is the identification and description of landmark activities that occur during an infant's early adventures. These landmarks are prevalent for locomotion and manual control.

Locomotion, for infants, includes crawling, creeping, and walking. Crawling is described as using the arms to pull and the legs to push oneself forward. During the crawling motion the infant's stomach stays in contact with the ground. Creeping is similar to crawling, but the infant's stomach and chest are off the ground. Walking is defined as a movement that shifts weight from one foot to the other, with at least one foot contacting the surface at a time. The occurrence of these forms of locomotion in the development of an infant is important. For example, Shirley (26) studied walking and offered a detailed description of the stages leading up to it. The infant first takes steps while being supported, than stands with support, then walks when led by an external source (e.g., a parent), and finally walks alone.

Similar to locomotion, manual control (movement of the hands and arms to manipulate an object) normally progresses in an organized fashion. The stages of manual control are reaching, grasping, and releasing behaviors. Infants generally move from simply moving the hand toward an object (reaching), to pressing against an object with the palm of the hand (early stage of grasping), to releasing the grasped object by dropping it, to releasing an object with fairly precise control. The learning of these stages in an elementary way generally takes about 14 months. Throwing, which incorporates more complex releasing techniques, generally requires 24 months.

CHILDHOOD   Childhood involves the improvements in fundamental movement skills and the practice of these movements for sports and recreational activities. During childhood, fundamental movement patterns are learned and refined from immature to mature levels. Fundamental movement patterns are common motor activities that involve specific movement patterns, such as walking, running, jumping, and throwing. Immature patterns are generally considered the minimal level of proficiency, whereas mature patterns are considered proficient enough to meet sports skill form (Fig. 16.9). By the age of three, most children display some level of funda-

Box 16.1
Examples of Primitive Reflexes for Infants

Reflex	Stimulus	Response
Sucking	Touch the face above or below lips	Sucking motion begins
Startle	Tap abdomen or startle infant	Arms and legs flex
Babinski	Stroke sole of foot from heel to toes	Toes extend
Asymmetric tonic neck	Turn head to one side	Same-side arm and leg extend
Palmar grasping	Touch palm with finger or object	Hand closes tightly

Practical Application 16.1

WHAT HAPPENS TO THE TONIC NECK REFLEX AS WE AGE?

Evidence of what happens with the primitive reflexes as we age can be found in a variety of sources. One such source is head and spinal injury patients. Many of these patients are unable to move voluntarily, and in some cases are not conscious. It has been demonstrated in a clinical setting that many of these patients demonstrate behavior similar to the primitive reflexes seen in infants. That is, when the central nervous system is compromised, the reflexes that seemed to fade out as we mature, now seem to reappear.

A second line of evidence comes from the laboratory. It was found that patterns consistent with primitive reflexes exist in the normal, mature CNS. If the head is turned to one side the limbs on that side extend more forcefully and the limbs on the other side contract more forcefully. That is, intact humans demonstrate a behavior consistent with the tonic neck reflex, but the effect is much more subtle than that shown in infants and spinal victims. This may be one reason why when one is performing a difficult biceps curl or is arm wrestling, it is best to turn the head away from that arm. Thus the answer to what happens to the primitive reflexes as we mature seems to be that they are integrated into our everyday movements.

mental movement patterns. Usually by six years of age, the child has refined these patterns to the extent that they would be classified as mature.

For the child to become aware of his or her shape, size, and capacity is critical at this point. In addition to being aware of one's body, basic mechanical principles of movement are being learned. A child may not know the formula for aerodynamics of an object, but he or she is starting to find out that changing the position of the hand held outside a moving car has interesting consequences. Furthermore, perceptual–motor integration is becoming better understood. The idea of a ball's flight toward the child and time to contact is starting to be understood, as is the idea of putting the hands out in coincidence with the ball's arrival.

ADOLESCENCE The research in regard to adolescence is fairly straightforward, but a bit controversial. Remember, much of this research is descriptive and, therefore, cannot explain why

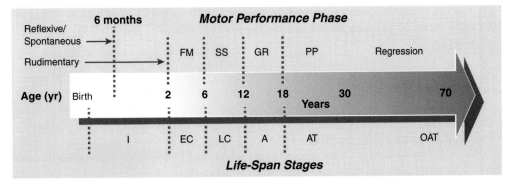

FIGURE 16.9 Stages of development and motor skill markers. *I,* infancy; *EC,* early childhood; *LC,* later childhood; *A,* adolescence; *AT,* adulthood; *OAT,* older adulthood; *FM,* fundamental movement; *SS,* sports skill; *GR,* growth and refinement; *PP,* peak performance.

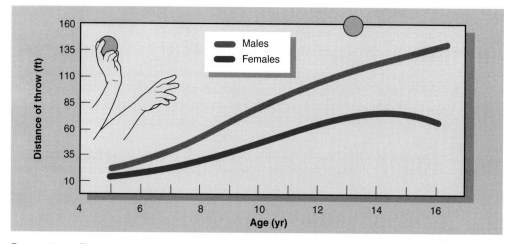

FIGURE 16.10 Change in motor skills for males and females over time. Reprinted with permission from Johnson WK, Buskirk ER. Science and medicine of exercise and sport. 2nd ed. New York: HarperCollins, 1974.

things happen. What is known is that as an individual moves from childhood through adolescence significant improvements in motor performance can be noted. Many of these changes are the result of body growth and changes in body structure.

At 10 to 12 years of age, there is a spurt in the child's growth, and male–female motor performance differentiation becomes apparent. Basically, through adolescence, males continue to improve their motor performance, but females level off at about 14 years of age (Fig. 16.10). This was true in 1974 when the original data were recorded and is generally considered true today.

Many of the sex differences seen in Figure 16.10 are the result of physical changes that give males an advantage over females. For example, males start to produce more muscle mass, and mechanical advantages developed, such as longer arms, narrower hips, and wider shoulders. However, some of the advantages may also be the result of societal pressures. Traditionally, females have been discouraged from several activities that could be beneficial to physical performance, such as weightlifting.

ADULTHOOD   Much of the specific information for adulthood has been covered in the previous sections of motor learning and motor control, so it will not be detailed here. In general, adulthood is seen as the time of peak performance. Generally, peak motor performance occurs at 22 to 25 years of age for females and around 29 years of age for males. There is a great deal of individual variation as to when individuals achieve peak performance, and the type of skill also plays a major role.

OLDER ADULTHOOD   Of all the areas of motor development, perhaps none is growing in interest as fast as is work with older adults. This is not surprising, considering that many of the 78 million baby boomers are already retiring (see Sidelight 16.1). Older adulthood is the largest-growing segment of the U.S. population. It is also estimated that the number of people over the age of 65 will double by the year 2040.

Gerontology, the study of the process and problems of aging, is the foundation for geriatrics, the branch of medicine concerned with the medical problems and care of the aged. Gerontology is not only a new addition to the study of motor development but a separate discipline in its own right. In this section, rather than discuss gerontology in general, the area known as **regression** by motor development specialists will be addressed.

BABY BOOMERS: THE GREAT BUMP IN CHILDBIRTHS

The fact that the population of the United States is growing older has been discussed for many years now. The first of America's 78 million baby boomers has already turned 50, and by the year 2000 the first wave of the boomers will have begun to retire. Baby boomers are individuals born between the years of 1946 to 1959. During that time, the birth rate in the United States increased to five times normal, coinciding with approximately nine months after the end of World War II.

The tremendous magnitude of this growth and the specific implications that the graying of America will have has recently been investigated from a variety of perspectives, including economic, sociologic, and psychologic. Findings from these investigations have led to the suggestion that it is time to revolutionize our thinking about aging, particularly in the most revered precinct, the human mind. It used to be thought that the negative consequences of aging, such as a loss of physical and mental abilities was inevitable. There is some truth in this statement, but we now know that the speed with which we decline can be attenuated by our lifestyle. In general, a sedentary lifestyle will speed the negative consequences, whereas an active lifestyle will slow the ill effects of aging.

Because of the graying of America, several aspects of exercise science will likely change. For example, the study of the older adult athlete should take on a more prominent stature in exercise science. Likewise, teaching motor skills will have to be tailored to older adults. Motor skills, such as driving, should be reinvestigated as a result of the abundance of older adult drivers in the near future. The increase in the number of older adults is likely to greatly affect the movement professions. For example, physical education could explore pedagogical techniques to target the older population. Other movement professions, such as physical therapy, will likely be quite busy. The effect the older population will have on exercise and movement science in the near future could be dramatic.

When motor development researchers refer to regression they are talking about a decrease in performance from peak. Decreases in performance are seen in three areas: cardiorespiratory function, muscular function, and **psychomotor function.** Older adults tend to decrease in physiologic function as they age. However, there are many things that can affect the rate of decline; one of the most important ways is to maintain a lifestyle characterized by physical activity. The bottom line to the regression stage of motor development is that the "Use it or lose it" adage holds true.

Cardiorespiratory function decreases about 0.75% per year after peak function. This means that a 70-year-old man will have approximately 30% decrease in maximal aerobic power and a 40% decrease in anaerobic power. As mentioned, there are considerable differences in cardiorespiratory regression. Figure 16.11 shows trends in the data for untrained individuals and trained athletes. The measure of interest is maximum oxygen uptake ($\dot{V}O_2max$) (27). Note the stunning difference between trained and untrained individuals of the same age. Regardless of the state of training, as individuals age, aerobic capacity declines.

There is a sex difference regarding muscular function regression. Males maintain peak force until they are about 45 years of age and slowly decline thereafter. Females start the regression much earlier. Some of this loss, for males and females alike, could be the result of a loss of muscle mass. However, the loss of muscle mass and the loss of strength are likely to be at least partially the result of less activity.

Psychomotor function can be defined as the ability to integrate cognition with motor abilities, for example, when communication is attempted with locomotion. Two common sayings regarding older adults are "With age comes wisdom" and "You can't teach an old dog new tricks." These two statements seem to contradict each other, but there is an explanation based on the distinction between **crystal intelligence** and **fluid intelligence.**

Crystal intelligence results largely from education and is information, such as word comprehension. Crystal intelligence can increase to about age 60, seemingly substantiating the first

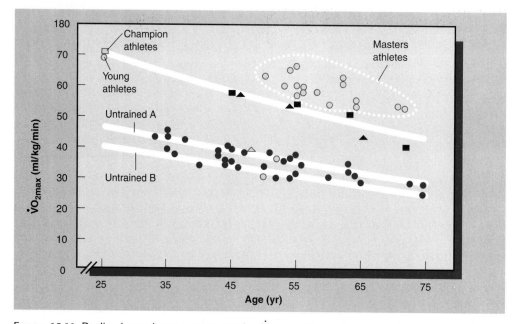

FIGURE 16.11 Decline in maximum oxygen uptake ($\dot{V}O_{2max}$) with age in groups of sedentary and physically trained men of varying age. Symbols are average $\dot{V}O_{2max}$ values for groups of men of different ages and training status. Closed circles are groups of untrained men from 9 studies. The open triangle represents a group of ex-champion athletes. Line A is lean untrained individuals and line B is overweight untrained individuals. The top line is trained individuals. The slope of the lines indicates that $\dot{V}O_{2max}$ declines 9% per decade of life regardless of current training status. People who continue to train, however, have higher $\dot{V}O_{2max}$ values. Adapted and used with permission from Heath GW, Hagberg JM, Ehsani AA, Holloszy JO. A physiological comparison of young and older endurance athletes. Jounal of Applied Physiology 1981;51:634–640.

saying. Fluid intelligence is reasoning and abstract thought, such as mental rotation. Learning is considered a mechanism of fluid intelligence. Essentially, fluid intelligence is a measure of the state of the brain, because it is a measure of our ability to make new and unique connections. Crystal intelligence is a state of the mind based on education, because it is a measure of well-established pathways in the brain not the formation of new ones. Fluid intelligence starts to decrease from the time we are in our middle 30s and declines as we age, thus seemingly substantiating the second saying.

The basic finding is that the elderly do not learn as quickly as younger adults do, but they can and do learn. Also, there is substantial evidence to suggest that the speed with which we lose fluid intelligence is related to the amount that we use fluid intelligence. The more we use our mind, just like with our body, the more intact it will stay for our entire life.

ADVANCES IN MOTOR BEHAVIOR

Motor behavior research has important implications throughout the life span. There have been numerous recent advances in the field; two of the most prevalent of these advances are technology and the application of research.

Technology

Throughout the years, the study of the brain and its functions has been complicated by the fact that the brain was not directly viewable, and therefore, inferences, rather than direct observations, were made to ascertain processes within the brain. Earlier, the chronometric method was mentioned as an indirect way to assess the speed of mental processing in the brain. Recently, with the advent of certain technologies, researchers are more able to view the brain and its functions directly. Two examples are positron emission topography (PET) and functional magnetic resonance imaging (fMRI).

In 1997, PET scans were used to investigate the change in active centers of the brain as individuals learned a motor task (28). Basically, the researchers found that during practice, several areas of the brain are used (e.g., premotor cortex). However, several hours after practice, the motor memory seems to consolidate in a few specific areas (e.g., cerebellum). Presumably, this suggests that memory for motor tasks is held in a few specific areas of the brain. Similar work could be done to investigate the similarity in learning among the brains of children, adults, and older adults. It is known that the learning patterns for these groups differ. One shortcoming to PET technology is that it requires the injection of radioactive isotopes in the brain, making the use of the technique in children somewhat controversial.

Like PET, fMRI allows researchers to identify brain areas that are activated during a cognitive task. Specifically, fMRI measures variations in cerebral blood flow by exploiting the fact that active brain regions have a higher ratio of oxygenated hemoglobin to deoxygenated hemoglobin than do nonactive regions. According to Guadagnoli, et al (29), the higher spatial resolution of fMRI allows more precise localization of brain activity than PET. Unlike the PET, the fMRI does not involve the administration of radioactive isotopes. An additional advantage is that fMRI allows researchers to rapidly alternate experimental and control conditions, and thus data from a single participant can be analyzed (rather than having to average across participants). Brain imaging studies in general have allowed researchers to study the relationship between cognitive processes and neural activity in the healthy living brain. More specifically, this research has increased our understanding of the brain mechanisms involved in such processes as speech perception, working memory, and attention.

Figure 16.12 shows an example of an fMRI. The bright areas are active parts of the brain when the subject is reading multidigit numbers. In general, systems such as the fMRI use various means to track blood flow throughout the brain. The presumption is that the areas where the blood is being used are the areas that are most active. A parallel to this idea can be found by exploring the periphery of the body. During the digestion of food we need blood to be concentrated in the area of the stomach and small intestine. Because of this, blood flow to other areas (e.g., the legs) cannot be provided efficiently soon after eating. The old adage that it is not good to go swimming directly after eating holds true, because of the competition between the muscles and digestive areas for the same blood. Typically, fMRIs of the brain have been used in clinical settings to assess brain anomalies, such as tumors or vascular problems resulting from a cerebral stroke. Recently their use has expanded into the research domain of motor behavior. Taken together, such techniques as the PET and fMRI are likely to be major players in the advancements of cognitive science.

Application of Research

A second advance in the field of motor behavior is that researchers have started to bridge the gap between theory and practice. One example is the work of Schmidt and Bjork (30), who have spent years of research examining the scheduling of feedback, the organization of practice, and the relationship between the learner and the task. These authors have consolidated the data in a manner that can be used by practitioners. The importance of this type of research is twofold. First, it allows practitioners, such as teachers, coaches, physical therapists, and athletic trainers, to benefit from the great deal of research in the field, which is typically written to be technically correct to practitioners. However, this style of writing is often difficult for nonspecialists to understand and use. Therefore, holistic applications of the theory-based work, such as that by Schmidt and Bjork, are valuable.

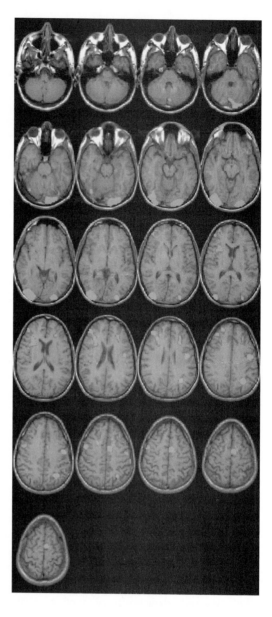

FIGURE 16.12 Functional MRI image of the human brain during number reading. Each of the 21 pictures corresponds to a horizontal section of a human brain as seen from below (looking up from the feet). The front of the head is at the top of each picture (e.g., the eyes and nose can be seen in the top row of pictures), the back of the head is at the bottom of each picture, the left side of the brain is on the right of each picture, and the right side of the brain is on the left. The pictures proceed from the bottom of the brain to the top of the brain as they are read left to right and top to bottom. The top left picture is the bottom-most image (closest to the neck), and the bottom right picture is the top-most image (closest to the top of the head). Differing densities indicate areas of the brain that were significantly more active when the subject read numbers than when the subject did nothing but stare at a fixation point. Reprinted by permission from Polk T, University of Michigan.

Second, applying this research can help with further theory development. When practitioners and individuals interested in applied research take laboratory-based research to the field, they find out the degree to which theory was correct. If the application is not in concert with the theory, it promotes an investigation of the theory and the specific parameters that may or may not cause the predicted effect. Essentially, theory and practice help each other to grow, and research that initially bridges the gap between theory and practice promotes this growth. One example of this is work investigating motor learning theory as it relates to the skill of putting (12). The findings in this study agree with the training wheels model described earlier. Consistent, repetitive practice—in this case putting to the same target repeatedly—yielded the best performance for both practice and learning; however, this was true only for novice golfers. For more experienced golfers, a randomized practice protocol—putting to different targets each time—yielded poor practice performance but efficient learning. Many more studies in the field of golf and other applied domains are now being published as a way to wed theory and practice.

SUMMARY POINTS

- Motor learning is the study of how one learns motor skills; cognition is important to this study.
- New models of learning have started to recognize that practice must change as the learner changes.
- Motor control often looks at the human as an engineered system and is interested in how this system is controlled.
- Motor development is concerned with cognitive, social, psychological, and physical changes associated with the life span.
- Research in the field of motor development is mostly correlational; therefore, we cannot conclude cause-and-effect relationships among the variables being studied.

REVIEW QUESTIONS

1. Why is the study of movement important?
2. What are the subcategories of motor behavior?
3. Name the areas of study of motor learning.
4. Explain three major findings in motor learning and how you can use this information.
5. Explain the major theories of motor control.
6. Name the areas of study of motor development.
7. Explain three major findings in motor development and how you can use this information.

References

1. Guthrie ER. The psychology of learning. New York: Harper & Row, 1952.
2. Hick WE. On the rate of gain of information. Q J Exper Psychol 1952;4:11–26.
3. Proctor RW, Reeve TG, eds. Stimulus-response compatibility: an integrated perspective. Amsterdam: Elsevier, 1990.
4. Klapp ST. Reaction time analysis of central motor control. In: HN Zelaznick, ed. Advances in motor learning and control. Champaign, IL: Human Kinetics, 1996:13–35.
5. Guadagnoli MA, Reeve TG. Movement complexity and foreperiod effects on response latencies for aimed movements. J Hum Movement Stud 1992;23:29–39.
6. Sternberg S. The discovery of processing stages: extensions of Donders' method. Acta Psychol 1969;30:270–315.
7. Sanders AF. Issues and trends in the debate on discrete vs. continuous processing of information. Acta Psychol 1990;74:123–167.
8. Atkinson RC, Shiffrin RM. The control of short-term memory. Sci Am 1971;225:82–90.
9. Baddley AD, Hitch G. Working memory. In: GH Bower, ed. Psychology of learning and motivation. New York: Academic Press, 1974:47–89.
10. Miller GA The magical number seven, plus or minus two: some limits on our capacity for processing information. Psychol Rev 1956;63:81–97.
11. Guadagnoli MA, Dornier LA, Tandy R. Optimal length of summary knowledge of results: the influence of task related experience and complexity. J Exer Sport Psychol 1996;67:239–248.
12. Guadagnoli MA, Holcomb WR, Weber T. The relationship between contextual interference effects and performer experience on the learning of a putting task. J Hum Movement Stud 1999;37:19–36.
13. Shapiro DC, Schmidt RA. The schema theory: recent evidence and developmental implications. In: JAS Kelso, JE Clark, eds. The development of movement control and coordination. New York: Wiley, 1982:113–150.
14. Battig WF. The flexibility of human memory. In: LS Cermak, FIM Craik, eds. Levels of processing in human memory. Hillsdale, NJ: Erlbaum, 1979:24–33.
15. Shea CH, Kohl RM, Indermil C. Contextual interference: contributions of practice. Acta Psychol 1990;73:145–157.
16. Shea CH, Kohl RM. Specificity and variability of practice. Res Q Exer Sport 1990;61:169–177.
17. Kerr B, Booth R. Skill acquisition in elementary school children and Schema theory. In: DM Landers, RW Christina, eds. Psychology of motor behavior and sport. Vol. 2. Champaign, IL: Human Kinetics, 1977:395–404.

18. Lavery JJ. Retention of simple motor skills as a function of type of knowledge of results. Can J Psychol 1962;16:300–311.
19. Adams JA. A closed loop theory of motor learning. J Motor Behav 1971;3:111–149.
20. Schmidt RA. A schema theory of discrete motor skill learning. Psychol Rev 1975;82:225–260.
21. Schmidt RA, Lange C, Young DE. Optimizing summary knowledge of results. Hum Movement Sci 1990;9:325–348.
22. Keele SW, Posner MI. Processing visual feedback in rapid movement. J Exper Psychol 1968;77:155–158.
23. Henry FM, Rogers DE. Increased response latency for complicated movements and a "memory drum" theory of neuromotor reaction. Res Q 1960;31:448–458.
24. Haywood KM. Life-span and motor development. 2nd ed. Champaign, IL: Human Kinetics, 1993.
25. Gabbard CG. Lifelong motor development. 2nd ed. Dubuque, IA: Brown & Benchmark, 1996.
26. Shirley MM. The first two years: a study of twenty-five babies. Minneapolis: University of Minnesota Press, 1931.
27. Heath GW, Hagberg JM, Ehsani AA, Holloszy JO. A physiological comparison of young and older endurance athletes. J Appl Physiol 1981;51:634–640.
28. Barinaga M. New imaging methods provide a better view into the brain. Science 1997;27:1974–1976.
29. Guadagnoli MA, Lance C, Kohl R. The degree of relationships between tests of cognitive ability. Under review.
30. Schmidt RA, Bjork RA. New conceptualization of practice: common principles in three research paradigms suggest important new concepts for practice. Psychol Sci 1992;4:207–217.

Suggested Readings

Fitts PM, Posner MI. Human performance. Belmont, CA: Brooks/Cole, 1967.

Magill RA. Motor learning: concepts and applications. 4th ed. Madison, WI: Brown & Benchmark, 1993.

Schmidt RA, Lee TD. Motor control and learning: a behavioral emphasis. 3rd ed. Champaign, IL: Human Kinetics, 1999.

Shea CH, Wright DL. An introduction to human movement: the sciences of physical education. Boston: Allyn & Bacon, 1997.

SOCIAL SCIENCE KNOWLEDGE BASE

Within the social science, knowledge base sports and exercise are studied from an intellectual base and not necessarily from a movement orientation. Although the subdisciplines presented in this section are not fields that deal directly with the science of movement that are important to health or the development of better athletes, these fields are important to students for gaining an understanding of the full scope of exercise science and its related areas.

The two subdisciplines covered in this section are important to understand our sporting past and the social forces that affect our behavior as we engage in exercise and sports as participants or spectators. Chapter 17 gives an overview of sports from a Western perspective in an attempt to show how these forces have helped shape modern-day practices. It not only relates events and notes important people who have played a role in sports' storied past but also provides important information to those students who may develop an interest in sports history and engage in researching and writing about sporting people and events. Chapter 18 focuses on the sociology of sports and particularly the roles that gender, race, ethnicity, religion, politics, economics, and social class play in our sporting world. Although sports history and sociology examine the same phenomena, the sports historian looks at the past, whereas the sports sociologist analyzes current trends.

17

Sports History

JOAN PAUL

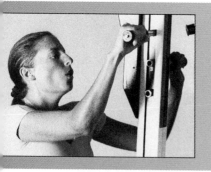

Objectives

1. Explain the role and place of sports history in exercise science.
2. What influences have shaped our past in sports?
3. Explain how and why men's and women's sports in America grew and developed differently.
4. What are the steps necessary for one to engage in researching and writing sports history?
5. Explain the differences in qualitative and quantitative research, particularly as they relate to historical research.

Sports **history** is a social science with its roots in the parent fields of history and sports studies. As an academic discipline, it is considered relatively new; it was formally recognized in 1973 with the establishment of the North American Society for Sport History (NASSH). However, people from many walks of life have written about sports and its history for almost as long as there have been written records.

The earliest foundations or history courses offered in the field of exercise science described the growth and development of the field of physical education. Courses in the history of physical education go back to the late nineteenth century, and their focus was on individuals who made major contributions in shaping the profession.

Today, sports history moves beyond the educational scope of this older approach and examines sports from educational, professional, and leisure pastime perspectives. It also investigates the social, religious, political, and economic effects of sport; it examines gender, class, ethnicity, and race in various sports settings; and it assesses how modernity has reshaped sports because of industrialization, technology, and urbanization. Sports history is concerned both with providing students knowledge and understanding of their sporting heritage and in teaching methods and techniques (**historiography**) of research that enable one to produce cogent and insightful accounts of sports from yesteryear.

The purpose of this chapter is not to identify the many sports historians who have shaped the field or to analyze their work; this information is available in the literature (1). The intent is to help students understand the nature of sports history as a subdiscipline of exercise science. In addition, the personal and practical information provided may encourage today's students to engage in sports history as a way of exploring the interconnectedness of sports' past with exercise science in early college and university programs.

DEFINITION, DESCRIPTION, AND SCOPE

History, whether of a social, intellectual, or political nature, is about re-creating the past. In descriptive and interpretative fashion, narrative sporting accounts tell stories that help one better understand how sports in its many forms has helped shape lives and influence culture. Sports historians seek to accurately depict the creation of organized sports and describe their growth and development. As historians, we examine the establishment of sporting institutions and organizations that have moved sports from pastime activities for children and youth to the highly organized and commercial enterprises they have become. Sports history inquires into the lives of the men and women who played active and varied roles in the creation, growth, and popularity of sports. Regardless of the direction one may take in examining sports, the researcher must pay attention to prejudice and discrimination, capitalism and monopoly, and power and intrigue.

> *History doesn't exist in a vacuum, and all societal relationships should be examined in the context of the time. It is also common practice today for historians to make value judgments about such happenings and point out injustices that are obvious.*

Its history reveals that sports has had both positive and negative influences in every age and on all cultures in the world. From the beginning of recorded time, sports and exercise have been used for military, health, social, political, religious, economic, and self-fulfilling reasons. Sporting events and the exploits of athletes have been written about by poets, playwrights, novelists, journalists, and academics.

Distinguishing Sports History from the History of Sports

Sports history and the **history of sports** are not precisely the same, yet these terms are often confused. The history of sports is the broad body of knowledge about the past practices and pur-

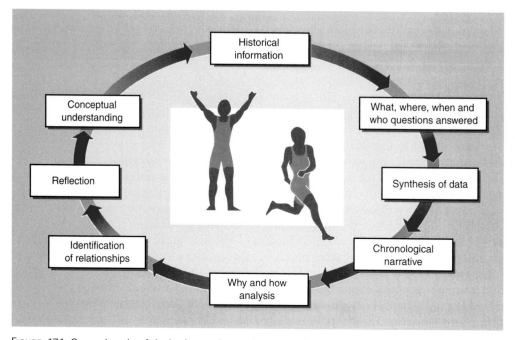

FIGURE 17.1 General cycle of desired experiences in sports history courses.

poses of sports, games, and exercise through the ages. The history of sports also includes descriptions of notable personalities who played various roles in the growth and development of sports, either as creators, players, or propagators. In contrast, sports history is a subdiscipline within the larger academic field that teaches students the history of sports while directing them in studies that produce new information about sports in earlier periods. It is through work in sports history that past sports events are studied and historical accounts of these events are produced (Fig. 17.1).

Scope and Description

Rowing, baseball, football, tennis, golf, track and field, boxing, wrestling, gymnastics, and almost all games had their roots in Europe. The modern martial arts of karate, judo, and aikido all come from Asia. American sports include basketball and volleyball as well as hybrid sports such as speedball, football (that grew out of soccer and rugby), and softball; but most of our sports are adopted from other countries of the world.

The history of sports in America is about how sports came here from other countries, how these sports grew and developed, and who the major characters were who helped in this process. In American sports history we study the organization and administration of athletic programs from community recreation to school and collegiate levels to professional leagues. Our scope in American sports history includes how religion, politics, social mores, and economics have shaped the growth of all of these programs. Sports history studies the growth of sports by gender, race, and social class. Analytical histories not only provide a description of an episode but critically examine purpose and outcome.

The scope of our history in sports is vast. It would take hundreds of books to hold summaries of the almost infinite historical works written on sports and exercise. This work would encompass sports from all ages and from all over the world. The various studies have been approached through traditional historical methods and through social theory and criticism and with different intents and purposes. Sports' past is a multifaceted past, and the following simple overview should give the novice a sense of U.S. sports history and its Western influences. Figure 17.2 illustrates how sports evolved in Western culture.

Ancient History: Prehistoric to Fourth Century B.C.

The history of sports begins with the funeral games of ancient times when sporting contests were held to honor celebrities at their burials. These games might consist of simple foot races or brutal contests that resulted in death. In early Roman times, two captives sometimes fought to the death over the grave of the deceased. Some early societies believed that blood was necessary for the second life. By sponsoring a blood-letting contest to pay homage to the deceased, the victim's body could then drain over the grave to provide the necessary blood.

The early histories of sports are glorious stories of ancient participatory Greek games and the brutal and degrading spectator sport of the Romans. Sports practiced by the early Greeks were track and field; wrestling; boxing; chariot racing, the precursor to horse racing and modern auto racing; and the pankration, the first version of today's ultimate fighting (2). Roman citizens were entertained by their prison captives in such life-threatening activities as gladiatorial combats and mock naval battles in the flooded Coliseum; sometimes boxers competed with *cestuses*

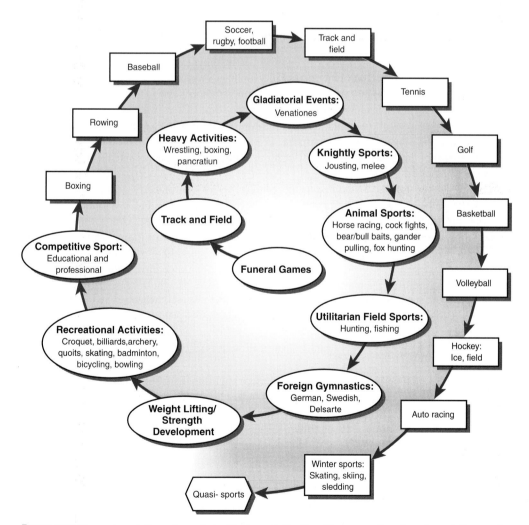

FIGURE 17.2 General evolution of sports in Western civilization. The examples given have influenced American sports and physical activity.

(similar to brass knuckles) on their fists (3). Some *cestuses* had metal spikes on them, and one solid blow to the throat or temple could kill the opponent.

There were also *venationes,* which were animal contests. These might be staged as animal against animal or man against animal. Some of the early *venationes* were sponsored by politicians as a way to garner votes from the Roman citizens. Caves, trees, and bushes were placed in the Roman Coliseum, and then the arena was filled with all manner of wild animals. Armed men would enter the arena and hunt before a full contingent of spectators. Later, to add excitement, unarmed men, and occasionally women and children, were placed in the arena; then wild animals were turned loose to attack the people.

Periods when sports were outlawed or otherwise rejected by the masses are also part of sports history. Such a vacuous era was the early middle period (fifth to ninth centuries), when sports fell into disfavor with the early Christians. Sports became antithetical to the Christian life because athletes often participating in the nude appeared to glorify the "sinful" body. An even greater influence in the demise of the ancient Olympics and other Panhellenic games was the pagan worship of Zeus and other gods through sporting contests. Paganism was so antagonistic to Theodosius' beliefs as a Christian emperor of Rome, that he terminated the Olympics in 393 A.D.

Later Middle Ages and the Renaissance: Tenth to Sixteenth Centuries

After sports' near demise for several hundred years during the early Middle Ages, military influence brought it back into society's good graces. The knights in the chivalric period used sports to prepare for war. They learned fencing, boxing, archery, swimming, horsemanship, gymnastic stunts, and other sports in their quest to become good soldiers. The idea of tournaments originated with the knights, who staged jousting and melee (type of free-for-all) contests in front of spectators. For many of the knights, the idea of competing in these tournaments became more important than the intended military purpose. In time, with the change in military tactics owing to the invention of gun powder, many of the military activities became accepted social and recreational pastimes (4).

From the Renaissance to the eighteenth century, sports continued to gain acceptance with the majority of the world's population. Certainly, the historical growth and development of sports was not uniform in any time period or among different countries. After the Protestant Reformation of the sixteenth century, Puritanism had a negative effect in the Western world on Sunday sports and on sporting activities thought to promote gambling, drinking, or other "licentious" activity. However, with Puritan acceptance of utilitarian activities, such as hunting, fishing, barn raisings, quilting, and cooking, the parameters of what might be classified as recreation or sports were probably extended. This is noted by modern colonial historians, who place activities such as women's weaving into the category of sports or recreation.

Colonial America: 1607 to 1776

In America's colonial period, the animal sports of cockfighting, bear baiting, gander pulling, and rat killing became common activities. This was a time when the work ethic, along with religious fervor, reigned supreme in the practiced activities of men, women, and children. Except for the most conservative religious sects—primarily Puritans with Calvinistic beliefs—sports themselves were not seen as sinful. It was the distraction from work or religious activities as well as the practice of betting and gambling that made sporting endeavors unacceptable to the early colonists.

Sports were seen as sinful by the early colonists only when people partook on the Sabbath, when people played when they should be working, when betting was part of the activity, and when participants or spectators drank alcohol.

However, by the eighteenth century, when religious restrictions were relaxing somewhat, holidays gave a welcome break to most colonists. These special days provided reasons to celebrate with feasting and engagement in games and other recreational activities, particularly in the South where the climate was more conducive to year-round outdoor activities. The fertile soil and the relief from labor (owing to slavery) afforded the southern landed gentry greater opportunity to engage in recreational pastimes than their northern counterparts. Tavern activities, such as card playing and dancing, developed in the upper south, whereas the more socially acceptable sports of horseracing, hunting, fishing, and boxing became popular in upper and lower regions.

Boxing was practiced on southern plantations where well-to-do landowners pitted slaves against each other in the ring. For some of the more skilled slaves, a string of victories could mean the reward of freedom. It was only in later years, when money, recognition, and status became associated with winning, that black boxers and jockeys were replaced with white fighters and riders. In 1875, 14 of the 15 jockeys in the Kentucky Derby were black. Issac Murphy, a black jockey won the Kentucky Derby three times. There were few black jockeys after 1894 and none after 1911 until more recent times.

Beginning of Organized Sports in America

The history of organized sport in the United States begins with the New York **Knickerbockers** in the 1840s. The Knickerbockers, a social club much like a modern country club, was composed of professional men (doctors, lawyers, and well-to-do entrepreneurs). In the early years, new members were voted in only by unanimous approval of the club's members. The group formed the first known baseball club; one writer stated, "This was the first time in American history that grown men put on costumes and played a child's game" (5). When competition and winning became more important to the Knickerbockers than social status, membership rules changed to allow working-class ballplayers free membership status and exemption from blackballing by other members (5). The importance of producing winners is obvious from the earliest accounts of sporting practices in this country.

Collegiate Sports

The history of collegiate sports in American life can be traced from Native Americans—who engaged in perhaps the first team sport on the continent, lacrosse—to the games and sports brought to North America by immigrants, especially Europeans, who settled in the New World. The earliest sporting practices in the United States, particularly in colleges, were most influenced by British sporting practices brought to this country by the colonists. The male students in colleges first played team games as extracurricular diversions from their studies and the rigid and confining rules of the mostly religiously oriented schools. The sports were usually played as class competitions; and although less organized and controlled than today's sports, they were similar to modern intramural sports programs. The earliest sports that developed in the male colleges were student organized, governed, and controlled. Because only the wealthier people could afford to attend college, it was they who were privileged to engage in sports. And because only males were allowed to attend institutions of higher education before the 1850s, sports for women developed later and with an entirely different purpose.

Intercollegiate sports for men began in 1852 with a rowing contest between Harvard and Yale (see Box 17.1). That first contest was sponsored by a railroad company, and men's intercollegiate sports from that first encounter have been as much related to commercial enterprise as to educational endeavor. After that Yale versus Harvard rowing contest, a New York newspaper predicted that intercollegiate sports would "make little stir in a busy world." The first collegiate baseball game was between Amherst and Williams in 1859, and the first football game was between Princeton and Rutgers in 1869.

Box 17.1
Harvard vs. Yale[a]

The first intercollegiate contest, a rowing match between Harvard and Yale, took place on August 3, 1852. The contest had been arranged through the efforts of James N. Elkins, superintendent of the Boston Concord and Montreal Railroad as a promotional activity for the summer resort area of Lake Winnipesaukee in New Hampshire. The fares for the student oarsmen were taken care of by the railroad, but there was a belief that parents and friends would attend the match, which would be of economic benefit to the railroad. This meant that the first intercollegiate contest ever was held away from home campuses, requiring players and spectators to travel more than 100 miles (over 200 miles for those from Yale) and to take room and board at the facilities of the resort area. Because the event was only moderately successful, the railroad company did not sponsor another contest the following year. It took a few more years before rowing as an intercollegiate contest was reinstituted.

[a]Rader BG. American sports: from the age of folk games to the age of televised sports. Upper Saddle River, NJ: Prentice-Hall, 1999.

Sports have evolved as rules have changed, placing American spin on the games. For example, in earliest baseball in the United States, there were rules that called for fielders to "plug" or "soak" (hit) the base runner with the ball to put him out, balls caught on the first bounce were outs for the batter, and bases were run in a counterclockwise direction. The first intercollegiate football game was actually a soccer contest with 25 men on a side. Running with the ball did not come into fashion until the 1870s after the Harvard College team met the Canadian McGill team, which played rugby instead of soccer-style football. The forward pass, seven men on the line of scrimmage, and the 10 yards required for a first down were not a part of football until early in the twentieth century, thus Americanizing the game.

From the 1870s through the end of the century, men's collegiate sports continued to expand on college campuses until its influence threatened to create an anti-intellectual climate in colleges around the country. It was only after there were many injuries and deaths in American sports, particularly football, that administrative control became imperative. There were also other problems associated with athletics that plagued college administrators, such as students missing class for games, students enrolling in only one class and being eligible to compete, and charges of cheating and professionalism that sullied colleges' reputations. In 1906 the National Collegiate Athletic Association (NCAA) was founded. It called for the formation of conferences, better equipment, rules and regulations for player eligibility, and educators as coaches.

In the earliest years of intercollegiate athletics, students had acted as their own coaches and managers. As spectators and gate receipts became a regular part of college games, more experienced and talented people were needed to direct the teams. Students were slowly replaced by temporary or professional coaches who were brought in only during the season of the sport, and most of these coaches were former athletes who had little if any educational background. These early coaches, usually hired by students, were eventually replaced by college professors. Administrative changes occurred when the early student coaches and graduate coaches were supplanted by part-time professionals, but the change to educators assuming control of intercollegiate sports had a more profound effect.

The NCAA played a role in bringing fledgling athletics into the physical education fold through its recommendation for coaches to be regular educators in the institution. These changes had an important effect on the field of physical education. Amos Alonzo Stagg became the first coach-physical educator when he was hired for both positions in 1892 by the University of Chicago.

> *Amos A. Stagg's hiring at the University of Chicago in 1892 set the precedent for hiring coach-physical educators, a practice that continues at the public school level and in some smaller colleges.*

Another effect was that the medical doctors who had become department heads of physical education academic departments in the late nineteenth century were replaced by athletic coaches early in the twentieth. It shifted the emphasis in curriculum from foreign gymnastics, anthropometry (taking structural bodily measurements), and formal drills to sports and games. And the objectives of the "new physical education" were broadened to extend beyond health and discipline as goals. Modern objectives embraced teaching sports skills, promoting character development through sportsmanship, emphasizing knowledge of sports, and continuing the focus on health through the promotion of physical fitness.

The emergence and growth of girls' and women's sports was quite different from that of boys and men. Society was much less accepting of the notion of women athletes. Whereas the highly skilled male athlete became a sports hero, the highly skilled female was more often ridiculed or scorned. In the mid-nineteenth century, sports outside the collegiate world for upper-class girls and women consisted primarily of proper activities, such as croquet, archery, and tennis. Women's sports were acceptable to society only if they were considered social affairs, promoted health, were noncompetitive, and were not strenuous enough to require a special costume. The bicycle, however, unleashed women from social restrictions in the late 1890s more than any sport. The bicycle demanded special attire to protect women's voluminous skirts from becoming entangled in wheel chains, and it also freed women to travel on their own without a male escort to drive the carriage. The bicycle, although approved more for the working girl than the debutante, promoted the divided skirt, which was the precursor to shorts and long pants that eventually freed women to become more active sports participants.

Whereas men's collegiate sports developed from student-governed activities outside the walls of academia, women's college sports began 40 years later as part of the educational curriculum. In the nineteenth century, sports were introduced to women in physical education classes in a basic noncompetitive format, but with emphasis on health and social interaction.

> *Sports were seen as desirable for developing red-blooded men, whereas women were accepted as sport participants only because of the health and social qualities they were thought to gain through friendly and cooperative activity.*

Men were getting their sports experiences outside the physical education world. From the mid-1860s, college women were instructed by physical educators in such sports as bowling, boating, ice skating, archery, swimming, and horseback riding. By the 1890s college women were playing class competitions in tennis, baseball, golf, track and field, field hockey, volleyball, and basketball. Basketball was the first intense team game that women played, and it quickly became both popular and controversial. The two women most prominent in the growth and development of girls' and women's basketball were Senda Berenson of Smith College and Clara G. Baer of Sophie Newcomb College. These women were generally responsible for the rules of the early game and did much to promote acceptance of the game (6).

Had the Vassar faculty not prevented it, Bryn Mawr and Vassar were scheduled to compete in a tennis tournament in 1894. Thus two intercollegiate basketball games that were played in 1896 mark the beginning of intercollegiate sports for women: The University of California at Berkeley competed against Stanford, and the University of Washington played Ellensburg

Box 17.2
Women Physical Educators

Women physical educators believed they were guardians of women's health, physically and morally, more than most educators in academic institutions. These educators were concerned with male coaches, who misunderstood women's limits; with the spectators, who they believed came to women's games primarily to see the players dressed in their playing uniforms; and with athletes' socially unacceptable behavior, which was promoted by serious competition. Sports for college women were taught as socially healthful activities that promoted cooperation, social interaction, and manners rather than a competitive spirit.

Normal School. Varsity athletics for girls and women were frowned on by almost all women physical educators at this time and for decades to come.

Educators were the leading opponents of intercollegiate sports and fought the notion of women copying the highly competitive men's programs (7) (see Box 17.2). Many articles appeared on the evils of men's athletics, and from the 1920s through the 1950s play days and sports days were promoted for women in place of interscholastic or intercollegiate sports (8).

Despite opposition, collegiate sports for women grew in the 1920s and 1930s, and other sports become as controversial as basketball. Track and field and softball were considered by society as too masculine for women who cared about their reputations. However, it was these three sports—basketball, softball, and track and field—that were adopted most often by working-class girls and women, who made up most of the commercially sponsored leagues across the country in the 1940s and 1950s. Although society as a whole was critical of women and sports, it was middle- and upper-class women who were most restricted. The more feminine and genteel sports of tennis and golf were approved, but masculine sports were highly criticized. Sports that promoted intense competition, required vigorous play or physical contact, and called for wearing revealing costumes were least approved. By the late 1930s, the opponents of highly competitive athletic programs prevailed in their opinion, and most high school and college programs were eliminated.

Until the passage of **Title IX** in 1972, which guaranteed no discrimination based on sex by any institution receiving federal funds, girls' school and women's college sports received little recognition or financial support. By the mid-1907s, after an uphill fight, women's programs began receiving funds for hiring coaches, buying uniforms and equipment, and paying for travel expenses. Provisions were made to share facilities with men's programs and/or to create new playing fields and buildings for courts, dressing and training rooms, and offices for coaches.

Women's sports were born and raised through the matriarchal hands of women physical educators whose objective was to promote recreational sports for all girls while prohibiting highly competitive sport for any. The women leaders in physical education proclaimed through the 1960s that their goal was "A sport for every girl and every girl in a sport." This motto was antithetical to highly competitive programs that promoted sports heroes and offered participation opportunities only to the gifted. Despite widespread opposition and proclamations about the dangers and pitfalls of male-modeled intercollegiate sports programs, young women wrenched loose from the grip of women educators and demanded equal opportunity. Women formed their first intercollegiate association in 1971, the Association for Intercollegiate Athletics for Women (AIAW). However, 10 years later there were contentious and bitter debates that led to the dissolution of the AIAW, because most of the women's programs moved their membership to the NCAA on promises of female governance, sponsorship of additional championships, and greater media attention (9).

Professional Sports

The United States was formed on capitalistic ideas, and certainly sports in America reflect the greater society. Payment to players has been used to distinguish amateurs from professionals in the United States. The earliest sign of professional sports in the United States was the baseball players of the mid-nineteenth century charging gate receipts to spectators and then dividing the money among themselves. Baseball and boxing were the front runners in organized professional sports in the United States.

Boxing matches between slaves became popular in the colonial period as entertainment for southern white landowners. White fighters became involved in the sport only when they saw there was money to be made. When this occurred, African American boxers were denied access to the heavyweight division until Jack Johnson, after trailing white champion Tommy Burns all around the United States and even abroad, was able to get a match. Johnson easily defeated the smaller and less-skilled Burns and became the first black heavyweight champion of the world in 1908. Johnson never allowed himself to be intimidated by white society, although he was considered a menace to humankind by some segments of the white population (10). There were a series of "white hopes," who were promoted as being able to take the championship from Johnson. However, as white fighters challenged and lost, Johnson continued to thumb his nose at society by dating and marrying white women and breaking many of the rigid social rules of the period. In 1910 Johnson was charged with violation of the Mann Act, a white slavery law that made it illegal for an African American to transport a white woman across any state line, so he left the country in an attempt to evade prison. In a fight in Havana, Cuba, in 1915, the much out-of-shape Johnson was defeated by Jess Willard. It wasn't until 1938 that an African American was again given the opportunity to fight for the heavyweight crown; that fighter was Joe Louis.

Baseball became the first professional team sport. Although it is known that some players received money under the table, the first recognized all-professional team in America was the Cincinnati Red Stockings of 1869. The Washington Nationals of the National Association of Base Ball Players (NABBP), an amateur league formed in 1857, beat the then-amateur Cincinnati Red Stockings 53-10 in 1867. This humiliation was one of the main reasons that the Red Stockings turned professional. They began hiring a few players that season; and by 1869, every player on the Cincinnati team was paid.

⚷ Professional sports was looked down on by educators and the more elite elements of society before the 1920s. This elitist idea about amateurism encouraged participation on teams only by the privileged minority. It was believed that if individuals who had to work to earn a living were allowed to devote themselves to sport, pleasurable sporting pastimes would turn into serious affairs.

In 1871, the NABBP changed its name to the National Association of Professional Base Ball Players (NAPBBP), reflecting the changing status of the once amateur game. Just 5 years later, it became the National League of Professional Baseball Clubs (NLPBC). This marked the change of power from players to owners and is the line of demarcation for sports being acknowledged as a commercial enterprise more than simply a pleasurable leisure pastime. Once it was evident that there was a profit to be made from sports, other short-lived baseball leagues appeared and failed or were integrated into the National League.

Because **Jim Crow laws** prohibited black and white players on the same team, African Americans formed their own baseball teams beginning in the 1880s. They barnstormed across the country, playing each other and occasionally having special games against the white leagues. Negro League baseball was successful by the 1920s, and by the 1930s both National and American Leagues were formed. Most successful of the Negro League teams were the Kansas City Monarchs and the Homestead Grays of western Pennsylvania. Although Negro League baseball never achieved the financial stability of white organized baseball, it produced some of the greatest players in history. Players such as Rube Foster, Satchel Paige, Josh Gibson, and Cool Papa Bell had baseball skills that equaled the white players of Ty Cobb, Babe Ruth, Walter Johnson, and Dizzy Dean.

In 1903, the American League won a long struggle with the National League over its professional status and became a part of organized baseball. Because baseball, as was most areas of society, was racist, the National and American Leagues were made up of only white players from 1897 until 1947, when Jackie Robinson was brought into the Dodgers' organization of the National League. The following year Satchel Paige at age 42, one of the Negro League's most famous players and baseball's oldest rookie, signed with the Cleveland Indians of the American League.

Once professional baseball was integrated, the only major changes in the sport were creating divisions in 1968, revoking the reserve clause in the 1980s, expanding the divisions in 1995, and allowing competition between the American and National League clubs before World Series play. Other than these changes, professional baseball remained much the same throughout the twentieth century.

While Rosie the Riveter was making her mark in industry during World War II, women entered another sacred male sanctuary. In 1943 when many of the male college and professional athletes were serving in the armed forces, Philip Wrigley, owner of the Chicago Cubs, collaborated with colleagues to form the All-American Girls' Professional Baseball League (AAGPBL) (11). This was the first professional league for women and, remarkably, it was in the man's world of baseball. The league began with 4 teams and first played by rules similar to softball. The league eventually expanded to 10 teams, base paths were lengthened, the pitching mound was moved back, and pitching was overhand.

Although the games were exciting and full of action, women were fully instructed on the importance of femininity in their every action. The women had female chaperones on trips, played in skirts, and abided by strict hairstyle and makeup regulations. The women were not allowed to wear slacks or shorts in public, and both smoking and drinking were forbidden. The league lasted until 1954, almost 10 years after World War II ended. After a 40-year lapse, a new semiprofessional women's baseball team was organized in 1995. Only time will tell if the Silver Bullets will succeed.

Football was the next sport to move into the professional arena, although college coaches did not support this move. Perhaps it was because football had been king of campus sports since the 1870s and professional football was seen as a threat to collegiate programs. Baseball players, unlike football, usually went directly to the professional leagues without attending college, and baseball also had gained an unsavory reputation. In fact, Gentleman Jim Corbett, first gloved heavyweight champion of the world, was a professional baseball player before turning to boxing. He claimed there was too much libation and swearing in baseball, so he preferred the sport of boxing.

Football, on the other hand, produced the much envied all-American sports heroes. College football was also becoming a cash cow, bringing money into the college institution coffers and funding other sports programs. Well-known and highly respected college coaches such as Amos A. Stagg, Pop Warner, and Walter Camp all decried professional football. Camp went so far as to proclaim that no gentleman would take money to play games (12).

Football's initial professionalization is said to have occurred in 1895 when Latrobe played Jeanette, both Pennsylvania teams with a few paid players. The first all-professional teams were Canton and Massillion of Ohio in 1902. These early professional teams were backed independently by wealthy men but had no organizational structure. There was corruption among these teams (e.g., coaches paid their own players to throw games and allowed college players to play under assumed names), and the sport developed the stigma of gamblers affecting game outcomes.

In 1920 the American Professional Football Association (APFA) was formed; "Papa" George Halas was the major catalyst. The first president was Jim Thorpe, tapped because of his famous name; he was replaced the following year. Because college coaches and administrators were so opposed to professional football, the APFA adopted two principles in an effort to appease the colleges. First, and most important, they agreed to keep their hands off players until their college eligibility expired. Second, was an agreement that teams would not steal other team's players so fans could recognize the players each week. The first principle was upheld in professional football until the United States Football League (USFL) broke the unwritten rule in 1983 by drafting Hershel Walker from the University of Georgia after his junior year.

The second principle was violated with great frequency those first few years, and yet teams went unpunished for pirating other team's players. In 1922, the APFA changed its title to the National Football League (NFL), and league rules were better enforced. However, with the commercial success of the NFL, a number of trade wars occurred for players when new competitive leagues were formed. Most of the fledgling conferences failed within a few years. In 1950, the NFL divided into the American and National Conferences, and this led to the inauguration of the Super Bowl in 1966.

Professional basketball for white males began in the 1890s, the same decade in which the sport was invented by James Naismith at Springfield College. It began like many of the early sports. There was barnstorming activity in which teams traveled around the country arranging games against any takers, and then passing the hat for what contributions the spectators might give. There was little formal organization until the National Basketball League was formed in 1898. After 5 or 6 years, the league folded and another was not organized until 1925. This, too, was short lived. In 1949 some measure of stability was achieved with the merging of the National Basketball League, formed again in 1937, with the Basketball Association of America to become the National Basketball Association (NBA). In 1967, the American Basketball Association was formed, and in 1976 it also merged with the NBA.

African American men had two well-known teams before the integration of professional basketball. They were the Renaissance, a traveling black team that usually played and beat white teams, and the Harlem Globetrotters. In 1950, the NBA began to draft black players; since that time, African Americans have increasingly dominated the sport.

Women's history in professional basketball in the United States is in its infancy. The only professional team for women until the 1990s was the Redheads, a barnstorming team formed in the late 1930s. This team played and most often beat men's college and semiprofessional teams, but this offered a chance to only a handful of women. Before the late 1990s, a woman's only reasonable choice to continue basketball careers beyond college was to play overseas. In 1996, professional basketball for women became a reality when two leagues were formed in the United States. The American Basketball League (ABL) began with 8 teams in two conferences (East and West), with plans to expand to 10. The Women's National Basketball Association (WNBA) played its first season in the summer of 1997, and although the salaries are lower and some of the players less known than those in the ABL, the initial interest shown through game attendance and television viewership has been excellent. For the first time, there is real hope that professional leagues for women will be successful.

During the 1970s when feminists were seeking to pass the Equal Rights Amendment to the U.S. Constitution, sports became a targeted area for greater equality. Title IX opened the door to school and college sports for girls and women, but professional sport remained primarily a male domain. There were a few female jockeys and even prizefighters, but the only professional sports that offered anything near equity to women were the traditionally feminine sports of tennis and golf. Professional volleyball and football leagues were begun that decade, but they failed commercially and folded.

Male and female golf and tennis champions received cash prizes in the 1920s, thus making them professionals as defined by American standards. The Professional Golf Association of America (PGA) was formed in 1916 for men only. The Ladies Professional Golf Association (LPGA) was organized in 1950, which eventually led to more substantial prizes for women's tournaments. Mildred "Babe" Didrikson Zaharias was instrumental in providing the excitement and the leadership in popularizing golf for women during this period.

Tennis was professionalized in 1926 when C. C. "Cash and Carry" Pyle, an American industrialist, persuaded some popular tennis players to join him in a national professional tennis tour. The biggest names were William "Bill" Tilden of the United States and Suzanne Lenglen of France. The tour was a financial success; but until the 1960s, most professional tennis was played in barnstorming exhibitions. When the World Championship Tennis circuit was formed in 1967, the same year that professionals were allowed to compete at Wimbledon, opportunities for professional tennis players increased. There was a great discrepancy between men's and women's championship purses until Billie Jean King and Rosie Casals organized a boycott of a Jack Kramer tournament over the disparity. Battles began in 1970 between and among the men and women players and the various professional tennis organizations until the war finally ended in 1973 when women's purses were raised to almost equal those of men's.

Golf and tennis, always recognized more as elitist sports because of their country-club background, have been dominated by white players. Althea Gibson in the 1950s, Arthur Ashe in the 1970s, and Venus Williams in 2000 won single titles at Wimbledon, the former two becoming the first highly recognized African Americans in the game of tennis. In golf, there have only been a handful of blacks who have made a name for themselves. However, Tiger Woods, who is of African and Asian heritage, among others, hit the professional circuit with a bang and became perhaps the biggest name in golf in the late 1990s. His credentials in amateur play rival if not better the great Bobby Jones; and if he lives up to expectations as a professional, he may eclipse both Arnold Palmer and Jack Nicklaus.

Prejudice and Discrimination

From the colonial period until the present, African Americans have been discriminated against in sporting arenas just as they have been in every dimension of American society—educational, political, social, and economical. African Americans who first made sporting reputations as outstanding boxers and winners of America's most prestigious horse races, such as the Kentucky Derby, suffered from the Jim Crow laws of the late nineteenth and early twentieth centuries that disenfranchised them from the dominant society. The *Plessy vs. Ferguson* case of 1896 made "separate but equal" the law.

The description that the United States is a melting pot is far from the truth. Although the South was the greater violator of human rights, with its policies of discrimination, America became a nation of distinct cultures. Many ethnic groups in addition to African Americans and Native Americans suffered from the prejudice and discrimination of the dominant groups, which scorned them as having inferior cultures. Ethnic and religious groups such as the Irish, Italians, Polish, other Euro-Americans, Catholics, and Jews were subjected to mistreatment in all spheres of American life. Women, too, were treated as second-class citizens by not being allowed to vote until 1920 and by being restricted in educational, vocational, political, and sports opportunities for a greater part of the twentieth century.

Far too many of the general books on the history of sports tell the story of white, Protestant, upper-class male athletes, as if this were the history of sports in the United States. Sports were exclusive because of social mores, bigoted beliefs, economic factors, and even misunderstood health issues. For example, white girls and women were often excluded from competitive sports before the middle of the twentieth century because of social issues relating to femininity, notions that a woman's place was in the home, and the misplaced belief that a female's health would be jeopardized by strenuous activity. African Americas were excluded from sports based on more perverse prejudice that classified them as almost subhuman and definitely inferior to whites. Other ethnic groups were also denied privilege into upper-class sports.

Lower-class white Americans also felt the sting of prejudice, because the amateur laws of the nineteenth and early twentieth centuries favored wealthier citizens who were not bound so tightly to working for a living. When the NABBP was formed in 1857, all players claimed to be amateur. The wealthy could take a leisurely approach to sports and games and meets could take place on weekday afternoons. The lower classes depended on jobs for their living, and their time for sports was limited to late evenings and Sundays, which made organized amateur sports for the laborer difficult before the 1920s. Beginning in the 1860s, labor unions formed to ease the harsh working conditions for American laborers. One goal was to establish the 8-hour workday; however, many employers did not conform until almost a century later. Although some textile mills and factories began sponsoring company sports teams for their employees, there were still many who required that their employees work 10- to 12-hour days, six days a week. The puritanical spirit of the day, particularly in small towns, meant that sports could not be played on Sunday. In nineteenth-century America, time, economics, discriminatory statutes, and social influence were the primary factors for the exclusion of African Americans, immigrants, and poor whites from organized sports.

We celebrate Jackie Robinson for breaking the color barrier in professional baseball. This was a tremendously important occurrence, but it was not the first racial barrier broken in professional sports. In the 1880s, Moses Fleetwood Walker, a bare-handed catcher, played with the professional Toronto team before Jim Crow laws ended his short career in white baseball in 1889. Furthermore, two African American football players were drafted by professional teams the year before Robinson was hired by the Dodgers. But it was the visibility and the media attention given to Robinson that were most instrumental in opening the sports door to other African Americans as well as to Cubans, Hispanics, Chicanos, and other nonwhite groups.

Today, most of us would like to think that walls of discrimination and prejudice are rapidly falling. Although there is evidence that sporting opportunities are greater for all groups today than at any other time in U.S. history, absolute equality has not yet occurred.

FOCUS ON SCIENCE

Research can be of a quantitative or qualitative nature. **Quantitative research** was long the technique most respected in the academic world as scientific, because it involves running tests (e.g., in a laboratory), collecting data, and then statistically analyzing the data (e.g., via computer programs). However, the value of **qualitative research** is now recognized for its ability to offer greater interpretation of the results; this has led to its respect in the academic community. Compared to quantitative, qualitative research requires clearer goals before the study begins, takes longer to complete, and forces the researcher to draw conclusions that cannot be supported with statistical data. As social scientists, historians engage in qualitative studies more often than quantitative. Although the historian goes through some of the same steps as other researchers, qualitative methods demand a different approach.

In quantitative research, a study is never designed to prove something, and objectivity must be upheld in formulating hypotheses and designing research techniques. Qualitative research, on the other hand, is rarely if ever approached without some biases on the part of the researcher. Sports historians do not begin their work with a conscious notion of proving something, but they will rarely if ever become engaged in a study without an opinion or bias connected to their research. Most people realize that girls and women have been discriminated against in sports because of the stereotypical and prejudicial attitude of society. Females have had fewer opportunities to be sports participants, have not enjoyed the economic opportunities of male athletes, and have been less appreciated for their sports skills than males. It would be impossible for a person to do a historical study about girls and women in sports without the knowledge of this discrimination having some effect on the work. This does not mean that researchers are dishonest when analyzing findings, but there is little doubt that some of the opinions and the research direction taken would be flavored by a bias against society's treatment of athletic girls and women.

To gain a clearer understanding of the practice of this subdiscipline, this section takes you on a personal walk through the practical steps of how research is conducted in sports history.

GEORGE BARKER WINDSHIP: STRENGTH SEEKER

The article "Autobiographical Sketches of a Strength Seeker"[a] relates the experiences of a boy, small for his 16 years, who attended Harvard College in the 1850s. George Barker Windship gave examples of how he was picked on by older and bigger students and how he was physically incapable of responding to their insults (see figure).

His first impulse was to challenge the bullies to a duel with pistols or swords; but not being skilled in either and loving his life, he quickly gave up that notion. He then described how he began an exercise program by lifting weights to gain the strength needed to defend his honor against the culprits who were playing pranks on him. He eventually became so strong that he could chin himself with either little finger, hoist a barrel of nails on his shoulders while talking to public groups, lift a weight of almost 3000 pounds by using a yoke on his shoulders, and pick up 1100 pounds with his hands alone. He explained how he experienced personal liberation and exaltation from his new reputation as being one of the strongest men in the United States by the time of his graduation. He never weighed over 143 pounds and was under 5 feet 8 inches tall at his largest!

In the 1980s I was in the library reading an 1862 issue of *Atlantic Monthly* and came upon Windship's story. Being fascinated with Windship, I decided to research his life and explore the role he played as a strength seeker and health reformer in the mid-nineteenth century. One problem with doing the research was that I was teaching in southern Louisiana, but Windship had lived, been educated, and worked (as a medical doctor and operator of a gymnasium) in Boston. I weighed the importance of the topic and believed it passed the So what? test. Windship was an influential man as a strength seeker and had affected medical and educational leaders through his work; and my interest in the topic was certainly substantial.

---

[a]*Windship GB. Autobiographical sketches of a strength seeker. Atlantic Monthly 1862;9:102–115.*
[b]*Paul J. The health reformers: George Barker Windship and Boston's strength seekers. J Sport History 1983;10:41–57.*

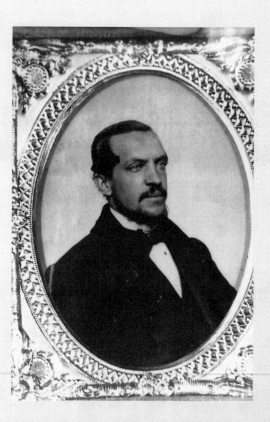

George Barker Windship after he had attained the reputation for being America's strongest man. Courtesy of Harvard Archives.

Because I was resolute about doing the research, I needed to travel to Boston to use the Harvard archives and do further work at the Massachusetts Historical Society. Selecting this topic meant travel expenses and extra time and effort to do the research, but the work was exciting and fun.[b] After I came to terms with the economic and geographic problems, I realized that the research was doable. You may need to answer such a location question, too, if your sources are not readily available.

Most college classes require outside papers and/or projects aimed at having students do basic research, use writing and reasoning skills, and gain a greater depth of understanding in an area than class time usually permits. The following discussion should be of great value to students with required historical assignments.

Steps in Historical Research

The following practical steps are placed in chronologic priority for engaging in historical research. Each step is important and somewhat time-consuming but is necessary for providing an orderly approach to setting up one's historical project.

Selecting the Research Topic

The first step in beginning a study in sports history is to define a problem you wish to explore. This should be a study of an area and in an era in which you have real interest. You then outline the purpose of your study and thoughtfully make a list of questions you wish to answer. The stated purpose and research questions serve as the framework to guide your research.

The topic selected to study should be significant enough to support the "So what?" question, i.e., put a judgment value on your project to determine if your projected discoveries and results would matter to you or to anyone. If your answer to the So what? question leads you to believe there is no relevance or general interest in the topic and that it would make no difference to anyone whether your questions were answered, then you may need to rethink the topic.

Framing the Study

This step helps you determine if your research project is feasible and defines the direction in which the topic should be pursued. It includes locating sources, limiting the time and space of the study, and forming an outline for the way the research should be approached.

LOCATING HISTORICAL SOURCES   Before beginning your research ask yourself whether the topic selected is manageable. An affirmative answer means that there are accessible libraries and archives where **primary sources,** period newspapers, and other documentary sources are available. Unless you have the time and financial means to travel in your research efforts, location of sources is an important, and maybe imperative, factor in settling on a topic (see Sidelight 17.1).

DELIMITATIONS OF THE STUDY   **Limitations** of a study are factors that affect your research over which you have no control. For example, if interviews are part of a study to determine the high school sporting experiences of adults over 50, you cannot be sure that the subjects' memories are reliable and that their depictions are accurate. These are limitations that you must acknowledge. A **delimitation,** however, is a boundary that you set for your research. Delimitation is used to set parameters for your study to keep it manageable.

The delimitations are often reflected in the title of the paper, and they are almost always noted in the stated purpose, which appears early in the paper. Once you have determined your topic and have ascertained that the resources are available for you to do the study, you set parameters of time and location.

For example, if you wanted to investigate the history of a particular sport, it would not be practical nor possible to examine the sport from its inception to the present. Using your research questions and your stated purpose, you must decide which time period to investigate and what geographic area to include in the study. For example, suppose that you wanted to examine how a world war affects the growth of sports. You might select one particular public school or university, focus on just one sport at the school, and then limit your time period to 1941 to 1945. These are the delimitations of your research study. Your research questions and the purpose of your work will then form the framework for your study within the parameters, or delimitations, you have established.

FORMULATION OF A THEORETICAL FRAMEWORK　After you have selected a topic and established parameters, you must form a set of research questions to direct the study toward obtaining the needed data. The set of questions identified at the beginning of a study may change or be expanded as the researcher becomes more familiar with the subject. The historian begins with the five Ws and an H—what, when, where, who, why, and how—when formulating research questions. The easiest parts of research are the what, where, when, and who. These questions allow the researcher to uncover verifiable facts, but they provide no significant interpretation in and of themselves. The more difficult questions to answer are why and how, but the answers to these questions provide the most important information.

> *The easiest research questions to verify usually provide the least important information for your study. The most important questions, which require analysis by the researcher, are the hardest to answer and to provide proof for verification.*

Sometimes in digging out the answers to why and how something transpired, the researcher will draw conclusions that are not concretely spelled out by the research. This is where the **analysis of the data,** based on as many facts as can be accumulated, depends on the skill and understanding of the researcher. Without answering the why and how questions, an historical research study provides only a descriptive chronicle of a period and offers no interpretation. Although previously unknown information provided by descriptive research is worthwhile, it is the simplest and most superficial historical work one does.

Getting Started

When a research project has been defined and the intent of the work is clearly outlined, the next step is to explore what has already been written on the selected topic. You will need to do much reading in the area, both on the specific subject and on the selected time period of your study. At this point, you will have identified the archival depositories, special collections, special museums, location of court house records, historic sites or organizations to contact, and other sources for collecting your data. You should have already found—and even read—the **secondary sources** that will guide you in providing context for your study.

The major sources used by historical researchers are written materials (primary or secondary), artifacts (e.g., pictures and equipment), and oral testimony. Sources categorized as primary or secondary, according to their time relationship to the subject being studied.

USE OF SECONDARY SOURCES　Secondary sources are written about a subject after it happened and by a person who was not an eyewitness to the occurrence; they include books, journal articles, newspaper articles, and other material. An extensive review of secondary sources is essential for gaining a full understanding of the subject you are researching. Reading secondary sources helps you find important primary works and gives direction to your research.

It is also necessary to do this reading to provide context for your work. If you are researching the early history of women's basketball, for example, you need to read in a number of different areas to become more familiar with your subject. There are many works written about women's early sports participation, general histories are available on basketball, and there are books and articles that discuss the 1890s when women first began playing the game. It is essential that you learn all you can about the early history of the game, why basketball was a controversial sport for women late in the nineteenth century, and the differences in societal expectations for men and women in that period.

The secondary sources will also provide notes and bibliographies of other books and journals you should read firsthand. They will often mention historical collections of archival material that should also be sought. And, most important, you will begin to feel comfortable with your research area as you learn more about it through reading secondary sources.

There are dangers in secondary sources of which you should be aware. Unless you are a discriminating reader who does not take as literal truth all that you read, you can accept fallacies and myths and become a party to perpetuating these untruths or half-truths. There are any number of myths perpetuated in sports history by researchers who have taken secondary sources at face value and repeated the previous writer's errors in their own works. For example, for more than a half century, sources referred to Abner Doubleday as the originator of baseball. Even in some modern books and in television commercials, references will be made to Doubleday and how he invented baseball in Cooperstown, New York, in 1839. See Sidelight 17.2 to find out how such a myth was created and why it has persisted so long.

USE OF PRIMARY SOURCES   **Primary sources** are usually written by an eyewitness at or near the time something occurred. These may be books, journal articles, and newspaper articles. Some important primary sources are diaries; scrapbooks; census reports; voter registration records; birth, death, and marriage certificates; church, court, and education records; correspondence; and personal memorabilia.

Primary sources are the most important sources for historical work; only primary works provide new information that can add to the cumulative body of knowledge. Through primary sources, the researcher is able to better understand the time period being studied and gain greater insight into the whys and hows essential to historical interpretation. Through primary research, myths can be corrected and the creation of new myths prevented. However, even the use of primary materials does not ensure that all errors will be avoided (see A Case in Point 17.1).

Interpretation of Data

At this stage, the writer of history becomes both scientist and artist. As a social scientist, you must be meticulous in the collection of information. This means writing down your information precisely if you are copying directly from a source. Be sure that you use quotation marks around anything that is copied so that you do not inadvertently commit plagiarism. When you paraphrase information, be sure that you accurately capture the meaning the author intended. It is only when there is fear of misinterpretation or for dramatic effect that direct quotations are used in finished papers.

Your interpretation of the results depends on your analysis of the data based on the theoretical framework established at the beginning of your study. It is important that the work be interpreted in the proper context, i.e., with the attitudes, customs, rules, and other nuances that apply to the time period in which your work is set. **Presentism** is the mistake of applying present notions to historical work, which can cause grave errors.

However, as an artist, you do have some liberty in your interpretations. As long as you do not stray beyond the implications of your researched data, you are obligated to make analyses that take your work beyond simple description. As an artist, it is also important to write in a style that is not only readable, but commands the attention of the reader. Whereas physical scientists

➤➤ Sidelight 17.2

THE FACTS BEHIND THE ORIGIN OF BASEBALL

Baseball was the first organized sport in America; and by the beginning of the twentieth century, it was being called our national pastime. Henry Chadwick, one of the earliest sports writers, refuted the notion in 1901 by writing an article and crediting baseball to British rather than American origin. Chadwick recounted playing a game called rounders as a boy growing up in England and stated that baseball was an offspring of this British game.

Albert Spalding, a former professional player and owner of a growing sporting goods business, established a commission in 1903 to pursue the origin of the sport. Abraham Mills, a past president of the National League, chaired the commission, which had two U.S. senators among the group's seven members. After 3 years of research, Mills concluded that the story told by an octogenarian about Abner Doubleday placing bases in a diamond shape and reducing the number of players to nine at Cooperstown, New York, in 1839 was the true origin of baseball.

The memory of Abner Graves was apparently never questioned by anyone on the commission or by Spalding. Personal testimony of others appears to be the total evidence used by the commission to uncover baseball's history. The problem with this story is that Doubleday was stationed at West Point in 1839 training to be an officer. A nationally known Civil War general, Abraham Mills met Doubleday once when he was a soldier in the Union Army. Perhaps Mills thought it logical that a man with military and tactical knowledge such as Doubleday could have invented a game that would become our national sport, but he failed to investigate any of his "facts."

If Mills had checked the story, not only would he have discovered that it would be impossible for Doubleday to have been in Cooperstown in 1839 but he would have found that Doubleday was a journalist who never once mentioned the word *baseball* in any of his writings. Mills, with a better investigation, would have also found that baseball was being played before Doubleday was born. Credit for the Americanization of the game's evolution from rounders goes to Alexander Cartwright and his New York Knickerbockers of the 1840s.

Why has the Doubleday myth persisted for so long? Because researchers perpetuated it by accepting a statement they read as truth without any verification. Testing results in qualitative works such as history cannot be done by using test tubes and statistics; it is through probing and checking facts that one verifies historical work. Researchers look for information to support the dates of events and to verify activities in people's lives. Historical research can be tedious, because researchers must follow leads to their extreme when checking information; but verification is a necessary step if the work is to be judged as reliable and honest.

often present their work in purely scientific nomenclature, which we sometimes think of as pedantic, the historian may write more like the novelist. Remember, history tells a story.

Historians can focus on various aspects of sports as they relay their stories. Experienced historians, although often approaching their study with some bias, are always meticulous in their attempts to capture the true essence of a past sporting event and to relay an accurate account. Sometimes the story is told through the athletic exploits of the participants, and sometimes the historical account may focus on the growth and development of a sport. The story may be on one narrow aspect of sports and highlight social, political, or economic factors. Sports are shaped by participants, coaches, spectators, managers, trainers, and entrepreneurs; and it is the job of the sports historian to relate such events in as honest a way possible (see Practical Application 17.1).

ADVANCES IN SPORTS HISTORY

Early histories of sports were most often written by newspaper sports writers and sports enthusiasts who had no academic training. Physical education histories were written by educators in the field early in the twentieth century as textbooks, but the recognition of sports history as a subdiscipline in our field is relatively recent. For that reason the establishment of a sports history organization and the academic specialization of the field of sports history represent advances in the field.

A Case in Point 17.1

THE IMPORTANCE OF PRIMARY SOURCES

A few years ago, I began research on Clara Gregory Baer, a woman who had taught physical education at Sophie Newcomb College, a Coordinate College of Tulane in New Orleans, from 1891 to 1929. The research was begun with little excitement, and if I had applied the So what?, I might not have done the work. I had been invited to speak at a national conference in a session on women in sports; but at the time of the invitation, I was between research projects with no new information to deliver. It was suggested that I look into Baer's development of the 3-division court for women's basketball, because she lived in southern Louisiana and New Orleans would be a close source for that information.

The research question seemed trivial to me, but reluctantly I agreed to do the research and speak on the topic. What I found was amazing.[a] Baer had initiated the first 4-year physical education degree program in the South in 1907, almost 20 years earlier than Peabody College in Nashville, Tennessee, which history credited. She published the first set of women's rules for basketball in 1895, although history credited Senda Berenson with the first published rules in 1901. Baer invented the game of Newcomb Ball, which may have laid the pattern for the game of volleyball credited to William Morgan.[b] Newcomb Ball is the only known game that became a competitive sports for boys and girls that was originated by a woman.

What Baer did not do was create the 3-division court for girls' basketball. Baer's earliest published rules called for an 11-division court, but she limited the divisions to 7 in her 1908 rules. Why was Baer credited with this bit of historical trivia, but nothing of more consequence? Because in James Naismith's[c] 1941 book on the history of basketball, written 50 years after his invention of the game, he credits Baer with devising the 3-division court. Until the 1980s, no one questioned Naismith's memory or investigated Baer's life to determine her role in the creation of women's basketball.

This, too, is a cautionary lesson in taking the written word as fact without investigation. Even though Naismith invented the game of basketball and is one of our heroes in sports history, he was subject to a faulty memory when recalling an incident that happened a half-century earlier. Accepting any statements without checking for accuracy is a practice that leads to myths and the perpetuation of fallacy in historical works.

[a]Paul J. Clara Gregory Baer: harbinger of southern physical education. Res Q Exer Sport 1985;46–55.
[b]Paul J. A lost sport: Clara Gregory Baer and Newcomb ball. J Sport History 1996;23:165–174.
[c]Naismith J. Basketball: its origin and development. New York: Association, 1941.

Organizational Recognition

With the founding of the North American Society of Sport History (NASSH) in 1973, scholars from physical education, history, English, classics, and other university departments in the United States and abroad came together to share their academic interests in sports history. Through this organization the subdiscipline of sports history received more attention, and the research and writing became more scholarly than before. The yearly conferences held in North America have sessions for the presentation of refereed papers, meetings at which the most important books in the field are critiqued, and sessions that focus on research techniques and the

SUMMARY POINTS

- Sports history is concerned with recreational, educational, and professional sports.
- Sports history is a social science that uses qualitative more than quantitative methods, although statistics about things such as numbers of spectators attending events, sporting goods sales, and volume of newspaper coverage can be used to provide quantitative data for historical works.
- Sports history must be studied in the context of local and world events.
- Sports history must be studied in the context of time and place.
- Sports history takes into account the effects of social, political, religious, and economic factors and how they affect the growth and development of sports.
- Gender, class, race, and ethnicity have almost always played a role of inclusion or exclusion in sports.
- Men's and women's sports developed in very different ways in the United States.

REVIEW QUESTIONS

1. How do sports history and the history of sports differ?
2. List and briefly explain the factors affecting the growth of women's sports in the United States.
3. Explain why it is said that men's intercollegiate sports are as much a commercial endeavor as an educational enterprise.
4. Give examples of how stereotyping, prejudice, and discrimination have played ominous roles in sports history.
5. List and briefly explain the steps for doing historical research.
6. Explain how historical research differs from experimental research.

References

1. Struna N. Sport history. In: JD Massengale, R Swanson, eds. The history of exercise and sport history. Champaign, IL: Human Kinetics, 1997:143–179.
2. Harris HA. Greek athletes and athletics. Bloomington, IN: Indiana University Press, 1966.
3. Woody T. Life and education in early societies. New York: Macmillan, 1949.
4. Baker WJ. Sports in the Western world, rev. ed. Urbana: University of Indiana Press, 1988.
5. Lucas JA, Smith RA. Saga of American sport. Philadelphia: Lea & Febiger, 1978.
6. Hult JS, Trekell M, eds. A century of women's basketball: from frailty to final four. Reston, VA: American Alliance for Health, Physical Education, Recreation and Dance, 1991.
7. Sefton AA. The women's division: National Amateur Athletic Federation. Stanford, CA: Stanford University Press, 1941.
8. Lee M. The case for and against intercollegiate athletics for women and the situation since 1923. Res Q 1931;2:122–123.
9. Morrison LL. The AIAW: governance by women for women. In: GL Cohen, ed. Women in sport: issues and controversies. Newbury Park, CA: Sage, 1993:59–66.
10. Roberts R. Papa Jack: Jack Johnson and the era of white hopes. New York: Free Press, 1983.
11. Pratt M. The All-American Girls' Professional Baseball League. In: GL Cohen, ed. Women in sport: issues and controversies. Newbury Park, CA: Sage, 1993:49–58.
12. Camp W. The book of foot-ball. New York: Century, 1910.

Suggested Readings

Berg BL. Qualitative research methods for the social sciences. Boston: Allyn & Bacon, 1995.
Eiser G, Wiggins DK, eds. Ethnicity and sport in North American history and culture. Westport, CT: Greenwood, 1994.
Reiss SS. The new sport history. Rev Am Hist 1990;18:311–325.

Smith RA. Sports & freedom: the rise of big-time college athletics. New York: Oxford University Press, 1988.

Smith RA. History of amateurism in men's intercollegiate athletics: the continuance of a 19th century anachronism in America. Quest 199;345:430–447.

Struna NL. People of prowess: sport, leisure, and labor in early Anglo-America. Urbana: University of Illinois Press, 1996.

Tygiel J. Baseball's great experiment: Jackie Robinson and his legacy. New York: Oxford University Press, 1983.

Vertinsky P. The eternally wounded woman: women, exercise and doctors in the late nineteenth century. Manchester, UK: Manchester University Press, 1990.

18

Sports Sociology

Joy T. DeSensi

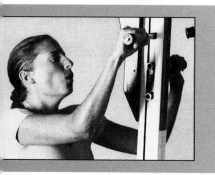

Objectives

1. Explain the relationship of sports sociology to exercise science, including the role sports sociology plays in the parent discipline.
2. Describe how the cultural values of sports influence the social institutions of sports and the relationship between these institutions and exercise science.
3. Identify the social theories and controversies in sports sociology that can affect the study of exercise science.
4. Explain the importance of a sociocultural approach to research in exercise science.

- **Definition, Description, and Scope**
  - Studying Exercise and Sports from a Sociologic Perspective
  - Cultural Values and Sports
  - Social Institutions and Sports
- **Focus on Science**
  - Social Theories and Sports
  - Issues and Controversies in Sports Sociology
- **Advances in Sports Sociology**

Summary Points
Review Questions
References
Suggested Readings

Although sports **sociology** is a subdiscipline of exercise science, it is also a part of the parent discipline of sociology, which is the study of human behavior and social interactions within particular contexts. Sports sociology examines sports as a part of cultural and social life, and adds a different dimension and perspective to the study of sports and exercise (see Practical Application 18.1). More specifically, sports sociology examines the relationship between sports and society and seeks answers to many issues and questions regarding sports and **culture** (see Box 18.1). Figure 18.1 illustrates the general content of sports sociology courses at most universities.

Sports are a pervasive part of culture and are considered to be social constructions within society created by groups of individuals and based on **values,** interests, needs, and resources (see Sidelight 18.1) (1). Sport forms are created by groups of individuals. Each culture creates and

Practical Application 18.1

THE LINK BETWEEN THE SOFT AND HARD SCIENCES OF EXERCISE SCIENCE

Exercise science has many specializations (areas of study) that contribute to the overall knowledge of movement. Studying sports sociology contributes to a wider understanding of exercise science by bringing forth a social awareness of the issues that affect our society and thus sports and general exercise behavior. This has the effect of broadening the knowledge base and thus our perspective. Exercise science students may study some subdisciplines more fully than others, but each subdiscipline affects the others, and the social issues we encounter are always relevant. Thus, although most of the subdisciplines of exercise science have hard science content, they do not exist in a vacuum but instead reflect the larger social world. It is at this point that the social science content of exercise science is most helpful for students.

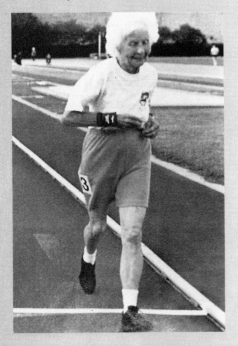

Senior games competition.

(continued)

Practical Application 18.1 (continued)

For example, in our society we can observe the increase in the numbers and types of different people who participate in physical activity. Sports and physical activity are no longer only for the able-bodied or the elite-level athlete. The increase in the number of individuals, especially young girls and women and older adults, participating in exercise and physical activity throughout their life spans has necessitated a greater need for the inclusion of these populations in research.

Specific questions that often arise regarding girls and women include the effects of exercise on the menstrual cycle and/or on the post-menopausal status of women. At the same time, questions regarding bone density and the effects of excessive exercise and training for girls and women are also being explored. In addition, we find more sports programs focusing on older adults and encouraging their participation in physical activity. The graying of the American society has a significant effect on the consumerism of certain physical activities. It is not uncommon to find older adults participating in both extreme competition and senior games (see figure).

The goal of sports sociology is to track these trends and to try to explain them in sociologic terms. Thus there is an established link between the contributions of hard and soft science, each having implications for future research in exercise science.

uses sports for its own purposes; therefore, sports take different forms from culture to culture. This directly relates to the concept of physical activity and exercise for different cultures. Because of various factors, such as religion, politics, and economics, certain groups of individuals may have limited access or be restricted or forbidden to take part in sports and/or exercise activities. Thus the value of sports takes on different meanings in different cultures. Other factors, such as who controls sports, what rewards (intrinsic or extrinsic) are received from sports participation, and the status of the athlete/participant have some effect on the value and place of sports in a particular society. The purpose of this chapter is to familiarize the student with the social issues that permeate society and thus permeate sports.

Box **18.1**
General Research Questions in Sports Sociology

How are sports related to other forms of social life, such as family, education, politics, religion, media, and the economy?

Why have some sports become a part of certain cultures and not others?

How do participation in sports and sports in general affect or create our beliefs regarding gender and the concepts of masculinity and femininity, the body, race, ethnicity, social class, ability and disability, competition and cooperation, and violence and aggression?

How are the meanings and value of sports in society associated with and how do they affect social relations?

How is the concept of power defined by sports?

How can individuals use sports and their knowledge regarding sports to effect social change?

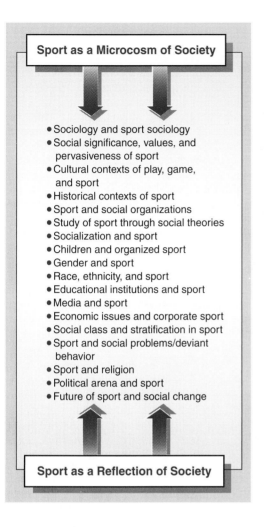

FIGURE 18.1 General content organization of a sports sociology course.

DEFINITION, DESCRIPTION, AND SCOPE

It is only since 1970 that sports sociology has gained significant attention as a serious area of study. This is in part owing to the increasing major role sports play in our lives and the intellectual traditions in both physical education and sociology. In 1978, the North American Society for the Sociology of Sport was organized as a professional association; and its scholarly outlet for research, the *Sociology of Sport Journal,* was established in 1984. The International Committee for Sociology of Sport is acknowledged within the International Sociological Association, and both groups co-sponsor the *International Review for the Sociology of Sport.* Another scholarly publication for sports sociology research is the *Journal for Sport and Social Issues,* thus confirming support for and the growth of this subdiscipline of exercise science (2).

Ways to study sociologic phenomena in sports rapidly became an issue with scholars as sports sociology was striving for legitimacy within the academic community. Kenyon and Loy (3) defined sports sociology as the "study of social order"; and in later works, Kenyon (4,5) set the tone for sociology of sports to take a positive perspective, noting that sports sociology is a "value-free social science" in which the researcher is to describe and explain values and attitudes, not shape them. However, value-laden research is also undertaken when various perspectives and theories are used to study sports. For example, the feminist perspective as a part of **critical theory** is obviously a value-laden approach, as is the conflict theorist's approach; but bias is recognized, acknowledged, and analyzed carefully within these approaches.

►► Sidelight 18.1

PERVASIVENESS OF SPORT

Whether as participants or spectators, people in North American society experience sports in some fashion in their daily lives. As a cultural phenomenon, sports are pervasive and reach us through print, broadcast, and computer-generated media; educational institutions; social organizations; work settings; religion; politics; and economics.

In addition to sports, varying forms of play and games also exist within cultures and are important parts of particular cultures. Play as an attitude, an activity free from rules, boundaries, and objectives helps socialize individuals into a culture. Games are developed and handed down from generation to generation within cultures, but generally differ from play in that games have objectives; require physical skill; and create a winner and loser, which have particular meanings regarding success and failure within the culture. With the creation and growth of television and other media and the affluence of industrial societies, sports have become a significant part of social life and are considered prominent social phenomena. The work ethic in Western cultures has made a distinction between work and play as well as between intellectual and physical activities. Play is considered as nonserious and nonproductive and as a lower form of culture; it is thus not given any significant academic attention.

Although play and games are important parts of a culture and significant within our socialization into sports, it is the concept of *sports,* or more specifically *organized sports,* around which this chapter is developed and about which ideas are expressed. Within organized sports, a high degree of physical skill is a predominant factor, along with competition that results in a winner and loser. In addition, organized sports are institutionalized, i.e., they take place within a specific structure, contain rules, have a regulatory agency that enforces the rules, require training, and are driven by extrinsic and intrinsic rewards. Spectators and sponsorship for teams play important roles in organized sports; and the economic effect of such activities is experienced, whether it be at the youth sport, amateur, interscholastic/intercollegiate, professional, or Olympic levels of competition. The study of sports sociology has grown significantly in recent years as have the prominence of sports and the recognition of the important influence of social issues dealing with social justice.

Sociology of sports poses critical and controversial issues. Because sports are considered a microcosm of society, the same social issues that exist in larger society also exist in sports. Sociology uses critical and conflicting approaches that force us to explore alternative ways to view the place and organization of sports in our society as well as how issues and problems presented by sports in society affect individuals.

Again, the issues and controversies that sports sociology uncovers are the same ones reflected in our society. Included in the numerous issues of sports are the concepts of values, race, gender, ethnicity, class, sexuality, age, ability, politics, religion, and economics. If, in fact, sports is a microcosm of society and/or mirrors society, we see an important reflection and thus must deal with the issues that are revealed. This chapter presents sociologic theories, or different approaches to thinking about sports and the issues that influence sports in our society. By becoming aware of these critical areas of sports sociology, students will

- Develop social awareness and social consciousness of factors and issues that affect sports.
- Be cognizant of the consequences of various forms of social organization.
- Be able to critically examine their own life experiences in relation to their own sports participation.
- Explore how sports, in whatever form, can be used to provide opportunities for those who lack access, power, and opportunity.
- Examine how social justice and social change can be achieved in sports settings.

As a result of gaining this knowledge and understanding, students will approach the scholarly study of exercise science via an inclusive perspective rather than a narrowly focused and exclusive one.

Studying Exercise and Sports from a Sociologic Perspective

The content of sports sociology comes directly from the parent discipline of sociology. Sociology is concerned with the social and cultural context in which behavior occurs and the connection between that behavior and the setting, and sports sociology specifically focuses on the relationship between sports and society. It gives us a closer look at human social behavior within the sports context. It is within sports sociology that the issues surrounding the relationships between individuals, groups, and sports are considered, explored, analyzed, and explained. From this view, a logical and scholarly critique of sports can be developed to set the stage for understanding potential social change.

To further clarify the definition and scope of sports sociology, specific factors must be considered (1):

- The relationship between sports and other areas of social life, such as family, education, politics, economy, the media, and religion.
- How sports and physical activity may impart knowledge regarding the body, gender, sexuality, social class, race and ethnicity, and disability.
- The social organization, group behavior, and social interactions that occur in the sports setting.
- The social processes that occur in sports, such as socialization, concepts regarding competition versus cooperation, social stratification, and the issue of social change.

Sports sociology is also defined as "the systematic study of human society and social behavior that interacts to produce social action" (6). Within the definitions offered thus far, the elements of social action and change appear, suggesting that, as a result of the careful study of sports sociology, individuals will have a strong foundation with which to effect change in society.

Culture is another important concept to be considered within the subdiscipline of sports sociology. Culture includes the established parts of life that are created by individuals in a specific society. It is the means by which society defines and perpetuates itself. By establishing and passing on shared values, beliefs, artifacts, norms, traditions, and appropriate behaviors of the group that have significant meaning, a culture affirms itself and is adopted by the individual participants of that group. Culture is also considered a patterned form of expression that becomes a product of habit rather than a conscious thought within groups of people. Culture is a human phenomenon that is diverse and has unlimited potential because of the creativity of people.

Although cultures are different, they also have common elements. For example, music, law, art, customs, and play forms seem to be shared phenomena. They may be different and expressed in different ways, but the phenomena still exist from culture to culture. Specific forms of play, games, and sports have distinct roles and importance within different cultures. Although play may be culturally universal, it differs in manner, style, and form across cultures. Games of chance may not exist at all in certain societies, yet games of strategy and physical skill are prevalent in achievement-oriented societies (1,7–9).

There is a need also to explore **subcultures** within society. Subcultures are subunits of culture that have a cluster of values that are different from the larger culture. Distinctions giving rise to subcultures can include gender, race, ethnicity, social class, religion, politics, physical ability, age, and sexual orientation. Each subcultural characteristic is important when applied to the study of sports, particularly when we realize that we each may belong to several subcultures. The diversity of groups of people is phenomenal; and this is important, particularly when exploring the purpose, value, and meaning of sports to individuals or groups representing each subculture.

It is difficult to study the issues associated with sports sociology without recognizing the historical context of sports (see Chapter 17). For example, without knowledge of the racial oppression and struggle for civil rights in our country, there is no foundation for understanding the racial segregation and background of the Negro Baseball League or the predominance of certain races in particular sports. Without knowledge of the history of the civil rights movement or the women's movement in our society, there would be no context for understanding the fight for equal rights for African Americans and women; subsequently, we would be blind to the need for laws guaranteeing civil rights and Title IX. This type of information, combined with the data secured in the hard sciences of exercise science, provides greater depth of understanding and more accurate basis for the overall discipline of exercise science. A multidisciplinary approach to the study of exercise science, therefore, is the most effective way to gain a breadth and depth of understanding of this comprehensive field of study.

Cultural Values and Sports

To understand the importance of sports, values within American culture must be understood. Values are based on a number of traditions that emanate from religion, race, ethnicity, and geographic location. The foundation of our values are the ideas and concepts about what is good, bad, right, and wrong and what is desired. Because our culture is diverse, incorporating numerous racial and ethnic groups, it is difficult to reach agreement on some factors. For example, in some cultures being thin is not valued, whereas in other cultures being thin is very important. Some cultures emphasize sports to a greater degree than others. The concepts of beauty and excellence also differ from culture to culture; therefore, finding a consensus on the issue is difficult. Whereas some of the core values may be contrary to those identified by specific cultural groups in our society, they nonetheless should be noted. Core values include achievement and success, activity and work, moral orientation, humanitarianism, efficiency and practicality, progress, material comfort, equality, freedom, external conformity, science and rationality, nationalism and patriotism, democracy, individual personality, and group superiority themes (10).

Values extend to sports and exercise as well (6,7) and include

- *Means to achievement:* discipline, hard work, and striving to meet a goal are valued.
- *Success:* measured by monetary or material possessions, power, and status.
- *Progress:* considered to be a look to the future, improvement of technology, and a means to make things better.
- *Individualism:* ingrained into American culture; overcoming adversity to rise above oppression.
- *External conformity:* the controlling factor within society; maintaining stability and abiding by societal expectations and established rituals.

These same values are reinforced through sports and exercise programs, and are further defined by functional attitudes. They include concepts such as building character, being self-disciplined, engaging in competition to achieve excellence, developing a healthy mind and body, and promoting nationalistic pride (Fig. 18.2).

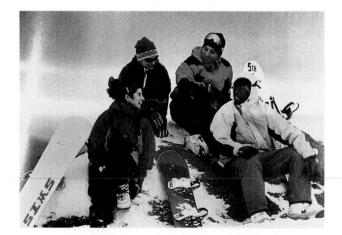

FIGURE 18.2 Cross-cultural values of sports.

Social Institutions and Sports

The social institutions of our society to which sports are closely linked are the family, education, the **media,** politics, religion, and the economy. Because sports are social phenomena, it is important to study them as they relate to other forms of social life.

Family

Organized youth sports play an important role in the life of the family in North America. They serve as a unifying agent, because they may bring the family closer together; parents and siblings support the athlete, taking him or her to practices and attending games. The family may unite as spectators, watching televised or live events and discussing the processes and outcomes. Today, the daily routine and/or weekend schedules of many families are geared around the children's involvement in sports. The social institution of the family, depending on the degree of support and encouragement offered, has the potential to be a socializing agent for children's participation in sports as athletes or spectators.

Education

Sports are inextricably intertwined with the institution of education in our society. At all levels of education, but particularly high school and college, high-level sports or varsity sports competition is present. Although the beginnings of interscholastic or intercollegiate sports are traced to physical education programs and recreational activities in North America, sports have developed a solid foundation within educational systems. The value of sports within education raises numerous questions, because they have become so important that a school's worth is judged by the success or failure of its athletic teams. Students have even been known to choose a college or university based not on the academic program in which they will enroll but on the success of the athletic programs. There is no question that sports afford positive values and opportunities for all students; however, we must carefully examine the extent to which the value of sports is placed above the value of education. Educational institutions need to address why varsity sports has become a marketable product instead of an educational program.

The Media

There has been phenomenal growth in all forms of the media in its relationship to sports. Television has virtually grown before our eyes as we have witnessed the addition of cable and satellite channels, sports programming, and the coverage of sports in general. Many millions of dollars have been paid for television rights for championship games, specific tournaments, special events, and especially the Olympic Games.

The future direction and success of college, professional, and Olympic sports have been paved by the broadcast media. However, the manner in which all forms of the media inform, interpret, create drama, and establish particular ideas about sports and society must be realized. For example, the media provide considerable knowledge about sports, and the ways in which the media choose to characterize or emphasize certain aspects of sports contribute to the mind-set of individuals in society. The media define the important sports as well as the importance of sports; interpret concepts such as the athletic body, femininity, and masculinity; and create sports heroes and antiheroes. For some, sports have become a form of entertainment and spectacle for the audience and for the purpose of extrinsic reward instead of being an activity characterized by intrinsic reward, enjoyment, fun, and challenge for the participant. The media have promoted sports as a product and the athlete as entertainer. There is no doubt that sports provide much enjoyment for the participants and spectators; however, the value of sports, how that value affects our culture and what role power plays in the representation of sports by the media cannot be overlooked.

Politics

Politics is another institution in our society that is linked to sports. Various theories (see below) propose how sports and politics use each other. Although countries use sports to enhance their image and power or that of their leaders, sports have also been used as peacemakers. The Goodwill Games, for example, served this purpose, and world leaders have used sports participants to engage in friendly challenges with athletes from other countries as a means of communication in the process of negotiation.

The display of flags and the playing of national anthems have raised controversy at Olympic and other international competitions, because of the interpretation that such displays promote political ideologies. Sports do offer a setting for national pride and unity in our society but at the same time raise questions regarding issues of power, particularly in regard to the selection of athletes for international competition and the control of sports events.

Religion

The institution of religion offers a strong setting for a relationship with sports in our society. Not only do churches sponsor leagues but athletes themselves publicly profess and promote religious beliefs. Organizations for Christian athletes in particular have been established for such purposes. Just as family schedules have been altered by sports participation, religious services have been changed to accommodate practitioners so that the start of a contest is not missed. College and professional athletes often openly engage in religious practices or rituals before, during, or after a contest. Such actions receive mixed reactions on the part of spectators. The sports sociologist raises numerous questions regarding the relationship between sports and religion and they use each other to promote their own purposes.

The Economy

The relationship between sports and the economy cannot be overlooked as we examine the other social institutions within society. The money spent by the consumers on tickets, concessions, club fees, membership dues, sports equipment and clothing, and gambling has a direct effect on the economy. The amount of money spent in any particular city on the weekend of a college or professional game ranges from millions to billions, because spectators spend money on hotel rooms, food, travel expenses, souvenirs, and other forms of entertainment over the span of 2 to 3 days. Corporations seem to have ever-increasing budgets for advertising and sponsorship of sporting events, particularly the Olympic Games; an advertiser may spend millions of dollars to have its name associated with such an event.

We have seen major corporations connected with college football bowl games and other contests. Even parts of a game have been sponsored by a particular company. The amount of money paid to some professional athletes and coaches is directly associated with the value and marketability of sports in our society. This issue raises numerous questions, particularly regarding the worth of entertainment and entertainers (sports and athletes) compared to other institutions within our society, such as education.

The political and economic ideologies of a country affect how its society regards the importance, value, and place of sports. We place much importance on the values of competition, hard work, and success. Sports, based on these concepts, has a critical and positive role in North American society.

FOCUS ON SCIENCE

This section focuses on the science of sports sociology, a field that is often viewed as an art. Coakley (1) discusses the concepts of the art and science of sports sociology and indicates that not all who study this field see things similarly. Sports sociology is both an art and a science, and critical questions are asked by researchers from both perspectives. However, before posing questions regarding how sports can be made better, it is important to understand what currently exists. Both qualitative and quantitative research have a role in answering specific research questions posed within sports sociology (see Chapter 17), and it is important to have a clear understanding of their purposes and potential within the field.

Social Theories and Sports

The value of theories is that they give us grounding, or a foundation, on which to build our positions and arguments. Theories offer a starting point from which we can address a particular issue within sports sociology. Although there are a number of theories from which sports sociologists draw, the most common are **structural functionalism, conflict theory,** critical theory, and symbolic interactionism.

Structural Functionalism

Structural functionalism maintains that sports are an inspiration in our society and that a systems approach (studying individual parts of society) is the best way to study society. Those who use this approach assume that society is composed of interrelated parts that are bound together by individuals who have the same values and processes, which produce consensus. Social order is maintained (balanced and functional) by individuals with shared values who work together toward consensus. When the balance is upset, dysfunction within the society occurs.

The system needs of society included in this theory are pattern maintenance and tension management, integration, goal attainment, and adaptation. It is the functionalist's contention that sports contribute to maintaining balance in society, because it requires that individuals work together to set goals and attain them. The functionalist notes that, because values and rules are taught within society, tension can occur and it is important to have a way to release it. Sports provide this catharsis. This theory contends that sports serve as a mechanism to bring individuals from different backgrounds together to work toward a common goal. Box 18.2 lists research questions formulated within the structural functionalist theory.

One of the limitations raised regarding this viewpoint is that it overstates positive comments regarding sports. Remember, to the structural functionalist, only that which is functional for society or is seen to contribute to order and efficiency is good. Therefore, if sports were dysfunctional they would not have lasted this long. Another limitation is that functionalists see the needs of all groups in society as similar.

Conflict Theory

Conflict theory envisions sports as an opiate of society, meaning that it deadens our awareness to social issues. Within this theory, society is not viewed as a stable system held together by com-

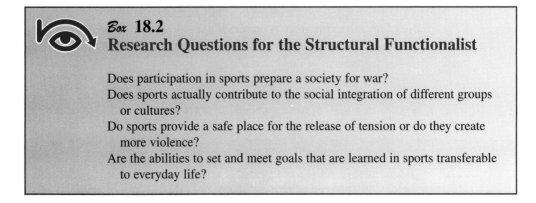

Box 18.2
Research Questions for the Structural Functionalist

Does participation in sports prepare a society for war?
Does sports actually contribute to the social integration of different groups or cultures?
Do sports provide a safe place for the release of tension or do they create more violence?
Are the abilities to set and meet goals that are learned in sports transferable to everyday life?

mon beliefs and values. Rather, society is a constantly changing set of relationships based on economics. Because some groups of individuals have resources or access to resources—and thus have a high economic class or status—they can manipulate and coerce others to accept their viewpoint. Class relationships are centered around economic power, the individuals who have attained it, and the manner in which they use it. Therefore, the process of change is based on these premises, which produces social inequality.

Categories of concern for the conflict theorists include the following:

- *Alienation:* how the elite athlete in high-level sports becomes alienated from his or her body, as if the body became separate from the self; includes the use of performance-enhancing methods to achieve better execution, higher profit, and heightened entertainment.
- *Coercion and social control:* those with resources and power focus the attention of society on the outcome of sports rather than on the important social, economic, and political issues of the society.
- *Commercialism:* promoting economic gain by encouraging individuals that consumption is a measure of self-worth and prestige; results in social injustice because those without means are excluded from high status.
- *Nationalism and militarism:* the extent to which sports promote a false sense of nationalistic pride and promote violence.
- *Racism and sexism:* reveals existing inequities; e.g., minorities do not have equal opportunity in sports administration (coaching and managing).

Important questions of conflict theorists are presented in Box 18.3.

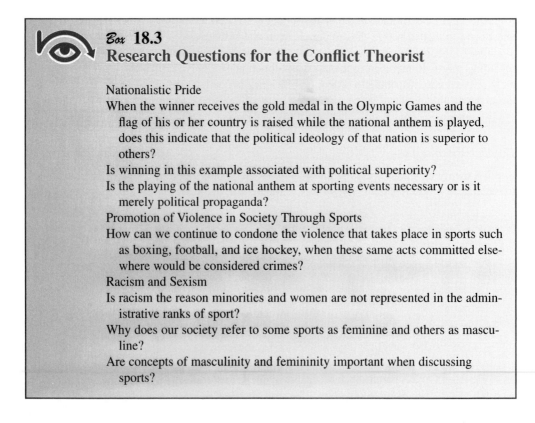

Box 18.3
Research Questions for the Conflict Theorist

Nationalistic Pride

When the winner receives the gold medal in the Olympic Games and the flag of his or her country is raised while the national anthem is played, does this indicate that the political ideology of that nation is superior to others?

Is winning in this example associated with political superiority?

Is the playing of the national anthem at sporting events necessary or is it merely political propaganda?

Promotion of Violence in Society Through Sports

How can we continue to condone the violence that takes place in sports such as boxing, football, and ice hockey, when these same acts committed elsewhere would be considered crimes?

Racism and Sexism

Is racism the reason minorities and women are not represented in the administrative ranks of sport?

Why does our society refer to some sports as feminine and others as masculine?

Are concepts of masculinity and femininity important when discussing sports?

> ### Box 18.4
> ### Research Questions for the Critical Theorist
>
> Why have sports undergone such drastic changes?
> Is there actual value to sports in capitalistic societies?
> Why are there specialized games for certain groups: e.g., ethnic groups
>   (Highland Scottish Games), older individuals (Senior Games), disabled
>   individuals (Special Olympics, Paralympics), and gays and lesbians (Gay
>   Games)?
> How do sports vary from one group to the other?
> How can sports be changed to be more inclusive?
> How can sports offer opportunities for interactions among people and poten-
>   tial changes in society?

Conflict theory also has some limitations. The economic basis is the theory's strongest argument but is also its weakness. This theory assumes that social life is driven only by economic factors and that people with resources are the ones who own and drive the market; people who are on the low end of the economic scale are victims of injustice and exclusion. Economic power certainly exists in society, but the conflict theory tends to focus on only individuals who lack or have such power. The theory does not address the fact that sports can be empowering for some individuals and groups. Economic forces are not the only relationships between groups of individuals, so to base arguments about sports solely on this premise is misleading.

Critical Theory

To understand the realities of sports and how they affect different groups and individuals in society, critical theories are employed. Not limited to one approach, but encompassing several, critical theories focus on the concepts of power, social action, and political involvement. It is important to understand that, when seeking answers to issues, critical theorists examine the sources from which power originates and how power changes and affects individuals. In an attempt to seek what is fair, equal, and inclusive, political action must be a part of this effort.

Critical theorists do not believe there is one broad explanation for the problems of society, but rather they believe a combination of history, social, and material conditions make up social life. As such, the issues and problems for which critical theorists are concerned involve "economic struggles over labor law, rights of workers, property ownership, and power structures in organizations . . . family violence, child and spousal abuse, and women's control over their own bodies" (1). Other inquiries regarding sports are addressed: Are certain individuals or groups privileged because of their sports excellence? What activities are regarded as sports? Why is violence in sports supported and considered part of the game? Box 18.4 lists additional research questions of critical theorists.

If it is important to explore sports within specific contexts, i.e., that sports is more than a reflection of society and that it is a socially constructed phenomenon, then critical theorists offer an excellent approach for such exploration. However, although the approaches to critical theory appear strong in their own right, one limit is that there are no clear guidelines for each approach. In addition, it is not certain at what point sports reproduce significant social relations and when they are or become a site for change (1).

Symbolic Interactionism

Interactionist theories offer another approach to the exploration of sports. These theories assume that our behavior involves choices that are based on the way we define our interactions in certain situations, allowing us to explore our identity. It is assumed that we behave according to the manner in which we envision the effect of our behavior on ourselves and others and thus develop a sense of who we are. Thus identity is paramount in the explanation of who we are in relation to sports or in a specific sports setting. Our identity is in a state of constant change, because each situation is different and the individual(s) with whom we interact can be different from setting to setting. Identity then influences how we behave or our choices of how to behave.

The interactionist studies actual occurrences or situations as they are created by individuals interacting with one another. An example of this type of study in sports is to examine how individuals develop meaning and identity associated with sports, such as what it is like for a child to participate on a Little League team. Other studies using interactionist theories have explored the meaning of pain in an athlete's life (11).

As with the other theories presented here, interactionist theory also has limitations. Personal definitions of the individual(s) and setting(s) are exclusive and do not seem to be related to the social structure of society as a whole. Although this is a valid criticism, the strength of this theory lies in the fact that individual meaning, identity, and interaction can be discovered, thus allowing the researcher greater insight into individual revelations and learning.

Explanations of social life have been pursued by numerous sociologists. These social scientists have collected data, challenged theories, and revealed findings regarding the social world. This pursuit to establish a general theory or foundation for the relationships and structures that enable individuals to live in cultures, subcultures, and societies has resulted in a number of truths rather than one general truth or theory. It is necessary, therefore, to consider the many diverse and complex factors that affect social life and consider the issues within sports sociology from various perspectives or theories.

Although researchers may argue over which theory is best, it is important to examine the strengths and weaknesses of each, considering, of course, the research questions to be explored and the perspective to be used. Each theory offers a different dynamic and potential for discovery. Further and extensive reading and study are needed within each theoretical framework to pursue questions regarding sports.

Issues and Controversies in Sports Sociology

Issues and controversies in sports sociology were presented earlier. It is also important to acknowledge the controversies created by the sociology of sports itself. Such controversy is created by the research produced in this area (1).

Because structural functionalists appear to like sports in its present form, their only suggestion might be to strengthen the foundation of what currently exists. Sports sociologists have, however, revealed that what exists in sports is not always good or fair. Challenging the structure of sports and calling for changes in laws and/or the addition of new laws that may give others more power, access, and freedom can be threatening to those who already possess power, access, and freedom. To explore in-depth each issue and controversy emanating from sports sociology is beyond the scope of this chapter; however, what follows is a brief introduction and the presentation of vital questions that should be asked within the social science knowledge base.

The issues presented here in the sociologic study of sports are media and sports; youth sports; education; gender and sports; race, ethnicity, and sports; politics and sports; and religion and sports. Although other areas can be examined from a sociologic perspective, these receive much of the attention in the sports sociology literature and are extremely relevant in understanding the relationship between sociology and exercise science.

Media and Sports

The media and sports share an unusual symbiotic relationship (see Sidelight 18.2). Each needs the other to survive, and although they may be each other's nemesis, they are also each other's savior. The media has a dual purpose within society (12). On one hand, based on economics and capitalism, they are basically profit-making industries that use the commodity of sports and exercise for their own gain. On the other hand, media play an important cultural role by reflecting social conditions and reinforcing the attitudes of society regarding sports. Here are some issues and controversies within the topic of the media and sports:

- Why do the media represent only what they consider the major sports played by men in our society?
- How do the media reinforce gender and racial stereotypes in our society?
- In what ways do the media influence social change within society?
- Can the media and sports exist without each other?

Youth Sports

Youth sports used to mean children playing in the backyard, on the playground, or in loosely organized leagues. Now concepts such as privatization, skilled performance, and adult-controlled games characterize youth sports. Private and commercial organizations have been added to the list of sponsors of organized youth sports activities along with tax-supported groups. Learning skills is an important component of this form of competition, and the child must evaluate and improve personal techniques to be successful. In addition, young athletes should be viewed as having certain rights; for example, they have the right to

- Participate in sports (all children, regardless of age, gender, race, or skill level have the right to participate in physical activity and to choose the activity in which they wish to participate) (Fig. 18.3).
- Participate at a level commensurate with their maturity and ability.
- Have qualified adult leadership.
- Play as children, not as adults.
- Share in the leadership and decision making of their sports participation.
- Participate in a safe and healthy environment.
- Have proper preparation for participation in sports.
- Have an equal opportunity to strive toward success.
- Be treated with dignity.
- Have fun in sports.

Adult control and participation as coaches have affected these games, making them resemble professional play; winning can replace the original objective of having fun and violence is often an outcome. This situation creates numerous questions: Is there too much pressure on children to learn competitive sports at a young age? Do children drop out of sports because of the emphasis by parents and coaches on perfecting skill and winning? Should young children specialize in a single sport, so that they can develop one set of skills well, rather than participate in a variety of sports?

The rights of young athletes offers pertinent points regarding the values, experiences, and potential outcomes for children in sports.

Education

The relationship between sports and education creates many conflicts. Athletic programs in North American society are generally linked to educational institutions and are thought to offer

►► Sidelight 18.2

THE SYMBIOTIC RELATIONSHIP BETWEEN SPORTS AND THE MEDIA

Although the effect of the media on sports has been established, particularly with commercial spectator sports, other forms of sports, known as noncommercial, still flourish, despite the lack of media coverage. The focus of the effect of sports on the media is worthy of exploration. The shared relationship, i.e., the media's dependency on sports and sports' dependency on the media, has created a symbiotic or mutually beneficial relationship. For example, the commercial success of both sports and the media depends on the need to sell the event both in broadcast and ticket sales as well as newspapers and magazines.

The place of sports and the media in popular culture is also established and maintained through this relationship. Economic factors have intensified the symbiotic relationship between sports and the media. Based on the concept of consumption by the public, corporations and businesses need to seek out ways in which their products, names, and images can be promoted and sold. With the worldwide attention that some sports are given, this need can be met quite easily by associating specific products with well-known and popular athletes. The buying of a product promoted and advertised by a popular professional athlete gives the consumer a source of identity, pleasure, and meaning associated with that individual.

Televised media coverage of events such as the Olympic Games has given legitimacy and power to sports and the media. As a result, higher TV ratings are experienced and more exposure and notoriety are given to the Olympic movement and individual athletes. The residual effects of winning a media bid to broadcast the Olympic Games make the bidding war to broadcast future games rewarding, because profits, status, and power are significantly increased for the winning network.

valuable positive learning experiences and opportunities for students. The controversy in this area is the reality of this statement for all students, high school and college students alike. The opportunity for professional success in sports is a dream, and in some cases a reality, for boys and men in team sports. With this goal in mind, many pursue sports with a seriousness that causes neglect of other areas of education that may prepare them for security over a longer term.

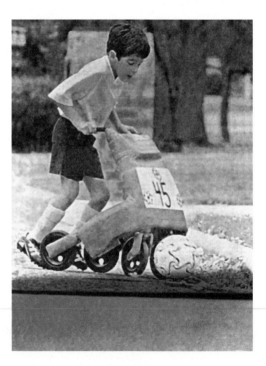

FIGURE 18.3 Differently-abled athletes competing in sports.

Girls and women, on the other hand, have not had this opportunity until recently, and certainly not to the same extent. Historically, women have been forced to play team sports abroad to have access to the professional level. Only recently has this situation changed with formation of the women's professional basketball league.

It is the big time or National Collegiate Athletic Association (NCAA) Division IA level of intercollegiate sports that raises many questions, because of the issues of recruitment, the awarding of scholarships, and the behaviors of donors to these programs. NCAA Division III athletics, although still very competitive, do not award scholarships and do not seem to have some of the major issues associated with their teams. This does not mean, however, that they are free from problems. Once again, the commercialization of Division IA programs and the need to obtain the best players have lead to competition both on and off the playing fields. They have paved the way for us to think about college sports as a major public relations tool.

Issues that are raised by conflict theorists also apply, e.g., does racism and sexism, coercion and social control, and alienation still occur in college sports? The answer to this question is contained in the mirror of society. Furthermore, if athletics are truly educational, are closely linked to the academic programs, and have a purpose within educational institutions, why aren't the profits gained by athletic departments shared more with academic units? Benefits in various forms should be realized by all involved in the educational institution, including all students, academic programs, and personnel.

> ⚷ *The relationship between academic and athletic programs and their values need careful philosophical examination to determine their missions within the educational institution, appropriate linkages, and objectives. Because athletic programs are public relations tools for the educational institution, they also serve a social and educational role.*

Gender and Sport

The concept of gender and sports invokes many thoughts and feelings regarding the ideas of **patriarchy,** maintaining feminine and masculine images, and sexuality. The topic of gender includes much more than equity. It is about history, socialization, humanness, opportunity, roles, expectations, and the future definitions and intersections of sports and gender. Social constructions or definitions of gender have controlled our thinking about these constructs. Women's position in society at large has been and still is in a transformational stage. There are ideologic struggles in efforts to improve the media coverage of women's sports and to change the cultural images regarding women and physical activity (13).

The advances made by women, however, have been significant. Many more girls and women have the opportunity and choose to participate in sports and physical activity than ever before, and certain positions are now open to women that were not previously available (Fig. 18.4). The top levels of sports are still not open to women and remain extremely difficult to access. Positions such as managers of exercise and fitness clubs, ownership of sports franchises, and political appointments within professional sports organizations are hard for women to attain. Even with the influx of women in sports owing to the passage of Title IX, the number of women who hold college coaching or athletic administrator positions has been decreasing (14). This situation is attributed to men's and women's athletic programs merging and retaining the male administrator.

Because women have less power, status, and resources in our society than men, and men possess political and social dominance, women are relegated to a secondary status. Patriarchy is a predominant controlling factor in society. As a result, patriarchal thinking labels specific sports and exercise activities as appropriate or inappropriate for males and females, thus restricting opportunity and a sense of freedom for participation in sports and physical activity (15). In addition, the naming of girls and women's teams as "lady" or with sexist terms such as "Pink Panthers" and

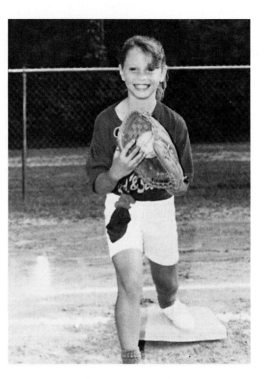

FIGURE 18.4 Title IX opens
the playing field to girls.

the practice of referring to women athletes by their first name only contribute to the perpetuation of gender bias and subordinate the status of girls and women to that of boys and men.

Here are some questions generated by gender issues and sports: In what ways has Title IX contributed to equality in sports participation? How have gender issues resolved the concept of gender-specific sports? In what ways are women in sports underrepresented or misrepresented in the media?

Race, Ethnicity, and Sports

The negative mind-set of individuals regarding race and ethnicity is unfortunately prominent. Opinions and biases regarding individuals of color or individuals from different cultures have been learned from our backgrounds as well as from the current media. For some, separating myth from reality regarding differences is difficult. We live in a diverse society; and to learn about others, we must first learn about ourselves and explore our mind-sets about those who are different from us. For example, the question of who we are in relation to race and ethnicity must be explored before any progress can be made in establishing cross-cultural understanding and relationships.

Biases regarding the physical and mental abilities or inabilities of whites and blacks have been at the center of debate for quite some time, thus creating even more tension between racial groups. Life decisions made solely on the basis of skin color rather than on true personal knowledge of and about those who are different from ourselves are at the heart of discrimination.

Because of racial stereotypes and biases on the part of a large segment of our society, a discriminatory practice in sports known as **stacking** has occurred. Stacking in team sports is considered the overrepresentation or underrepresentation of racial or ethnic groups in certain positions. Generally, the underrepresentation is noted in what are considered central positions or leadership/strategic positions within team sports. Biologic, psychologic, and sociologic myths regarding differences between racial groups are noted for the practice of stacking, and such myths are perpetuated today.

Stacking occurs when coaches say, for instance, that they want to recruit blacks for positions that require quick reactions, fast sprinting, and intricate movements and to reserve whites for positions that require thinking.

Whereas questions associated with race and ethnicity are imbedded within the brief description of this issue, additional controversies to examine include How do the sports experiences of black men and women differ regarding stacking? What discriminatory practices exist in front office positions? Why should racial and ethnic differences be considered when discussing sports? A related research issue is the need to distinguish between biologic and cultural explanations for the dominance of black athletes in certain sports.

Politics and Sports

Because they do not exist in a cultural vacuum but rather are part of the social world, sports are influenced by many different societal and cultural forces. One important force is that of politics. Politics deals with the concept of power, how it is obtained, and how it is used. Whether we examine settings such as the local high school football game, the women's Final Four Basketball Tournament, Wimbledon, the Olympic Games, or the Paralympic Games, politics are involved. At a local level, decisions regarding facility use by organizations and city sanctions and ordinances must be considered. At national collegiate competitions, the NCAA governs and controls events.

At the international level, governments choose the coaches who in turn select the athletes who will compete in the Olympic Games. Governments also use sport in these ways: as a political tool, e.g., Olympic boycotts by the United States (1980) and the former Soviet Union (1984); as a propaganda showcase, e.g., the 1936 Olympic Games in which Hitler demonstrated his military power; and as an economic and national showcase of a host nation. Sports serve as a sociopolitical mirror reflecting the state of a nation, its political ideology, and power. Laws have been passed by our government to specify regulations regarding the Olympic ideal. The Amateur Sports Act and Title IX of the Educational Amendments Act specifically address laws regarding opportunity and the regulation of sports in the United States.

Some controversies involving politics and sport are In what ways are sports effective or ineffective tools of political propaganda? How are the Olympic Games separated from concepts of politics? In what ways can sports be used as integrating and truly peaceful endeavors? How can international competitions be changed to be friendly rather than hostile encounters (see A Case in Point 18.1)?

Religion and Sports

Religion and sports might be considered an unusual combination, but the concept offers some interesting comparisons. As individuals attempt to explain sports and religion as similar to or different from each other, the comparisons show that both institutions are cultural practices in our society. There may well exist the practice of religion in sports and/or the practice of sports within religion, but saying that they are the same sparks debate (Fig. 18.5).

Similarities and differences between sports and religion need to be determined before any conclusion can be drawn. One such comparison is shown in Table 18.1 (16). It is agreed that both sports and religion have places for communal gathering; drama is linked to both settings; there is a hierarchical structure in both sports and religion; they both have special celebratory days, heroes and saints, choirs, hymns, chants, sermons, joining of hands, and revered objects; and there are special ceremonies within both realms. Both of these institutions emphasize self-sacrifice. Comparisons, however, need careful consideration.

A Case in Point 18.1

DOES INTERNATIONAL SPORTS COMPETITION ESTABLISH UNITY?

When considering politics, international competition, and the establishment of unity between nations, the concepts of power and political ideology must be understood. Because there is a winner and loser in competition, the winner is envisioned as powerful and the loser as weak. In international competition, the awarding of medals to a specific country, the raising of its flag, and the playing of its national anthem have the potential to lead viewers into believing that the country possesses a superior political ideology to that of other countries. Thus the political ideology of the specific country being awarded the medal takes on an aura of superiority and dominance over other nations, if only for a limited time. Such was the case during the 1980 Olympic gold medal ice hockey match between the United States and the former Soviet Union. The contest was often referred to as a war of political ideologies. This point is further evidenced during the opening ceremonies of Olympic Games. During the entrance and parade of athletes, the flag of the United States is never dipped to recognize the dignitaries of the nations in which the games are held.

The boycotts, terrorist killings of athletes, demonstrations, protests, threats, and other incidences that have occurred during Olympic Games have been initiated for political reasons to show political superiority; to demonstrate military power; and to protest against communism, military invasion of countries, and apartheid. Again, the question arises, Does international competition actually establish unity?

Christian organizations such as Athletes in Action or Jocks for Jesus, for example, do attempt to combine sports and religion, but some professional athletes have admitted to using such organizations to promote themselves and do not really adhere to the tenets of the organization or the religion. Others are true believers in the Christian sport organizations and demonstrate their convictions by praying publicly before, during, and/or after contests. Because much of sports takes place on the campuses of public schools and colleges, issues surrounding the separation of church and state are raised. If we have public prayer or team private prayer before sporting events in these settings, how is the separation of church and state reconciled? In this example, both political and religious issues are posed. Questions regarding religion and sport include the following: How are the concepts of intrinsic and extrinsic rewards evaluated within sports and religion? In what ways do individuals receive reconciliation through sports? What role does the congregation or fan play in sports and religion? Should team members be forced to take part in prayer before games? What are the consequences if an athlete refuses to pray at the coach's request? What religious beliefs are or should be promoted by a team?

ADVANCES IN SPORTS SOCIOLOGY

Although sports sociology has always been inclusive in its population considerations (i.e., race, gender, ethnicity, age, sexuality, ability, and class) and in the diverse issues it covers, there seems to be a globalization or broader realization and outreach of the applications and implications of the effect sports are making on the world.

With the increased interest, participation, and spectatorship of sports and physical activity by girls, boys, women, and men of all age levels, cultures, and abilities, the value and meaning of sports have assumed more significant places in our lives and society. Sports and physical activity are not just acceptable for a chosen few, but for all.

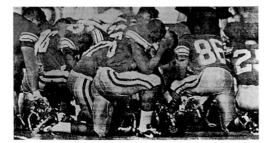

FIGURE 18.5 The practice of religion in sports.

The effect of political, economic, and social theories and subsequent studies have defined additional ways to study sports sociology. Research has broadened considerably in sports sociology, and this area of study has taken on the characteristics of a cultural studies approach. That is, sports sociology and its many issues can be explored from not only a cross-disciplinary perspective but from a multidisciplinary one. As a result of the multidisciplinary approach to sports sociology, the extent to which qualitative methodology is being used has increased, giving a broader perspective and data interpretation. Studying the athlete as a potential agent for societal change, exploring the concepts and meanings of power and oppression in sports, and examining the potential of the cyborg athlete are but a few examples of the ways in which broader cross-disciplinary and multidisciplinary perspectives of sports may be gained.

Coakley (1) discusses the potential of the college and/or professional athlete serving as agents of social change. The athlete should have the freedom (i.e., experience no coercion or social control imposed by organizations or coaches) to openly support political and social issues, such as affirmative action, equal rights, and other antidiscrimination movements. Tiger Woods is a prime example of the athlete as an agent of social change. In various television advertisements and broadcast interviews, he has supported the concept of multiracial identification by referring to himself not as only African-American but as Caublinasian (a combination of Caucasian, black, Indian, and Asian). He has also referred to the exclusion of blacks from playing at some private golf courses. By raising these issues via the media, he has created an opportunity to increase the awareness of the public regarding these forms of oppression and may affect social action (17).

The relationship between humans and technology (i.e., the cyborg athlete) is another intriguing area that is expanding the research in sports sociology. Although elite athletes already perform at high levels, the challenge exists for them to exceed their previous performance levels to the degree of extraordinary. The multitude of ways in which technology (e.g,. performance-enhancing drugs, psychological interventions, enhanced equipment, and genetic alterations) can assist the athlete to perform at such levels and the meanings attached to this type of performance are raising many questions in cross-disciplinary and interdisciplinary studies of sports. This is a relatively new area of study, but it is one that will continue to challenge the scholarly study of sports from a sociologic perspective (18–20).

Table 18.1 COMPARISON BETWEEN SPORTS AND RELIGION[a]	
Sports	**Religion**
Profane and material	Sacred and supernatural
Pursuit of fame and fortune in the here and now	Pursuit of goals in the afterlife
Rooted in specific rules and relationships	Rooted in the concept of faith
Competitive	Noncompetitive
Instrumental and goal oriented	Rituals are expressive and process oriented
Clear-cut and crude	Mystical and pure

[a]Hoffman SJ. Sport and religion. Champaign, IL: Human Kinetics, 1992.

Other advances in sports sociology include the development of critical and interpretative theories. These theories offer the researcher a way to construct, deconstruct, and critique sports in ways that, it is hoped, will lead to social activism and potential change.

SUMMARY POINTS

- Sports sociology examines the relationship between sports and society and focuses on behavior and social processes in sports, which are then described within the structure of sports and the social structures in which sports exist.
- Sport sociology is concerned with explaining how individuals are affected by the world and how they can effect change.
- Theoretical frameworks establish the foundation for research in sports sociology.
- The issues, controversies and questions about sports in society that are derived from the various theories address the structures of sports and the relationships of individuals to each other and call for either maintaining the status quo or taking social action for changes in society and sports.
- As a social science, sports sociology uses both qualitative and quantitative methodology.
- With the increase in the production of research involving critical theoretical and methodologic analysis, sports sociology has taken on a broad framework, making it appropriate and more relevant to the study of sports and exercise science.
- The broader perspective of sports sociology appears to be taking on characteristics of the cultural studies tradition, thus giving it even more prominence in the analysis of societies and cultures in relation to sports and exercise and in explaining concepts such as power, social class, race, and gender.
- The issues that evolve from the study of sports sociology, like sports history, must be studied within contexts of time and place but also in relation to the global concerns of politics and economics.

REVIEW QUESTIONS

1. Define sports sociology and explain the aspects that are included in this area of study.
2. Discuss the ways in which sports are a microcosm of society.
3. Define and discuss one social institution associated with sports in society.
4. Discuss the relationship between culture and sports.
5. What is the value of using theoretical perspectives to study sports?
6. In what ways are religion reflected in sports?

References

1. Coakley JJ. Sport in society issues and controversies. 6th ed. Boston: McGraw-Hill, 1998.
2. Sage GH. Physical education, sociology, and sociology of sport: points of intersection. Sociol Sport J 1997;14:317–339.
3. Kenyon GS, Loy JW. Toward a sociology of sport. J Health Phys Educ Recreation 1965;36:24–25.
4. Kenyon GS. A sociology of sport: on becoming a subdiscipline. In: RC Brown, BJ Cratty, eds. New perspectives of man in action. Englewood Cliffs, NJ: Prentice-Hall, 1969:163–180.
5. Kenyon GS. Aspects of contemporary sport sociology. Chicago: Athletic Institute, 1969.
6. Bryant JE, McElroy M. Social dynamics of sport and exercise. Englewood, CO: Morton, 1997.
7. Eitzen S, Sage G. Sociology of North American sport. 6th ed. Dubuque, IA: Brown, 1996.
8. Harris JC. Suited up and stripped down: perspectives for sociocultural sport studies. Sociol Sport J 1989;6:335–347.
9. Roberts JM, Sutton-Smith B. Child training and game involvement. Ethnology 1962;2:166–185.
10. Williams R. American society: a sociological interpretation. New York: Knopf, 1970.

11. Curry T. A little pain never hurt anyone: athletic career socialization and the normalization of sports injury. Symbol Interact 1993;16:273–290.
12. Hallin DC. The American news media: a critical theory perspective. In: J Forester, ed. Critical theory and public life. Cambridge, MA: MIT, 1985:121–146.
13. Theberge N, Birrell S. Structural constraints facing women in sport. In: D Costa, S Guthrie, eds. Women and sport: interdisciplinary perspectives. Champaign, IL: Human Kinetics, 1994.
14. Acosta R, Carpenter L. Women in intercollegiate sport: a longitudinal study and fifteen year update, 1977–1995. Unpublished manuscript, 1995.
15. Messner M, Sabo D. Sport, men, and the gender order: critical feminist theory. Champaign, IL: Human Kinetics, 1990.
16. Hoffman SJ. Sport and religion. Champaign, IL: Human Kinetics, 1992.
17. Giacobbi PR, DeSensi JT. Media portrayals of Tiger Woods: a qualitative deconstructive examination. Quest 1999;51:408–417.
18. Cole CL. Resisting the canon: feminist cultural studies, sport, and technologies of the body. J Sport Soc Issues 1993;17:77–97.
19. Cole CL. Addiction, exercise and cyborgs: technologies and deviant bodies. In: G Rail, ed. Sport and postmodern times. Albany, NY: State University of New York Press, 1998:261–275.
20. Hoberman J. Sport and the technological image of man. In: WJ Morgan, KV Meier, eds. Philosophic inquiry in sport. Champaign, IL: Human Kinetics, 1995:202–214.

Suggested Readings

Ashe AR Jr. A hard road to glory: a history of the African American athlete. New York: Warner, 1988.
Brooks DD, Althouse RC, eds. Racism in college athletics: the African-American athlete's experience. Morgantown, WV: Fitness Information Technology, 1993.
Coakley JJ. Burnout among adolescent athletes: a personal failure or social problem? Sociol Sport J 1992; 9:271–285.
Eitzen DS, Zinn MB. The de-athleticization of women: the naming and gender marking of collegiate sport teams. Sociol Sport J 1989;6:363–370.
Lever J, Wheeler S. Mass media and the experience of sport. Commun Res 1993;20:125–143.

PART THREE

FUTURE DEVELOPMENT

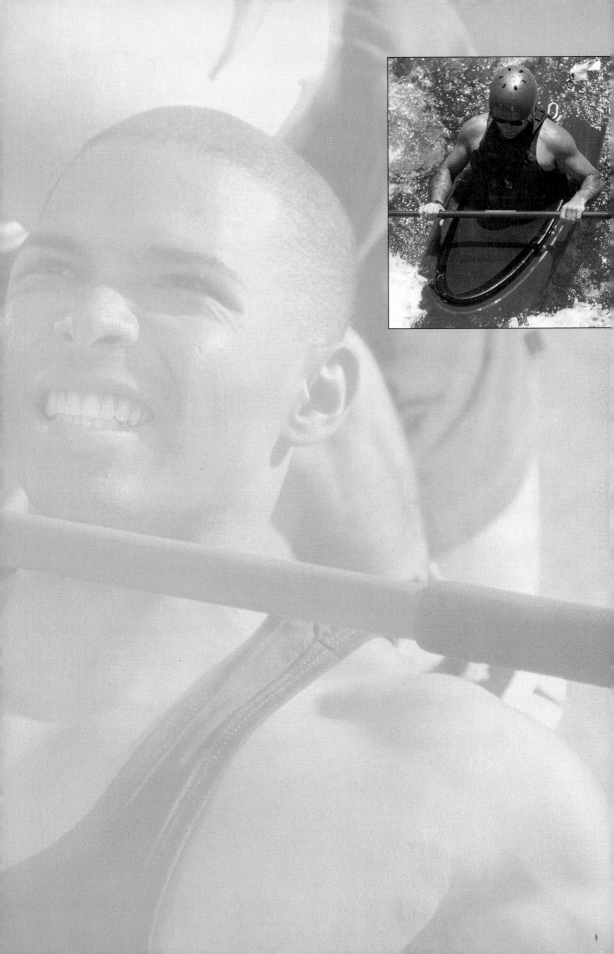

Section 8

EXERCISE SCIENCE IN THE TWENTY-FIRST CENTURY

At the close of the twentieth century, the field of exercise science continued to evolve in scope and focus. Since the 1970s, the refinement of exercise science as an academic discipline coincided with the emergence of a variety of subdisciplines. The 1990s saw the emergence of new subdisciplines and significant advances toward the development of exercise science as an academic discipline. Associated with the development of exercise science subdisciplines is the explosion of scientific and scholarly findings that have given the field a substantive foundation that did not formerly exist.

How will exercise science continue to change as we move further into the twenty-first century? Will exercise science have a larger or smaller effect on the culture? Anticipating future directions is an important exercise, because we will all be there to experience it. At the beginning of this text it was noted that as we approach the new millennium the science of movement—*Exercise Science*—will continue to develop, expand, and become even more significant to the human experience. The exercise sciences are still evolving, and new avenues of scientific inquiry that are sure to come with emerging technologies will likely lead to further significant changes in the discipline. This last section of *Introduction to Exercise Science* takes a "look" forward to what the future may hold for exercise science. What new directions exercise science takes because of emerging technologies, and how future scientific developments may influence the professional fields related to the movement knowledge base is something that awaits both exercise science students and professionals.

19

Future of Exercise Science

J. LARRY DURSTINE AND STANLEY P. BROWN

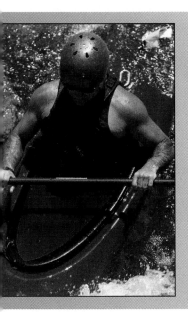

Objectives

1. Explain the paradigm shift associated with the development of exercise science as an academic discipline.
2. Describe two important distinctions between a profession and a discipline.
3. Explain how modern technology may continue to affect exercise science into the twenty-first century.

- **A Paradigm Shift**
- **Basic Science Effects**
- **Disciplinary Versus Professional Concerns**
- **Future Perspective**
  Exercise Science in the Twenty-First Century
  Future Trends

A PARADIGM SHIFT

We undertake our daily lives in a set pattern, an established way of viewing life or perceiving the world in which we live. This is true not only for individuals, but for large and small groups of people. A set pattern such as this is the definition of a **paradigm.** As we live our lives, we often do not consider the possibility of other ways of thinking. Paradigms are powerful in that they often preclude the possibility that any other worldview is conceivable. However, paradigms can and often do change. After years of small often unnoticed adjustments, the once well-established daily patterns undergo complete modification, usually as a result of far-sighted thinking by a few individuals, which then becomes established in the larger culture. The resulting new pattern is often much different from the original. These changes in a set pattern are viewed as a paradigm shift, which occur over time and after the initial fear of change has subsided.

An example of a paradigm shift often cited is the switch that occurred in the 1970s from the popularity of the mechanical watch made by the Swiss to the electronic watch made by the Japanese and Americans, which subsequently captured the vast majority of the world's watch market. When the electronic watch was first proposed, the idea was met with disdain by those who, at that time, held 70% of the world's market share of watches. Over time, this new way to make watches caught the public's imagination, and the paradigm shift was under way.

The emerging exercise science discipline is another example of a paradigm shift. Over the years the focus surrounding the study of physical education changed as a result of the desire to bring academic respectability to the study of human movement. This shift is still occurring, and is expected to broaden later in the twenty-first century.

The physical activity paradigm has undergone many changes since humans first started to walk the earth. Accounts of human movement have been highlighted throughout history. The ability to plan and properly execute movement have always been two of the most basic survival skills. Early civilizations emphasized in one way or another physical activity and/or physical training. Movement skills were practiced and incorporated into competition, tribal rituals, and war. Although some cultures promoted physical training, a few cultures, such as the Chinese, believed that disease could result from inactivity. The Greeks became the first to keep a scholarly account on how human movement was accomplished. Later, Leonardo da Vinci studied in detail human movement and described muscle origins, insertions, and actions throughout a range of motion. Advancement in the way we viewed physical activity and studied human motion during the twentieth century began to occur in a variety of different disciplines, including physiology, engineering, and psychology.

BASIC SCIENCE EFFECTS

The changes that took place in the late twentieth century resulted in a number of profound contributions. Two contributions were an increase in the growth and development of scientific-based curricula and an increase in the number of laboratories studying human movement. These have led to increased opportunities for graduate study and research. Graduate and undergraduate students finishing exercise science programs have a stronger science understanding and are better equipped to contribute to the scientific study of human movement than earlier students. This contribution was perhaps the single most important one, because the addition of a strong scientific knowledge base for all the subdisciplines involving the study of human movement was foremost to the growth of the discipline.

The last half of the twentieth century saw many technologic advances. This age of technology also helped make advancements in the various exercise science subdisciplines. Respiratory gas analysis was once completed with complicated hand-operated apparatuses that exposed expired air to several chemicals. This process was at best tedious, requiring large amounts of time

A Case in Point 19.1

HUMAN MOVEMENT STUDIES IN SPACE

On April 17, 1998, the space shuttle *Columbia* was launched from Kennedy Space Center. On board was Neurolab, a series of complicated experiments that were carried out during the 16-day mission. These experiments were designed to study how the nervous system develops and functions in space. This significant research effort is thought to have important consequences for humankind's hope to develop long-duration space flights. James A. Pawelczyk, payload specialist, NASA astronaut, and professor of kinesiology, was on board to conduct some of these experiments (see figure); Pawelczyk was the first exercise scientist to fly in space. Interest in space research is now international in scope. The Neurolab investigations were supported by the National Institutes of Health; the Office of Naval Research; the National Science Foundation; the Spanish Ministry of Education and Culture; and the Canadian, European, French, German and Japanese space agencies. As humans continue to take bold steps into space, our understanding of movement in this environment will have to increase. Exercise science will continue to play a large role in this important undertaking.

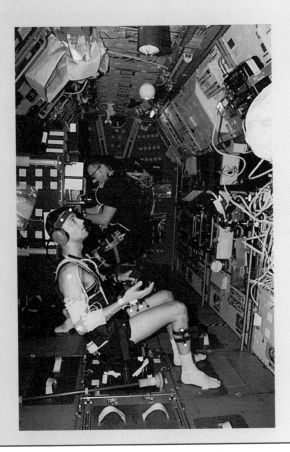

Payload specialist James A. Pawelczyk prepares to catch a ball as part of the ball-catching (Kinelite) experiment. On Earth, the ball would fall based on the acceleration of gravity; but in space, the ball is propelled at a constant velocity. During this experiment a spring-loaded apparatus measures the anticipatory contraction of his muscles. The Kinelite experiment is designed to investigate how catching (representative of a stored complex motor response) changes in microgravity.

►► Sidelight 19.1

MOLECULAR BIOLOGY AND EXERCISE SCIENCE

Since the 1980s, the discipline of molecular biology has revolutionized our understanding of living organisms. Molecular biologists study the structures that ultimately determine the physical appearance and function of cells. All human cells contain between 75,000 to 100,000 genes, and in each cell, 500 to 1,000 of these genes are expressed. Each gene participates in the synthesis or expression of a single type of protein, which performs some critical function for the cell. Intercellular and extracellular signals regulate the amount of protein synthesized, depending on the metabolic and environmental demands placed on the cell. Understanding those factors that regulate the expression of genes is a major goal of modern molecular biology. The signaling pathways that regulate gene expression are also of enormous importance to physiologists and exercise scientists.

Exercise training causes well-described adaptations to a host of cells, allowing better tolerance of the imposed metabolic stress. Indeed, it is known that endurance training increases the intracellular density of energy-producing organelles called the mitochondria. Hence the molecular biologist working in conjunction with an exercise scientist can unravel the question of how exercise regulates the expression of the genes that make the mitochondrial proteins. Results from this type of scientific collaboration might allow the exercise scientist to design the most effective training regimen to achieve a desired performance benefit (the dose–response relationship is an important concept in exercise prescription).

Recent studies have shown that physical activity is associated with a decreased incidence of certain diseases. The mechanism by which this potential health benefit is acquired is not yet clear. One of the more revolutionary tools available to the molecular biologist is called polymerase chain reaction (PCR), for which its developer, Kerry Mullis, won the 1995 Nobel prize. With this technique, differences in the concentration of messenger RNA (mRNA), an index of gene

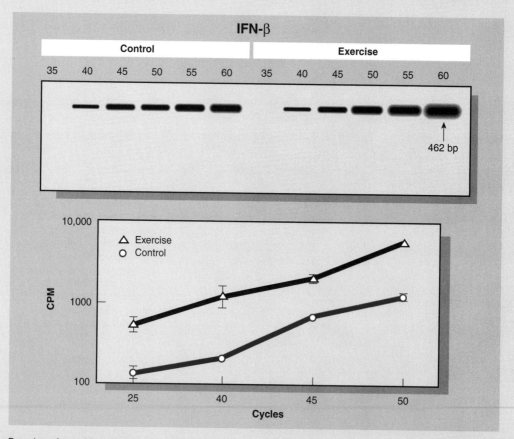

Beta interferon blots before and after exercise.

expression, can be determined by how much time it takes (number of cycles) to make a certain amount of mRNA. Using reverse transcriptase (RT-PCR) it has been possible to measure minute levels of mRNA in difficult-to-obtain populations of immune cells in lung tissues (see figure). After exercise, there is a greater amount of mRNA (*black bands*) that codes for beta interferon (β-IFN) after 60 cycles than in control groups. β-IFN is a cytokine protein that, when expressed at higher than normal levels in the lung immune cells, improves the defense against infections. Thus with the help of molecular biologists, exercise scientists may one day be able to explain how regular physical activity improves the functioning of the immune system as well as other physiologic systems.

to analyze one sample. Today, this same measure (although based on the original procedure) can be accomplished by using electronic instrumentation, and the measurements are completed almost instantaneously. The space program brought about the use of radio-transmitted signals. Space itself is proving to be a wonderful medium for the scientific study of human movement (see A Case in Point 19.1).

Technology of this type is now common in exercise science laboratories. Another important addition in the last 20 years of the twentieth century to all science laboratories is the computer. This once large apparatus is now quite small, very powerful, and an essential piece of laboratory equipment. These technologic and equipment advances have reduced the labor associated with data collection and, at the same time, increased the amount of data compiled and the precision accumulated. These technologic advances, however, did not change the scientific inquiry process or the direction in which each exercise science subdiscipline was moving; they did, however, shorten the time necessary to complete the inquiry. Although variables such as oxygen consumption, heart rate, and blood pressure remain important, cellular and molecular mechanisms for exercise responses and adaptations have become the principal variables of inquiry (see Sidelight 19.1).

DISCIPLINARY VERSUS PROFESSIONAL CONCERNS

After World War II people interested in studying human movement were found in academic settings such as departments of physical education. Traditional physical education programs focused on teacher preparation for elementary, middle, and secondary schools. Nonetheless, undergraduate academic physical education preparation since the 1970s has changed considerably. Presently, in addition to the traditional teacher education approach, there is an in-depth scientific, knowledge-base approach concerning human movement study. The present trend in exercise science is toward undergraduate programming requirements that include calculus, chemistry, physics, biochemistry, anatomy, physiology, exercise physiology, biomechanics, and nutrition. There is now, as a result, little difference between the general academic course requirements for physical therapy, medicine, and exercise science. This approach, in conjunction with the increased awareness for the need to be physically active to improve health, has opened many professional opportunities previously not available for students in exercise science.

Many students interested in professional careers, such as occupational therapy, physical therapy, and medicine, are now using exercise science as preprofessional training. Other allied health fields also incorporate exercise science principles. New career opportunities in clinical exercise settings such as cardiac and pulmonary rehabilitation programming have been formed. National associations such as the American College of Sports Medicine (ACSM) and, more recently, the American Association for Cardiovascular and Pulmonary Rehabilitation (AACVPR) have been founded. The transition from a traditional teacher education approach to a science-based approach reflects a paradigm shift: A transition from a discipline that emphasized teacher preparation to a new discipline that emphasizes science-based preprofessional preparation. This new approach is the discipline of exercise science, which exists alongside its sister discipline of physical education.

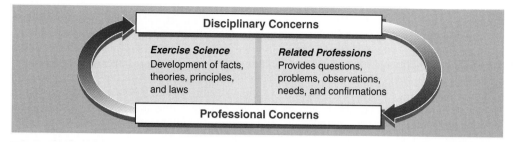

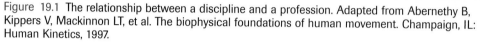

Figure 19.1 The relationship between a discipline and a profession. Adapted from Abernethy B, Kippers V, Mackinnon LT, et al. The biophysical foundations of human movement. Champaign, IL: Human Kinetics, 1997.

The refinement of exercise science as an academic discipline effectively leads to a refocusing of physical education. Although physical education retains the status of academic discipline, its activities, to a large extent, have taken on the characteristics of a profession. The relationship between an academic discipline and a profession is illustrated in Figure 19.1. Academic disciplines are chiefly concerned with providing definitions, descriptions, and cause–effect relationships of variables (1). These are research-based activities that seek to add to the body of knowledge of the discipline. Professions (using physical education as an example) are concerned with objectives, programs, teaching, learning, and evaluation. In addition, clinical professions are concerned with diagnoses, therapies, prescription, rehabilitation, and prognoses.

The knowledge derived from the discipline of exercise science is translated into practice by the profession. As can be seen in Figure 19.1, the relationship between an academic discipline and a related profession is symbiotic. That is, the flow of information occurs in both directions. Professions often function as a guide for the discipline, which may lead the discipline to alter a theory, based on observations made in the day-to-day practice of the profession. The comments of Abernethy and co-workers (1) are key to understanding the interrelationship between discipline and profession:

> The principal function of a discipline is therefore to develop a coherent body of knowledge that describes, explains and predicts key phenomena from the domain of interest (or subject matter). In contrast, professions, as a general rule, try to improve the conditions of society by providing a regulated service in which practices and educational/training programs are developed that are in accordance with knowledge available from one or more relevant disciplines.

Disciplines seek to understand subject matter and professions to implement change based on this understanding. Many professions use knowledge about human movement in their practices. Examples besides physical education include medical doctors, nurses, physical and occupational therapists, and individuals in the field of ergonomics (human factors). Increasingly, the core content of exercise science is becoming the core content of professions that rely on a fundamental understanding of human movement. This use of the core content of exercise science in the practice of many different professions will continue in the next century.

FUTURE PERSPECTIVE

Prediction of the future of human enterprise with any degree of success is at best tenuous. But at the same time prediction of possibilities or trends frequently materialize in small or altered forms. Knowing our past does not always help in an attempt to predict the future, but by knowing history we may gain an appreciation for where we might go. An important activity in any disciplinary field of study is to attempt to predict the future courses and directions. This has been largely neglected in exercise science. Swanson and Massengale (2) explain that

> the process of creating alternative futures, studying them, and then selectively choosing the most appropriate future is not currently being done in the field of exercise and sport science.

The leadership of the field needs to focus attention upon the creation of alternative futures, the selection of one, and then take the necessary steps to make that future come true.

A complicating factor is that the future will not be like the past, regardless of accurate trend extrapolation; it will be far more complex. New data that are yet to be established may not be like current data. Frames of reference will probably change. Demographics will change, as will science and technology. Social norms, cultural norms, and political institutions will vary independently of one another, as well as independently of science and technology.

Leaders in the field of exercise science can forecast many possible alternatives for the future. The question is which alternative will be the correct one, if any, or will new unforeseen alternatives be created? Reviewing the historical development of exercise science reveals two consistent points: *(a)* the direction and growth of the profession must continue to be assessed and it must be determined whether the present curricula are meeting this growth and *(b)* possibly the most important consideration is the continued development of a science-based exercise science curriculum so there is continued training of undergraduate and graduate students in the scientific subdisciplines of human movement and performance.

Exercise Science in the Twenty-First Century

The journey that was begun in the twentieth century will lead inextricably to exciting new avenues of growth in the next. How will exercise science continue to develop? What will be the relationship between the discipline of exercise science and new and existing professions with human movement as their knowledge base? Will our understanding of human movement continue as rapidly as the pace of technologic advancement? As was alluded to earlier, predicting the future is best left for prophets, but some interesting possibilities might be helpful for exploring this point.

As we begin to think prospectively about the possible or even probable future exercise science may have, it is important to note that this is the type of intellectual activity that makes up a field of study known as futures studies (3). As we begin this exercise in prospective thinking, the student should keep in mind that what is presented is only one of the many possibilities for the future of exercise science. However, what is clear at the outset is that for any future to be bright it takes hardworking people with a vision to make it happen.

> ⊶ *The purposes of futures studies are to discover or invent; examine and evaluate; and propose possible, probable, and preferable futures (3).*

Future Trends

Recent demographic projections of the U.S. population show that by the middle of the twenty-first century approximately 70 million Americans will be over the age of 65, and the number older than 85 years will increase to nearly 12 million (4). Owing to modern medical advances and future technologic advancements, the older population will have a greater chance to be healthier than any person of similar age in previous generations. But at what cost to the healthcare industry? What is inevitable as any population ages is that healthcare costs rise. It has been projected that the graying of the American population, and that of all industrialized nations, will bring with it severe economic burdens, if these increasing costs are sustained into the future (4). Furthermore, barring some great advance in genetic engineering that ameliorates aging and its attendant diseases, the evidence points to lifestyle interventions as being the best method for optimizing health and reducing healthcare costs (5,6). Sidelight 19.2 presents one vision of the future course of the movement profession.

►► Sidelight 19.2

ANOTHER PARADIGM SHIFT FOR EXERCISE SCIENCE?

According to Booth, "The 21st century will mark individualized exercise prescription for the prevention of disease using polymorphisms in disease susceptible genes. It will mark the identification of molecular linkages of exercise to disease prevention. These events will encourage policy makers to further emphasize physical exercise in lifestyle in order to maintain health."[a] And according to Roberts, "Medical care must integrate physical activity to maximize health. As health care technology and expense of medical care expands, the most cost effective strategy to improve public health is getting sedentary individuals to become active. If primary care clinical providers make the paradigm shift to approach every patient as an athlete, we will achieve great improvement in the health of individuals."[a] These cogent predictions, made by two prominent exercise scientists at the end of the twentieth century regarding the future of exercise science, may indeed foresee a paradigm shift that could take place early in the next. Like the one that occurred in the late twentieth century, which saw exercise science become a respectable academic discipline, the next shift may well see exercise science and related movement professions take on a much more prominent role in society. But, how might it happen?

Market forces that were driving healthcare policy at the end of the twentieth century are likely to become more intense in the first decade of the twenty-first century, leading to more reliance on the movement professions. As the population ages, exercise and physical activity will play larger roles in both medical and movement dysfunction diagnoses and treatment. It is not hard to envision that with the first decade of the twenty-first century, the economic burden of the graying population could drive healthcare costs up to unforeseen heights. How the national economies of Western nations are to be sustained in the face of this kind of economic strain is difficult to tell. Because of this and because of tremendous political pressures from the ever-

[a]Blair SN. Sports medicine and exercise science in the 21st century. Sports Med Bull 1999;34:8.

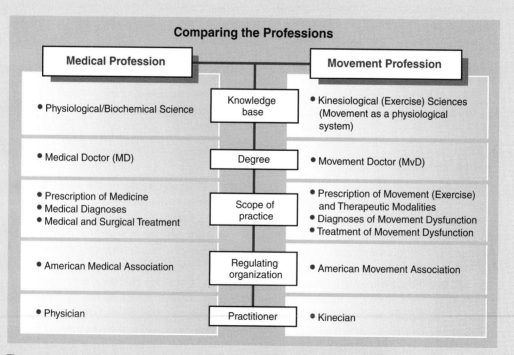

The movement profession juxtaposed with the medical profession in the year 2015.

increasing national debt, a decision could be made to restructure healthcare delivery. Research has shown, mostly based on molecular biologic evidence, that physical activity prevents potential medical problems from reaching an overt clinical state; thus the prediction may not be far-fetched.

The fact that the healthcare delivery mechanism is ill-equipped to adequately prescribe and implement physical activity interventions may prompt state legislators, lobbied by activists from the movement professions (mainly physical therapy and physical education) and exercise science, to begin funding a radically new vision of what healthcare could eventually become by 2015. As is usually the case with major change, this radically new approach to healthcare could start in progressive regions of the country (on the West coast, for instance) and slowly move to the rest of the country. The federal government is also likely to be involved when an understanding is reached that the new structure could save a tremendous amount of money.

The figure (previous page) shows the way the movement profession may be juxtaposed with that of the medical profession in the year 2015. The evolution of the movement profession to a status equal to that of the medical profession would lead to notable changes. For example, the earning power of movement profession practitioners could more than double once their field moves from an allied health profession to the doctoral level practitioner. These professionals would practice in private offices, clinics, and medical centers. The movement profession, like the medical profession, would include specialties, including those left over from the restructuring of academic programs in occupational therapy, physical therapy, and exercise science. Therefore, the future landscape of the movement profession would mirror that of the modern medical profession; the majority of kinecians (movement doctors) would be in general practice and others would be in specialized fields, often working closely with medical specialists.

Although the vision presented in the sidelight may or may not come to pass, clearly futurists see value in this endeavor to enable people to make informed decisions about their lives (3). One of the most important research directions exercise science will embark on is to determine the medical value of exercise for preventing, managing, and treating disease and rehabilitating patients. As more data substantiate the important roles of exercise and nutrition on health, exercise science will continue to gain acceptance in the medical and allied health professions. In addition, as the evidence concerning the scientific basis of movement continues to grow, society will begin to expect individuals who work in some aspect of exercise science to be knowledgeable, certified, and academically prepared. The following predictions, made by prominent exercise scientists at the end of the twentieth century, should help students of exercise science think about future directions (7).

- *Claude Bouchard:* "Daily energy expenditure will continue to decrease leading to a growing proportion of children and adults who will be in positive energy balance most of the time. This will be accompanied by an increasing prevalence of overweight and obesity, leading to dramatic increases in obesity-related diseases. We will see the development of the field of molecular exercise science, which will permit classifying individuals by genotype and the identification of those most at risk of sedentary habits and those who will gain most from becoming physically active."
- *Barry A. Franklin:* "Courses in exercise and nutrition counseling will assume an increasingly important role in medical school curricula and in the training of physicians. This should prompt an explosion of hospital and medically based fitness centers. Additionally, the over 85 age group is the fastest growing segment of our society. The socioeconomic ramifications of keeping older adults self-sufficient through physical activity programs will represent important opportunities in gerontology."

Whether these predictions and other predictions of the future of exercise science come about remains to be seen. What is clear is that, in this century, exercise science and those professions relying on the movement knowledge base will play an important role in the lives of us all.

SUMMARY POINTS

- The development of the subdisciplines produced a great increase in the scientific and scholarly findings concerning human movement.
- The development of exercise science as an academic discipline during the last quarter of the twentieth century represented a paradigm shift in the scientific study of human movement.
- Concerning the future development of exercise science two points are important: *(a)* the need to continue assessing the direction and growth of the profession and to determine whether the present curricula are meeting this growth, and *(b)* the continued development of a science-based exercise science curriculum.

REVIEW QUESTIONS

1. Why is the emergence of the discipline of exercise science considered a paradigm shift?
2. Explain the relationship between a discipline and a profession.
3. Give one example of a technologic advance that has helped the discipline of exercise science.

References

1. Abernethy B, Kippers V, Mackinnon LT, et al. The biophysical foundations of human movement. Champaign, IL: Human Kinetics, 1997.
2. Swanson RA, Massengale JD. Current and future directions in exercise and sport science. In: JD Massengale, RA Swanson, eds. The history of exercise and sport science. Champaign, IL: Human Kinetics, 1997:439–450.
3. Bell W. The purposes of futures studies. The Futurist 1997;31:42–45.
4. Brock D, Guralnick J, Brody J. Demography and epidemiology of aging in the U.S. In: E Schneider, J Rowe, eds. Handbook of the biology of aging. San Diego: Academic, 1990:3–23.
5. Hurley BF, Hagberg, JM. Optimizing health in older persons: aerobic or strength training? In: JO Holloszy, ed. Exercise and sport sciences reviews. Baltimore: Williams & Wilkins, 1998:61–89.
6. Buchner D, Wagner E. Preventing frail health. Clin Geriatr Med 1992;8:1–17.
7. Blair SN. Sports medicine and exercise science in the 21st century. Sports Med Bull 1999;34:8.

Suggested Readings

Massengale JD. The unprepared discipline: selection of alternative futures. Quest 1988; 40:107–114.
Shea CH, Wright DL. An introduction to human movement: the sciences of physical education. Boston: Allyn & Bacon, 1997.

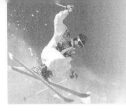

APPENDIX A: EXERCISE SCIENCE JOURNALS

JOURNAL TITLE/INTERNET ADDRESS	PRIMARY FOCUS
ACSM's Health & Fitness Journal www.health-fitjrnl.com/	Health and fitness
Acta Physiologica Scandinavica www.blackwell-science.com/~cgilib/jnlpage.bin?Journal =APS&File=APS&Page=aims	Exercise physiology
American Journal of Health Behavior 131.230.221.136/ajhb/	Health
American Journal of Health Promotion www.healthpromotionjournal.com/publications/ journal.htm	Health
American Journal of Sports Medicine www.sportsmed.org/j/j.htm	Athletic training; sports medicine
Applied Ergonomics gort.ucsd.edu/newjour/a/msg02560.html	Biomechanics
Athletic Insight - The Online Journal of Sport Psychology	Sports psychology
Aviation, Space, and Environmental Medicine www.dciem.dnd.ca/ASEM/	Exercise physiology
British Journal of Sports Medicine www.hbz-nrw.de/elsevier/03063674/	Athletic training; sports medicine
Canadian Journal of Applied Physiology www.humankinetics.com/products/journals/ journal.cfm?id=CJAP	Exercise physiology
Clinical Biomechanics www.elsevier.com/inca/publications/store/3/0/3/9/7/ index.htt	Clinical biomechanics
Clinical Exercise Physiology www.humankinetics.com/products/journals/ journal.cfm?id=CEP	Clinical exercise physiology
Clinical Journal of Sports Medicine www.lww.com/cgi-bin/wwonline.storefront/286276921/ Product/View/1050-642X	Athletic training; sports medicine
Clinics in Sports Medicine 167.208.232.26/catalog/wbs-prod.pl?0278-5919	Athletic training; sports medicine
Ergonomics www.taylorandfrancis.com/JNLS/erg.htm	Biomechanics
European Journal of Applied Physiology link.springer.de/link/service/journals/00421/	Exercise physiology
Exercise Immunology Review www.humankinetics.com/products/journals/ journal.cfm?id=EIR	Clinical exercise physiology
Exercise and Sport Sciences Reviews www.lww.com/cgi-bin/wwonline.storefront/885249558/ Product/View/0091-6331	Exercise science
Gait and Posture www.elsevier.com:80/inca/publications/store/5/2/5/4/4/2/	Clinical biomechanics

JOURNAL TITLE/INTERNET ADDRESS	PRIMARY FOCUS
Human Movement Science www.elsevier.nl:80/inca/publications/store/5/0/5/5/8/4/	Motor behavior
Human Performance www.erlbaum.com/Journals/journals/HP/hp.htm	Exercise science
International Journal of Epidemiology ije.oupujournals.org/	Health; epidemiology
International Journal of the History of Sport www.frankcass.com/jnls/ihs.htm	Sports history
International Journal of Sports Medicine www.thieme.com/onGJIJIAFFEHEGM/display/762	Exercise physiology
International Journal of Sports Nutrition www.humankinetics.com/products/journals/ journal.cfm?id=IJSN	Sports nutrition
International Review for the Sociology of Sport www.sagepub.com/Shopping/Journal.asp?id=4579	Sports sociology
International Sports Journal scolar.vsc.edu:8005/VSCCAT/ACP-9227	Exercise science
Isokinetics and Exercise Science athene.hbz-nrw.de/elsevier/09593020/	Clinical biomechanics
Journal of Aging and Physical Activity www.humankinetics.com/products/journals/journal.cfm? id=JAPA	Exercise physiology
Journal of Applied Biomechanics www.humankinetics.com/products/journals/ journal.cfm?i=JAB	Sports biomechanics
Journal of Applied Physiology jap.physiology.org/	Exercise physiology
Journal of Applied Sport Psychology www.aaasponline.org/journal.html	Sports psychology
Journal of Athletic Training users.media5000.net/jat/	Athletic training
Journal of Biomechanics www.elsevier.com/inca/publications/store/3/2/1/index.htt	Biomechanics
Journal of Cardiopulmonary Rehabilitation www.lww.com/cgi-bin/wwonline.storefront/1269793696/ Product/View/0883-9212	Clinical exercise physiology
Journal of Electromyography & Kinesiology www.elsevier.com/inca/publications/store/3/0/4/4/2/ index.htt	Clinical biomechanics
Journal of Exercise Physiology www.css.edu/users/tboone2/asep/fldr/fldr.htm	Exercise physiology
Journal of Motor Behavior www.heldref.org/html/body_jmb.html	Motor behavior
The Journal of Performance Enhancement: Practical Exercise Science members.tripod.com/JPE_Sportscience/	Sports fitness
Journal of the Philosophy of Sport www.humankinetics.com/products/journals/ journal.cfm?id=JPS	Sports philosophy
Journal of Science and Medicine in Sports www.humankinetics.com/products/journals/ journal.cfm?id=JSMS	Exercise science

JOURNAL TITLE/INTERNET ADDRESS	PRIMARY FOCUS
Journal of Sport and Exercise Psychology www.humankinetics.com/products/journals/ journal.cfm?id=JSEP	Sports and exercise psychology
Journal of Sport History www.aafla.org/SportsLibrary/JSH.htm	Sports history
Journal of Sport Management www.humankinetics.com/products/journals/ journal.cfm?id=JSM	Sports management
Journal of Sport Rehabilitation www.humankinetics.com/products/journals/ journal.cfm?id=JSR	Athletic training/sports medicine
Journal of Sport and Social Issues www.sagepub.com/Shopping/Journal.asp?id=4711	Sports sociology
Journal of Sports Sciences www.tandf.co.uk/journals/routledge/02640414.html	Exercise physiology
Journal of Strength and Conditioning Research www.nsca-lift.org/publications.htm	Exercise physiology
Measurement in Physical Education and Exercise Science www.erlbaum.com/Journals/journals/MPEE/mpee.htm	Exercise science
Medicine and Science in Sports and Exercise www.lww.com/cgi-bin/wwonline.storefront/509708572/ Product/View/0195-9131	Exercise physiology
Medicine and Sport Science www.biomednet.com/library/mss	Exercise physiology
Motor Control www.humankinetics.com/products/journals/ journal.cfm?id=MC	Motor behavior
Pediatric Exercise Science www.humankinetics.com/products/journals/ journal.cfm?id=PES	Exercise physiology
Physician and Sportsmedicine www.physsportsmed.com/	Health and fitness
Research Quarterly for Exercise and Sport www.aahperd.org/aahperd/publications-rqes.html	Exercise science
Science and Sports www.elsevier.com:80/inca/publications/store/5/0/5/8/2/2/	Exercise physiology
Sociology of Sport Journal playlab.uconn.edu/ssjedit.htm	Sports sociology
The Sport Journal sportsmedicine.miningco.com/health/sportsmedicine/gi/ dynamic/offsite.htm?site=www.thesportjournal.org/	Exercise science
The Sport Psychologist www.humankinetics.com/products/journals/ journal.cfm?id=TSP	Sports psychology
Sport History Review www.humankinetics.com/products/journals/ journal.cfm?id=SHR	Sports history
Sports Marketing Quarterly www.fitinfotech.com/smq/smqpage.html	Sports marketing
Sports Medicine www.adis.com/	Exercise physiology

JOURNAL TITLE/INTERNET ADDRESS	PRIMARY FOCUS
Sports Medicine, Training, and Rehabilitation www.gbhap-us.com/journals/353/index.htm	Exercise physiology
Strength and Conditioning Journal www.nsca-lift.org/publications.htm	Sports fitness

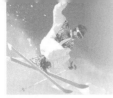

APPENDIX B: REVIEW QUESTIONS WITH ANSWERS

CHAPTER 1: THE EMERGENCE OF EXERCISE SCIENCE

1. List the subdisciplines of exercise science.

    Answer: Exercise physiology, sports nutrition, physical activity epidemiology, clinical exercise physiology, sports biomechanics, clinical biomechanics, athletic training, exercise and sports psychology, motor behavior, sports history, and sports sociology.

2. What are the major areas of motor behavior? What is the major focus of each?

    Answer: Motor control (neurophysiologic), motor development (maturational changes across the life span), and motor learning (processes in acquiring motor skills).

3. What events precipitated the reforms that led to specializations in graduate physical education programs?

    Answer: Conant's suggestion that graduate physical education programs should be eliminated caused the profession to undergo self-examination. Henry and other physical education leaders responded to this challenge by changing graduate curricula from sports and games to a more scientifically oriented focus.

4. Describe how individuals outside of physical education played such an important part in establishing the foundation on which the exercise sciences would later be developed.

    Answer: The first people who applied science to movement and sports were scientists and engineers who happened to be interested in exercise and how their particular specialty might contribute to understanding or improving performance. Physiologists, physicists, psychologists, engineers, chemists, and a host of others carried out the earliest studies that laid the strong foundation used by physical educators in more recent times.

5. How did World Wars I and II affect the exercise sciences?

    Answer: These wars unveiled a general lack of physical fitness in recruits and were responsible for a general focus on the need for attention to components of fitness in school physical education programs. The Harvard Fatigue Laboratory was the site of much research on nutrition, fitness, and training. Psychologists were actively involved in working on the problems of motor learning related to pilot training; and engineers concentrated on problems related to ergonomics, a field that was later examined by biomechanists.

6. Give a hypothetical example of an interdisciplinary approach to a research problem.

    Answer: [Example; answers will vary.] Suppose we wish to determine the effects of proper and improper weightlifting techniques on subsequent motor performance. A specialist in biomechanics would determine the two procedures to use in lifting; an exercise physiologist might quantify performance in terms of volume of work, lactic acid production, heart rate, and blood pressure; and a motor behavior specialist would contribute by selecting or designing the motor performance criteria to be used.

7. List six individuals who have been important to exercise science in a historical sense, giving a very brief description of the contribution of each.

    Answer: [Example; answers will vary.] (a) Bruce Dill directed the prestigious Harvard Fatigue Laboratory; (b) T. K. Cureton directed an excellent graduate program, taught, and published research in fitness and kinesiology at the University of Illinois; (c) Franklin Henry was a leader in physical education reform that resulted in graduate specialization and published the important memory drum paper; (d) Steve Horvath headed the Institute of Environmental Stress in Santa

Barbara and was a prolific scholar in aging and environmental research; *(e)* Robert Singer wrote a landmark text on motor learning; *(f)* Per-Olof Åstrand is representative of the many individuals from other countries who contributed much of the early research literature in exercise physiology; *(g)* John Basmajian's use of electromyography in the study of anatomical kinesiology.

8. What is the relationship between exercise science, its subdisciplines, and the body of knowledge?

Answer: Exercise science is the academic discipline that is composed of several distinct subdisciplines. Through scientific inquiry within the domain of particular subdisciplines, movement (the body of knowledge of exercise science) is further described and explained from the unique perspectives of the various subdisciplines.

9. How are physical education and exercise science related?

Answer: Exercise science emerged out of physical education and is a separate discipline. The two are related in that each has movement as their body of knowledge. Exercise science seeks to expand our knowledge of movement by conducting research within the subdisciplines. The goal of physical education is pedagogical, teaching about movement, and doing related research.

CHAPTER 2: EXERCISE AND SOCIETY

1. What are some differences between modern and postmodern exercise? Identify some additional differences that are not discussed in this chapter. Provide some critical analysis of the differences between modern and postmodern exercise.

Answer: [Example; answers will vary.] Modern exercise took canonical form, such as football, basketball, track, hockey, and baseball. Modern exercise was often blatantly sexist and racist, such as in the segregation of Major League Baseball. There was a means to an end, and the definition of *exercise* was not vague. Professional athletes in modernity were rarely superstar celebrities; the heroes of modernity were often statesmen, soldiers, and writers. In postmodernity, athletes implode into virtually all segments of society and celebrity culture; superstar athletes like Michael Jordan are identified as heroes and role models. In postmodern exercise, there are often different means and ends and a seemingly infinite selection of exercise. The term *exercise* is vague and all-encompassing in postmodernity. Ironic and performative sports, such as American Gladiators, Sumo diving, and dwarf bowling appear in postmodernity, as do extreme/x sports and alternative sports. The human body was natural and performed in real time in modern exercise; in postmodern exercise, the body takes on cyborg form in the use of exercise machines, microsurgery, specialized clothing, technology, and virtual performance. Sports are transnational and driven by the market economy. Super slow motion and other technologic innovations are used to screen exercise. The medical profession is highly involved in all aspects of postmodern exercise for a large proportion of the population. In modernity, only specialized athletes consulted the medical profession. There is a phenomenal growth of female, disabled, and senior participants in postmodern exercise. The couture of exercise influences all aspects of society in postmodernity.

2. Identify a binary that is associated with the broad understanding of exercise. Be creative and discuss which part of the binary is subtly considered to be deviant and, if applicable, point out how a part or parts of the binary are made the subject of social policy or how it has been subordinated by society's values about that particular binary.

Answer: [Example; answers will vary.] Fast versus slow runners: Slow is considered deviant; fast runners stand out as athletes and make the team. Slow runners are mediocre athletes and get cut from the team. Fast runners are made part of public policy when they are identified and given special coaching, training, and performance enhancers. Slow runners are subordinated by society's values when they are ignored in advertising and in contests.

3. What are some of the sociologic reasons forwarded by scholars for why people feel nostalgic and are obsessed with collecting exercise-related things?

Answer: *(a)* In postmodernity, people are alienated from family and close friends because everything is moving so fast. They gather an artificially constructed community around them in the form of things such as baseball cards or closely following their favorite team. *(b)* People want closure, because it assures them that they are powerful and that they will have a sort of immortality. The collection provides the collector with safety and control. It concretely memorializes the collector's interests and joy. *(c)* Exercise-related memorabilia highlights the very best of human performance; it makes collectors feel good to be close to this perfection. Such memorabilia showcases what humans are capable of. It provides a dramatic story of winning and losing, surprising endings, and a cast of fascinating and unique players. *(d)* In collecting, the person, instead of merely watching, makes history and participates in the making of history. *(e)* If economic capital is lacking, collections provide cultural capital.

4. Why do some scholars say that exercise is the foundation of civilization?

Answer: Based on the long history of humanity, it seems that exercise is universal to all times and places of human community. Through exercise, language and the great institutions of humankind are built.

5. What are some of the main ideas of cultural studies? Give specific exercise-related examples.

Answer: (a) Conjunctural analysis: Untangle the complex origin of the Olympic flame ceremony. *(b)* Hegemony studies: Focus on studying the history of the women's marathon or how sexism excluded female participation for many years. *(c)* Political action: While studying the subcultures of inner-city basketball, one might also launch a campaign to eliminate billboards in the vicinity that further racist beliefs about athletic success and poverty.

6. Characterize some styles of postmodernity. Provide examples from exercise and sports screened specifically on television, film, video, and video gaming, articulating how these exemplify particular postmodern style.

Answer: Kitsch, hyper-reality, pastiche, imperialist nostalgia, super slow motion, and holography.

CHAPTER 3: PROFESSIONAL ORGANIZATIONS

1. List the eight leading exercise science professional organizations.

Answer: American College of Sports Medicine, American Association of Cardiovascular and Pulmonary Rehabilitation, American Society of Biomechanics, National Athletic Training Association, National Strength and Conditioning Association, North American Society for the Psychology of Sport and Physical Activity, North American Society for Sport History, and North American Society for Sport Sociology.

2. Briefly explain why membership in a professional organization is important for professional growth.

Answer: It brings a sense of belonging as well as other more concrete rewards. Examples of these are opportunities for participation in meetings, voting rights, publications, and networking opportunities.

3. List two organizations with and two without a scholarly mission.

Answer: (a) With: American Alliance for Health, Physical Education, Recreation and Dance and the National Strength and Conditioning Association. *(b)* Without: American Council on Exercise and Aquatic Exercise Association

CHAPTER 4: EXERCISE SCIENCE AND FITNESS CERTIFICATIONS

1. What is professional certification?

Answer: The process by which an individual, institution, or educational program is evaluated and recognized as meeting certain predetermined standards through successful completion of a validated, reliable examination.

2. What is the typical process of becoming certified?

Answer: The acquisition of a core of knowledge and skills through formal educational and/or professional experience; completion of an application form and submission of candidacy credentials (e.g., letters of recommendation and documentation of professional experience or degrees); review of prerequisite knowledge and skills through the use of study guides, review courses, and/or workshops; selection of an examination date and site; and passing the certification examination.

3. What are the purpose and rationale for becoming certified?

Answer: To ensure within a profession or service that standards are being maintained to guarantee safe and ethical practice. It indicates that the person has mastered the expertise, advanced knowledge, skills, and/or proficiency necessary to practice in a particular area of specialty identified by the administering organization.

4. What are the major professional groups that provide certification for exercise science professionals?

Answer: American College of Sports Medicine, National Strength and Conditioning Association, National Athletic Trainers' Association, Board of Certification in Professional Ergonomics, Young Men's Christian Association, American Council on Exercise, Aerobics and Fitness Association of America, and Association for the Advancement of Applied Sport Psychology

5. What are the recommended certifications for aerobic dance and exercise leadership, personal training and health fitness instruction, strength and conditioning, directing health fitness and wellness programs, sports medicine, exercise testing, special population rehabilitation, kinesiology and biomechanics, and sports psychology?

Answer: See Table 4.2.

6. Describe some of the benefits of certification.

Better job opportunities, credibility, an expanded level of competence and qualifications, self-confidence, and greater income.

CHAPTER 5: JOB ACTIVITIES AND EMPLOYMENT

1. Describe the expanding role of the exercise science professional.

Answer: The exercise science graduate plays a key role in assessing, interpreting, prescribing, and designing health and physical activity programs for a variety of levels of health status and in a number of settings, including schools, community health agencies, fitness clubs, work sites, and medical settings.

2. Name and describe four evolving employment areas of growth in the field of exercise science.

Answer: (a) Health and fitness: delivery systems that encompass the fitness industry, corporate wellness, wellness programs, spa fitness, and personal training. *(b)* Health rehabilitation: an alliance of specialists working with people who have unique needs or are at high health risks. Special intervention training is required for individuals who have neurologic, orthopedic, muscular, and cardiorespiratory deficiencies. *(c)* Teaching and higher education: encompass teaching and/or conducting research; opportunity to teach health and physical activity courses at a variety of educational levels. Most of these opportunities require a master's degree in the field. Advanced expertise usually leads to employment at universities, colleges, national institutes, hospitals, and medical research centers. *(d)* Fitness specialties: a multitude of nontraditional opportunities. Because the training of professionals is quite diverse, a number of specialty tracks are open for careers, some of which may entail additional education or training.

3. Identify and describe the different career paths that may be pursued in the health and fitness domain.

Answer: (a) Fitness industry: fitness club owner or manager, fitness director, aerobics director, special programs director, teacher, exercise physiologist, and personal trainer. *(b)* Corporate wellness: addresses the needs of the constituents in the corporate setting. The goals of these programs are to positively influence the development of good health practices and supportive environments. *(c)* Wellness programs: work in a variety of settings including schools, medical sites, YMCAs, YWCAs, YMHAs, Boys and Girls Clubs, community centers (religious and nonaligned) and communities. Employment opportunities can also be found in colleges, long-term care facilities, recreation departments, aquatic centers, health management systems, and lifestyle management organizations. *(d)* Residential spas: fitness director, health and fitness instructor, and personal trainer. Spa programs are quite diverse with interest areas in many aspects of mental and physical well-being. *(e)* Personal training: helping people improve the quality of their lives through a personalized approach to exercise participation; must be able to promote, market, and sell ones services as well as learn business skills.

4. Explain where the exercise science professional may work within the area of health rehabilitation.

Answer: Occupational therapy, physical therapy, clinical exercise physiology, dietetics, and athletic training. These positions will require further academic preparation and credentials beyond the undergraduate degree in exercise science.

CHAPTER 6: MANAGEMENT AND MARKETING CONCERNS

1. What are some of the roles of the manager?

Answer: Planner, organizer, leader, controller, and implementer.

2. Explain the program development cycle.

Answer: It begins with an understanding of the purpose, or mission, of the organization. Once the mission is understood, needs are assessed to address any weaknesses. Once the needs have been identified, goals and objectives that are designed to correct any weaknesses are established. Plans must then be developed to effectively and efficiently meet the goals and objectives. The plans must be implemented, and the program must be evaluated.

3. What is leadership?

Answer: There are many definitions; but it is safe to say that it is a process that involves influencing others to facilitate the achievement of personal and organizational goals.

4. What are the differences among the autocratic, democratic, and laissez-faire leadership styles? Which is the best style?

Answer: (a) Autocratic leaders: believe in a strict chain of command; generally do not elicit much input before making decisions; expect that their wishes (orders) will be promptly carried out. *(b)* Democratic leaders: usually elected or chosen by the group; often elicit some input from the individual group members, but ultimately make the final decisions by themselves. *(c)* Laissez-faire leaders: tend to guide the group; elicit group input; group consensus is sought whenever possible; characterized by group decision making; communication is wide open, with little regard for any chain of command.

There really is no best style. The situation dictates which style is most effective. When decisions must be made rapidly, autocratic leadership is best. When the decision does not need to be made right away, the laissez-faire approach is more creative and involves a greater knowledge pool. Thus assembling a group of experts to generate a consensus-type decision is desirable. Most situations do not require immediate decision making but are restricted by some time frame. Thus the democratic, or participatory, style is usually employed.

5. What are the essential differences among the great man theory of leadership; the contingency model theory of leadership; the path–goal theory of leadership; and the life cycle theory of leadership?

Answer: (a) Great man theory: focuses on the individual leader, fails to consider the characteristics of the follower, fails to consider situational variables. *(b)* Contingency model: recognizes the importance of leader characteristics, recognizes the importance of the leader–follower relationship, recognizes some situational variables (e.g., the nature of the task), fails to recognize the need to evolve as the followers mature. *(c)* Path–goal theory: implies that the role of the leader may be to work for the follower, the leader helps the follower achieve goals by keeping the path to the goal clear of obstacles. *(d)* Life cycle theory: recognizes that leader characteristics are important, recognizes that the maturity level of the follower is important, recognizes that the style of the leader must evolve as the follower matures.

6. What is risk management?

   Answer: Involves the planned and organized techniques used to provide a systematic reduction of the probability that one will be successfully sued for negligence.

7. What is negligence?

   Answer: A tort that involves the breach of legal duty, which is determined to be the direct cause of an actual injury. Managers, leaders, and coaches are expected to act reasonably and prudently when dealing with clients and players.

8. Describe the search and experience qualities customers may associate with a fitness center or club. When do customers assess each of these qualities?

   Answer: (a) Search qualities: aspects of the service that can be examined before using the service: promotional materials (pamphlets, fliers, TV ads), price lists for various memberships or programs, and exterior facility appearance (and whatever else customers can observe before buying). *(b)* Experience qualities: aspects of the service or event that can be evaluated only after the experience is over: the way the workers and facility made customers feel (excited, relaxed, distressed), evaluation of the service quality provided by employees, evaluation of the quality of the equipment used, and evaluation of whether the price paid for membership is worth what the customers get in return.

9. Why is sports marketing different from many other types of product and service marketing?

   Answer: The uncontrollable nature of the primary service offering makes it more difficult than other businesses. The myriad circumstances that can influence individual or team performance makes it difficult to promise fans that the team or individual will win. The primary service is made up of individuals (players) who are inconsistent and difficult to predict.

10. Outline a marketing strategy for a local sports team or fitness center, including explanations of each of the five components of a marketing strategy.

    Answer: [Answers will vary.] Your answer should include a thorough description of the target market(s), the product or service offering (primary and secondary services), promotion (image presented), pricing (relative perceived value), and distribution (facility, TV contracts).

11. If you were managing a snow skiing resort, how would you price lodging and lift tickets according to demand fluctuations? When would be a good time to maintain or even increase prices? Cut prices?

    Answer: [Example, answers will vary.] Ski resorts experience demand fluctuations on a daily, weekly, monthly, and seasonal basis. Prices can be adjusted accordingly to maximize revenue: daily (daily passes vs. after 5 p.m. passes), weekly (Monday to Thursday rates vs. weekend rates), monthly (specials for weeks not close to paycheck days), and seasonal (increased Christmas rates; lower January rates). Ski resorts will also have to schedule enough personnel to deal with the fluctuating demand.

12. Using Figure 6.3, rate a local fitness center or sporting event or stadium. What changes would you make to serve customers better?

    Answer: [Answers will vary.]

CHAPTER 7: PROFESSIONAL ISSUES

1. What six criteria does Flexner include as characteristics of the professions?

Answer: Essentially intellectual operation, continual flow of new knowledge, activities of a practical nature, representative professional organization, communication, and altruism.

2. What five characteristics do Purtillo and Cassel list as important for health professions?

Answer: Self-governed autonomy, social value, specialized knowledge, representative organization, and lifetime commitment.

3. What is role delineation?

Answer: The process of defining the specific responsibilities of the professional within the context of a job description written relative to the responsibilities of others with whom the professional is working. For the student of exercise science, the role is usually dictated by the local organizational structure and responsibilities of others who may be licensed.

4. What is encroachment?

Answer: Occurs when one member of the healthcare delivery team performs the skills and techniques of another healthcare provider.

5. What is the difference between certification and licensure?

Answer: (a) License: provided by state law; usually preceded by a standard of practice and a specific description of the responsibilities of that professional within the context of the responsibilities of others who may also have a license to practice. *(b)* Certification: awarded to a professional, usually by a nationally recognized organization, after the completion of an examination. Although a certification examination can be used as a licensing examination, only the state can award a license to practice.

6. Which state is currently the only one to offer a license for clinical exercise physiology?

Answer: Louisiana (since 1996).

CHAPTER 8: EXERCISE PHYSIOLOGY

1. Define exercise physiology.

Answer: The study of how our bodies' structures and functions are altered when we are exposed to acute and chronic bouts of exercise.

2. List five activities each that can be classified as power, speed, and endurance activities.

Answer: [Example; answers will vary.] *(a)* Power: kicking a football, pole vault, weightlifting, 40-yd sprint, shot-put. *(b)* Speed: 200-m sprint, 100-m swimming sprint, body building, 400-m sprint, speed skating. *(c)* Endurance: marathon run, triathlon, 5- to 10-K run, ice hockey, 400-m swim.

3. Using the activities listed in question 2, identify the predominate metabolic pathway.

Answer: (a) Power: phosphagen system. *(b)* Speed: lactic acid system. *(c)* Endurance: aerobic system.

4. Explain the differences between acute and chronic exercise.

Answer: (a) Acute: an individual bout of exercise; exercise physiologists study the body's responses during exercise. *(b)* Chronic: repeated bouts of exercise; exercise physiologists study the body's adaptations (changes) as a result of exercise training.

5. Describe how the body uses energy to produce movement. What is the relationship between muscle contraction and energy production?

   Answer: Muscles need energy to contract. This energy comes in the form of ATP, which is made in the cell (including muscle cells) as energy nutrients are catabolized in metabolic processes. Depending on the type of exercise, ATP is made from carbohydrates, fat stores, or both.

6. Explain how the cardiorespiratory system is coordinated with energy production.

   Answer: These processes require a steady supply of oxygen to make ATP. At the beginning of aerobic exercise, there is an initial imbalance between the demand the working muscles have for oxygen to support their heightened metabolic activity and the ability of the cardiorespiratory system to supply oxygen. This initial imbalance occurs because heart rate and cardiac output take a while to increase at the start of exercise. After 3 to 5 min of aerobic exercise, supply and demand are equalized. At this point a steady state is said to exist, which lasts for as long as the exercise continues.

7. Explain the importance of thermoregulation during exercise.

   Answer: During aerobic exercise a tremendous amount of heat is generated. This heat must be released so that the core temperature does not increase too much. The thermoregulatory system does this primarily via the evaporation of sweat off the skin. Without the thermoregulatory system, death would ensue owing to excessive heat buildup.

CHAPTER 9: SPORTS NUTRITION

1. What is the main focus of the field of sports nutrition (and hence, a sports nutritionist)?

   Answer: How nutrition affects exercise performance at all levels (novice to elite athlete), how nutrition affects physical performance (e.g., in individuals who have jobs that require a great deal of physical exertion), and the effects (including dangers) of ergogenic aids on nutrition and physical performance.

2. Why are carbohydrates important?

   Answer: They provide blood glucose, which is necessary for the brain and central nervous system; they maintain muscle glycogen stores, which are important for exercise and activities of daily living.

3. List five complex carbohydrates.

   Answer: [Example; answers will vary.] Barley, whole wheat pancakes, pasta, baked potato, cereal.

4. Why should a person limit his or her saturated fat intake?

   Answer: Saturated fats increase low-density lipoprotein cholesterol levels in the blood, which increase the risk of coronary heart disease.

5. Do athletes need a higher percentage of fat in their diets than do nonathletes?

   Answer: Although some research has been done in this area, athletes do not need more fat in their diets than nonathletes. It is recommended that 30% of the total caloric intake be from fat.

6. How much protein do endurance athletes and strength athletes need, respectively?

   Answer: (a) Endurance: 1.0 to 1.4 g/kg/day. *(b)* Strength (e.g., body builders): 1.1 to 1.7 g/kg/day.

7. What are some of the roles of minerals in exercise?

   Answer: Working in combination with enzymes in the body, becoming part of the organizational matrix of cells, speeding up reactions in the body, and being part of the antioxidant system of the body; may also act directly in many of the reactions involved in energy metabolism, such as glucose, lipid, and protein metabolism.

8. List the water-soluble and fat-soluble vitamins.

Answer: (a) Water-soluble vitamins: B_6, B_{12}, folate, thiamin, riboflavin, niacin, pantothenic acid, biotin, C, and choline. *(b)* Fat-soluble vitamins: A, D, E, and K.

9. What are some signs of dehydration?

Answer: Impaired muscular endurance, impaired aerobic exercise performance, and decreased mental functioning.

10. What is a safe amount of body weight to lose per week if a person is trying to lose weight?

Answer: Between 1 and 2 lb; this regimen results in little muscle tissue and water loss.

11. What are the effects of caffeine on endurance performance?

Answer: It spares muscle glycogen by increasing free fatty acids into the blood for use as energy.

12. Will chromium picolinate increase muscle mass?

Answer: Most studies have shown that it has no effect on muscle mass or weight loss.

CHAPTER 10: PHYSICAL ACTIVITY EPIDEMIOLOGY

1. Why are physical activity surveys a popular measure of physical activity?

Answer: Because of their nonreactiveness, practicality, applicability, and accepted accuracy.

2. What objective measures of physical activity are used in epidemiologic studies?

Answer: The doubly labeled water technique, respiratory chamber, activity monitors, pedometers, heart rate monitors, graded exercise tests, field tests, and observation.

3. What are the two major types of study designs used in epidemiologic studies?

Answer: Observational and experimental.

4. What are the three major types of observational studies?

Answer: Cross-sectional, case-control, and prospective (or longitudinal).

CHAPTER 11: CLINICAL EXERCISE PHYSIOLOGY

1. What role does a clinical exercise physiologist play in healthcare?

Answer: He or she uses fundamental principles of exercise physiology in clinical settings to minimize the risk of chronic diseases associated with physical inactivity and to treat those already afflicted.

2. List three unique contributions of the clinical exercise physiologist in healthcare.

Answer: The ability to use exercise as a means of evaluating functional capacity and assisting physicians in diagnostic testing; the expertise to prescribe exercise based on individual patient needs and abilities; and the skills to instruct, supervise, and monitor exercise programs in clinical settings.

3. How does a diagnostic exercise test differ from a functional exercise test?

Answer: (a) Diagnostic: performed to uncover underlying disease. *(b)* Functional: performed to determine aerobic exercise capacity.

4. What physiologic measurements are taken during an exercise test?

Answer: Resting and exercise electrocardiogram, blood pressure, heart rate, rating of perceived exertion, and oxygen consumption.

5. What chronic diseases and conditions are commonly treated by clinical exercise physiologists?

Answer: Cardiovascular, pulmonary, metabolic, rheumatologic, orthopedic, and neuromuscular.

6. Give two examples of how basic research may be applied in a clinical setting.

Answer: [Example; answers will vary.] The discovery of immunosuppressant drugs has helped overcome critical problems associated with rejection of donor hearts, and 1-year survival rates for heart transplantation are now greater than 80%. The recent isolation of the *ob* gene in mice has given greater insight into the pathophysiology of human obesity and may someday be used to help with weight control.

CHAPTER 12: CLINICAL BIOMECHANICS

1. Explain the effects of a muscle that pulls perpendicular to the bone to which it is attached compared to a muscle that pulls more parallel to the bone.

Answer: (a) Muscle that pulls perpendicular to the bone: provides the greatest rotatory component; is the most efficient angle of muscle pull. *(b)* Muscle that pulls parallel to the bone: has a very small rotatory component; the angle provides more compression or distraction to the joint.

2. Explain the effect of a load applied to the limb when the limb is positioned at 0°, 30,° 45°, 60,° and 90° to the horizontal.

Answer: When the limb is horizontal (0°), the load from gravity is 100%. As the limb moves from the horizontal position, the rotatory component of the gravitational load decreases by the cosine of the angle. At 90°, the gravitational moment is 0.

3. How does the resultant change as the angle between two concurrent forces decreases?

Answer: As the angle between two concurrent forces decreases, the resultant increases. As the angle between two concurrent forces increases, the resultant force decreases.

4. What type of lever is the most common in the human body? What are the advantages and disadvantages of this anatomic arrangement?

Answer: Third-class lever. *(a)* Advantages: provides longer excursions of the distal end of the limb, allows greater speed of the distal end of the limb, allows for a hand or foot to be at the distal end of the limb. *(b)* Disadvantage: more effort force (E) is needed to hold or move a resistance.

5. Discuss the importance of Wolff's law and how an exercise professional can use this law.

Answer: Body tissues respond to the loads placed on them. Generally, too much load or too little load can retard growth of connective tissue. Within limits, increased loading of the tissues will increase the size and strength of the tissues. Little or no load will cause the tissues to atrophy and become weaker.

CHAPTER 13: SPORTS BIOMECHANICS

1. Define sports biomechanics.

Answer: The application of the principles of biomechanics to activities including sports, exercise, and recreational activities. Biomechanics is the study of human motion; it uses applied anatomy and mechanical physics to assess techniques employed by the individual. Sports biomechanics concerns itself with the in-depth study of the forces and motions associated with sporting techniques, including the roles of the musculoskeletal and neuromuscular systems; its emphasis is to improve an athlete's performance while minimizing the potential for injury.

2. Discuss the biomechanical concepts and variables of kinematics and kinetics.

Answer: (a) Kinematics: the study of the temporal and spatial aspects of motion in which displacement, velocity, and acceleration of an object or body are quantified. (b) Linear kinematics: the point to point motions of an object as measured within the quadrants of a Cartesian coordinate system. (c) Angular kinematics: the rotation of a lever around an axis as measured within a polar coordinate system. (d) Kinetics: the study of forces and torques that create the kinematics of a body. When a force is applied to a body it will, if sufficient in magnitude to overcome the body's inertia, cause the body to increase or decrease linear and/or angular velocity. To change the body's angular velocity, the force must be applied at a distance from the body's or body lever's axis of rotation (lever arm) so that a torque is generated. The greater the magnitude of the applied force or torque and the longer the force or torque is applied, the greater the change in linear and/or angular velocity of the body or body segment.

3. List several sports activities for each of the following variables. In each case, the variable is the most important biomechanical principle for the production of a successful performance.

Answer: (a) Horizontal velocity of the body: running sprints, swimming sprints, speed skating, downhill skiing. (b) Vertical velocity of the body: high jump, standing vertical jump, jumps in basketball (shooting and rebounding), jump to spike in volleyball, pole vaulting, platform and springboard diving. (c) Horizontal velocity of an object: baseball pitch, softball fast pitch, football pass, team handball goal throw. (d) Resultant velocity (combination of horizontal and vertical) of a body or object when angle of takeoff is important: running long jump, triple jump, outfield throw in baseball or softball, basketball shot, javelin throw, shot-put, discus throw, hammer throw, gymnastics tumbling. (e) Horizontal force application involving an impact: baseball and softball batting, tennis strokes, golf shots, hockey, soccer kick, football blocks and tackles, volleyball spike.

4. For the following activities indicate which form of kinetic link is used in performing the skill and briefly discuss why.

Answer: (a) Golf swing: movements occur in a sequential fashion. In the downswing, as the club is accelerated toward the ball, the lower body works first, followed by the hips, upper trunk, arms and wrists. (b) Standing vertical jump: movements occur simultaneously. Because the jumper is moving a large mass, it is important that the major muscles of the body work at the same time to overcome the body's large inertia and cause a sufficient vertical acceleration to enable a jump to occur. The greater the rate of acceleration and the longer the force is applied, the higher the jump. (c) Javelin throw: movements occur in a sequential fashion. Toward the end of the running throw, the athlete generates motions in the lower body that are transferred through the hips to the trunk to the shoulder to the elbow and, finally, to the wrist near the point of release. This sequence leads to a high-end velocity of the hand/javelin at the release point. (d) Free throw (arm actions): low-velocity sequential activity in which control is of great importance. After the contribution of the legs, the velocity in the shooting arm flows from the shoulder, to the elbow, to the wrist, with release occurring as the fingers make their contribution to the ball's velocity and angle of release. (e) Overhead (military) press (arm actions): simultaneous kinetic link activity, because the major muscles involved around the shoulder and elbow fire concentrically. If the magnitude of the forces are sufficient to overcome the inertia of the barbell, the lifter may then generate the vertical momentum necessary to complete the exercise.

CHAPTER 14: ATHLETIC TRAINING

1. Define athletic training.

Answer: The allied health profession that deals with the prevention, recognition, and care of injuries to physically active individuals.

2. List each domain of athletic training and identify the principal activities associated with that domain.

Answer: (a) Prevention: conducting preparticipation physical examinations; running physical conditioning programs; educating athletes, coaches, and parents; establishing safe practice and competition sites; and minimizing environmental risks. *(b)* Recognition, evaluation, and immediate care: systematically evaluating injuries, which includes a primary survey (life-threatening situations) and a secondary survey (history, observation, palpation, and special testing to establish the nature and extent of the injury); initiating emergency care and referral to other medical professionals. *(c)* Rehabilitation and reconditioning: using therapeutic modalities and exercise (isokinetic, isotonic, and isometric) to restore normal function, range of motion, and strength; scheduling the progression to return to play. *(d)* Healthcare administration: managing personnel and the facility and its design; budgeting; keeping medical records; dealing with insurance, public relations, and control of legal exposure. *(e)* Professional development and responsibility: remaining current in the profession, mentoring and educating student athletic trainers.

3. In what settings are athletic trainers employed?

Answer: Sports medicine clinics, educational institutions, and industry.

4. Explain the difference between a sign and a symptom.

Answer: (a) Sign: observable, quantifiable piece of data; objective. *(b)* Symptom: something related by the athlete; subjective.

5. Explain the differences between a strain and a sprain.

Answer: (a) Strain: a stretch beyond normal limits of a muscle, tendon, or both. *(b)* Sprain: stretch beyond normal limits of a ligament or joint capsule.

Chapter 15: Exercise and Sports Psychology

1. What are the primary research objectives in the exercise and sports psychology area?

Answer: Determination of the psychological antecedents of participation in sports and physical activity and determination of the psychological consequences of participation in sports and physical activity.

2. What has been the most commonly used measurement strategy in exercise and sports psychology?

Answer: The self-report, which usually involves the use of standardized questionnaires or psychological inventories.

3. *Answer:* What is the primary difference between exercise psychology and sports psychology?

(a) Exercise psychology: concerned with the application of the educational, scientific, and professional contributions of psychology to the promotion, explanation, maintenance, and enhancement of behavior related to physical work capacity. *(b)* Sports psychology: concerned with the educational, scientific, and professional contributions of psychology to the promotion, maintenance, and enhancement of sports-related behavior.

4. Which dispositional theory of personality has been used to study personality in the physical activity domain?

Answer: Eysenck's trait theory, which is composed of the extroversion–introversion, stability–neuroticism, and superego–psychoticism dimensions.

5. How are personality states and traits distinguished?

Answer: (a) Traits: relatively enduring dispositions that exert a consistent influence on behavior in a variety of situations. *(b)* States: psychological reactions to a particular situation that are consistent with the individual's traits.

6. What is meant by the term *self-serving bias?*

   Answer: Winners tend to attribute success to ability or effort; losers tend to attribute failure to situational causes (e.g., "the sun was in my eyes").

7. What are the two most prominent models for studying arousal–performance relationships?

   Answer: Drive theory and the inverted-U hypothesis.

8. What are the ways in which attention can be studied?

   Answer: Behaviorally (via dual-task paradigms and self-reports) and physiologically (responses known to be related to attention).

9. Of the various hypotheses for explaining why exercise might lead to improved mental health, which is focused on brain neurotransmitters?

   Answer: The monoamine hypothesis.

10. Are endorphins responsible for the feel-better phenomenon associated with exercise? Why or why not?

   Answer: Current evidence is inconclusive; data exist that both support and refute this notion.

CHAPTER 16: MOTOR BEHAVIOR

1. Why is the study of movement important?

   Answer: Movement is essential to everything we do, including locomotion, communication, and basic needs like eating and procreating. Understanding motor learning can help us become more efficient learners of both everyday and sports skills. Understanding developmental patterns can help us evaluate our progress. Understanding motor control can help us diagnose problems and make advances in human factors engineering.

2. What are the subcategories of motor behavior?

   Answer: Motor learning, motor control, motor development.

3. Name the areas of study of motor learning.

   Answer: Memory, information processing, practice organization, and learning; the paradox principle encompasses all these areas.

4. Explain three major findings in motor learning and how you can use this information.

   Answer: Appropriate KR is important to learning and depends on the level of the performer and the complexity of the task (paradox principle). Research on memory and information processing tells us that we have a finite ability to process information and, therefore, the organization of information is important. Practice organization should be matched to the learner, which implies that it should change as the learner changes.

5. Explain the major theories of motor control.

   Answer: (a) Locomotion: studies the direct links between perception and action. *(b)* Reaching and grasping: includes writing and drawing, keyboarding, and sign language; studies the integration of vision and other sources of feedback. *(c)* Vision: includes eye movements (blinking, pupil constriction, etc.); studies the eyes' role in balance, the vestibular-ocular reflex, and movement perception. *(d)* Speech production: output is auditory rather than visual or proprioceptive and is usually carried out for purposes of communication (other activities are only occasionally performed with the direct aim of communication); vocal tract and articulary dynamics are important from a physiologic and engineering standpoint; studies speech in relation to hearing (we may recognize speech sounds by recruiting knowledge about how they are produced), speech programming (it may use perceptual representations of likely auditory consequences), co-articulation (planning one movement while considering the next movement), and sentence construction.

6. Name the areas of study of motor development.

Answer: Infancy, childhood, adolescence, adulthood, and older adulthood; each of these areas can be examined from physiologic, cognitive, and social standpoints.

7. Explain three major findings in motor development and how you can use this information.

Answer: [Example; answers will vary.] *(a)* Older adults: cardiovascular function and mental function are affected by activity; in other words, use it or lose it. *(b)* Children: specific stages of development for motor skills exist. *(c)* Adolescence: some sex differences are societal and some are physical.

CHAPTER 17: SPORTS HISTORY

1. How do sports history and the history of sports differ?

Answer: (a) Sports history: an academic subdiscipline concerned with the production of historical accounts of sports and a social science that studies the sporting lives of men, women and children; the origin, growth, and development of sporting institutions; and the political, social, economic, class, ethnic, racial, and sex factors that have influenced sporting outcomes. *(b)* History of sports: accumulative body of knowledge produced by sports historians on the past accounts of exercise practices, leisure and recreational activities, school athletics, physical education activities, and amateur and professional sports.

2. List and briefly explain the factors affecting the growth of women's sports in the United States.

Answer: Women were first introduced to sports by women physical educators in the middle to late nineteenth century, who presented sports as educational activities. The major factors affecting the growth (or lack thereof) of women's sport were public attitudes that viewed sports as masculine and outside the sphere of girls and women. Until relatively recently, it was believed that social interaction and health promotion were the only defensible reasons for women's engagement in sport. Women physical educators introduced sports emphasized that women should not engage in highly competitive interscholastic or intercollegiate sports, that becoming a sports heroine was inappropriate for women, and that their sports participation should be lady-like and moderate. It was only after the passage of Title IX in the 1970s that girls and women were given opportunities to become athletes and enjoy some of the same sporting privileges that boys and men had enjoyed since earliest recorded times.

3. Explain why it is said that men's intercollegiate sports are as much a commercial endeavor as an educational enterprise.

Answer: From the first intercollegiate contest in 1852, money and prestige have played major roles in men's athletics. That first rowing contest was sponsored by a railroad company with the intent of making money. Since then, athletics have been responsible for spending and bringing in more money than almost any other division within colleges and universities. The cost of equipment, facilities, recruitment, travel, scholarships, and other expenses have made athletics at major universities big-time business enterprises. Coaches are paid higher salaries than most, if not all, professors, and usually more than university presidents. Because gate receipts are so important to the success of athletic programs, a business approach is essential to keep programs fiscally solvent.

4. Give examples of how stereotyping, prejudice, and discrimination have played ominous roles in sports history.

Answer: Women, African Americans, and other minorities have suffered at the hands of society in amateur and professional sports. Sports were first perceived as benefiting well-to-do, white, Protestant males more than any other group in America. White males were privileged to engage in sports, and minority groups were often barred from team membership.

5. List and briefly explain the steps for doing historical research.

Answer: Select a topic that is of interest, is worthy of research, and for which resources are available. Frame the study by asking research questions that deal with who, where, what, when, why, and how. Collect data from secondary and primary sources. Check and recheck the data for accuracy. Analyze the data for meaning. Write up the results.

6. Explain how historical research differs from experimental research.

Answer: History is a social science; historical research looks for meaning in descriptive accounts more than in quantitative data, which may be subjected to statistical analysis. Historical data cannot be verified in the same ways as experimental data. Historians cannot claim to be objective or able to produce the truth. Historical research is as much an art as it is a science.

CHAPTER 18: SPORTS SOCIOLOGY

1. Define sports sociology and explain the aspects that are included in this area of study.

Answer: Examines sports as a part of cultural and social life, focusing on the relationship between sports and society, for example: *(a)* the ways in which sports are related to other forms of social life such as family, education, politics, religion, media, and the economy; *(b)* how some sports have become a part of certain cultures and not others; *(c)* how participation in sports affects or creates our beliefs regarding gender and the concepts of masculinity and femininity, the body, race, ethnicity, social class, ability and disability, competition and cooperation, violence, and aggression; *(d)* how the meanings and value of sports in society are associated with and affect social relations and how the concept of power is defined within sports; and *(e)* how people can use sports and knowledge about sports to effect social change.

2. Discuss the ways in which sports are a microcosm of society.

Answer: As social institutions, sports reflect similar values, issues, and controversies that are found in society. For example, the concepts of family, education, religion, politics, and the economy as well as the issues of sexism, racism, homophobia, nationalism, and power are prevalent within sports settings.

3. Define and discuss one social institution associated with sports in society.

Answer: [Example, answers will vary.] Social institutions include family, education, politics, the economy, and religion. Family: Informal and formal sports are linked to the family as a unifying agent. Sports bring family members closer together to share in watching televised and live sports events, participating together in sport activities, and/or supporting family members who are involved in sports activities. In this context, sports may well serve as the socializing agent for children into and/or away from sports.

4. Discuss the relationship between culture and sports.

Answer: Culture encompasses the established parts of life that are created by individuals in a specific society. It is the means by which a society defines and perpetuates itself. Culture is a patterned form of expression that becomes a product of habit rather than conscious thought among groups of people. Play is one element that different cultures share; thus the games and sports that develop out of play are inextricably linked to culture.

5. What is the value of using theoretical perspectives to study sports?

Answer: They serve as a foundation on which to base discussion, exploration, and potential research. Theories lend support to or refute an individual's opinions regarding sports and serve as a starting point or basis for the formulation of arguments.

6. In what ways are religion reflected in sports?

Answer: Consideration of sports as religion; differences and similarities between the two social institutions; praying at games; the involvement of athletes in Christian evangelical organizations; and the types of ceremonies, rituals, and taboos with which sports, athletes, and coaches are associated.

CHAPTER 19: FUTURE OF EXERCISE SCIENCE

1. Why is the emergence of the discipline of exercise science considered a paradigm shift?

   Answer: Because it has led to a profound deepening and broadening of our understanding of human movement by using sciences in a way that was not formally done on a large scale. This paradigm shift has led to the formation of the subdisciplines.

2. Explain the relationship between a discipline and a profession.

   Answer: (a) Disciplines: develop a certain body of knowledge. *(b)* Professions: use the outcomes of disciplinary knowledge in practice.

3. Give one example of a technological advance that has helped the discipline of exercise science.

   Answer: [Example; answers will vary.] Computers.

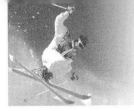

GLOSSARY

Absorptive. Ability to absorb; the body absorbs the majority of nutrients in the small intestine, the more absorptive a food is, the more readily the body absorbs that food.

Acceleration. The rate of change of velocity. Acceleration is directly proportional to the applied force and inversely proportional to the mass of the object.

Action potential. A brief reversal of the electrical charge in the membrane of nerve and muscle cells allowing an electrical signal to be transmitted throughout the membrane.

Adenosine triphosphate. ATP; the energy currency of the cell, responsible for delivering free energy to accomplish cellular activity.

Adiposity. The relative amount of body fat being carried by an individual.

Aerobic. With oxygen, especially referring to a class of exercise using aerobic metabolic processes.

Amine. A nitrogen-containing compound that has gone through a slight chemical alteration.

Anabolism. Bodily chemical reactions resulting in the buildup of large molecules from smaller molecules.

Anaerobic. Without oxygen, especially referring to a class of exercise using anaerobic metabolic processes.

Analysis of the data. Drawing theoretical conclusions from a collection of findings to answer questions of meaning associated with past events.

Anatomic kinesiology. Emphasizes the study of muscles, bones, and joints as they are involved in movement.

Angina pectoris. Heart pain that occurs whenever the blood supply to the heart muscle cannot meet the muscle's need for oxygen.

Angle of takeoff. The projection angle at the instant of release or takeoff of an object or body as measured relative to the horizon at the instant of release (e.g., throw, kick, jump).

Angular motion. The rotation of a lever—e.g., body segment, sports or exercise implement (bat, barbell)—about an axis (joint) in a circular path.

Anthropometry. Measurement of the size and proportions of the human body. Anthropometric (adjective).

Antioxidant. Compound that prevents the oxidation of substances in foods or in the body; examples are vitamins A, C, and E and the mineral selenium.

Arousal. Responsible for energizing an individual; ranges from deep sleep to extreme excitement.

Assumption of risk. A common defense against negligence. It states that activities often have inherent risks and that the participant knew of the risks and freely chose to participate despite the risks involved.

Atherosclerosis. A progressive, degenerative disease that leads to a gradual blockage of arterial vessels, thereby reducing blood flow through them.

Atherosclerosis susceptibility gene. A gene located on chromosome 19 that is linked to an increased predisposition for atherosclerosis.

Athletic training. The allied health profession dealing in prevention, recognition, and treatment of injuries to athletes.

Autocratic leadership. A style that is task oriented, expeditious, and inflexible. It is the "my way or the highway" approach.

Autoimmune disease. Disease in which the body produces antibodies against its own tissues, resulting in tissue injury.

Axial loading. Situation in which the load is placed over the center or axis of an object.

Bending loading. When an object is distorted because of a force. For example, a load placed on a beam that is located between two supports may cause the beam to curve.

Beta adrenergic blocking agents. Medications that interfere with the transmission of nerve signals in the heart, thereby decreasing heart rate, blood pressure, cardiac muscle contractility, and oxygen demand.

Beta-oxidation. A metabolic pathway that catalyzes fatty acids.

Binary. Made of two things or parts. Humans structure (invent) their world, goods, language, thoughts, fears, hopes, etc., into taxonomic categories.

Bioenergetic. Energy processes in living organisms.

Biologic plausibility. The facts that a hypothesis and the relationship that it proposes are in harmony with existing scientific information.

Biomechanics. Application of mathematics and principles of physics to the study of human movement.

Blood glucose. Blood sugar; glucose is a simple sugar and is the breakdown product of carbohydrates.

Blood-borne pathogens. Disease-causing agents carried in the blood. For example, hepatitis-B and HIV.

Braking force. A force applied to the body by the ground, a person or an object that causes it to slow down.

Cantilever loading. For example, a beam has one end firmly supported, and a load is placed on the unsupported end, as when a person stands on the end of a diving board.

Capacity. The amount of information that a memory store can hold.

Capillaries. Smallest blood vessels in the body; they participate in oxygen and nutrient exchange with tissues.

Carbohydrates. Energy nutrients that include sugars, starches, and cellulose.

Cardiac output. The volume of blood pumped by the heart per minute

Career. A field for the pursuit of progressive achievement in public, professional, or business life.

Case-control study designs. Also known as retrospective study designs; for example, individuals with and without a specific disease or condition are asked questions about their past, particularly their exposure to a specific risk factor, to determine whether a relationship exists between the risk factor and the disease or condition.

Catabolism. Bodily chemical reactions resulting in the breakdown of large molecules to smaller molecules.

Causal attributions. Reasons given for a particular outcome

Cellular respiration. A series of metabolic processes involved in the aerobic production of ATP.

Central nervous system. CNS; the brain and spinal cord.

Certification process. Involves acquisition of a core of knowledge and skills through formal educational and/or professional experience; completion of an application form and submission of candidacy credentials (e.g., letters of recommendation and documentation of professional experience and degrees); review of prerequisite knowledge and skills through the use of study guides, review courses, and/or workshops; selection of an examination date and site; and passing the certification examination.

Certification. The process by which an individual, institution, or educational program is evaluated and recognized as meeting certain predetermined standards through successful completion of a validated, reliable examination.

Challenge point. The point at which the learner is being optimally challenged to enhance learning.

Chronometric method. Using reaction time to analyze a person's behavior between the presentation of a stimulus and their response.

Circadian dysrhythmia. Disruption of daily sleep–wake cycles, usually owing to travel across time zones

Clinical biomechanics. Application of biomechanics to the treatment of patients, e.g., by orthopedic specialists or physical therapists.

Clinical exercise physiology. Application of exercise physiology to the treatment of patients, as in cardiac rehabilitation.

Clinical trial. Individuals free from a specific disease or condition are randomly assigned to receive either an intervention or no intervention (the control group). Subsequent follow-up determines if the groups differ by the percent of individuals who eventually develop the disease.

Closed kinetic chain. Physical activity in which the terminal end of a body segment is involved in functional forces

Closed loop. Receiving feedback (i.e., sensory information) during the movement that helps us control the movement.

Cocking phase. The extreme rotational position (externally rotated) of the upper arm around the shoulder joint during a throwing motion. In tennis, this position is called the "backscratch position."

Cofactors. Chemicals that are part of a reaction and are necessary for a reaction to move forward (they may be part of an enzyme). Minerals and vitamins may act as cofactors.

Collinear. Acting along the same line.

Composition. The process of combining forces to obtain one representative or resulting force. The forces tend to press on the object.

Compression. Process in which two forces act along the same line in opposite directions toward each other.

Compressive force. A force that squeezes an object's surface(s) together and causes its mass to bulge.

Concentric contraction. A muscle action in which the muscle force exceeds the load and the muscle shortens.

Concurrent. Meeting at the same point.

Conflict theory. A theory that contends that sports is an opiate of society, deadening our awareness to social concerns.

Confounder. A variable whose effect is entangled with the effect of the risk factor of interest (e.g., physical activity). The variable must be related to the disease or health outcome of interest and be related to the risk factor.

Consumption. The processes by which consumer goods and services are created, acquired, purchased, and used.

Consumptivity. The process in postmodernity by which market and other forces influence us to consume more than we need. First, we become aware at a very young age that we have purchasing power, or the ability to consume. Second, through advertisements, our value and belief systems, and everyday socialization, we are taught to desire things we don't really need and to buy the "right" brand. Third, we are socialized by a multitude of cultural beliefs and marketing about how to consume. Our passions are educated and our tastes are refined.

Contextual interference. Describes the interference that results from practicing a variety of tasks within the context of a single practice situation.

Contraindications. Any condition, especially any condition of disease, that renders some particular line of treatment improper or undesirable.

Contusions. Bruises, usually caused by direct blows

Coplanar. Acting within the same plane.

Core temperature. Deep internal temperature of the body; usually measured rectally. Normal is 37°C, but may easily exceed 40°C during heavy aerobic exercise.

Couture. The business of designing, making, and selling fashionable clothing. Today, exercise couture is high fashion and worn as global streetwear.

Creatine phosphate. High-energy phosphate molecule that serves as a reservoir of phosphate units to resynthesize ATP from ADP.

Creep. Progressive deformation of a material caused by a constant load over an extended period of time.

Critical theory. Focuses on concepts of power in social life and explains action and political involvement.

Cross-sectional studies. The investigator collects information about the health outcome and the potential risk factor at the same time within the same group to determine if a relationship exists between the two variables.

Cross-sectional method. Requires data collected on individuals of different ages, who represent different samples of the life span.

Crystal intelligence. Results largely from education; is information, such as word comprehension; and generally increases with age until the later stage of life.

Culture. The patterns of life that individuals create in a society through interacting with each other; it consists of behaviors, feelings, beliefs, norms, objects, values, and other shared characteristics of a group of people

Cultural studies. Cultural, interpretive, philosophical, anthropologic, sociologic, and semiotic study of exercise and culture; made up of many parent disciplines (e.g., literary criticism, sociology, economics, political science, history, psychology, anthropology, English, and pedagogy). Some major categories of work include gender and sexuality, nationhood and national identity, identity politics, colonialism, aesthetics, popular culture, narrative and rhetoric, and transnational economies.

Deductive. Reasoning from a general principle to an unknown.

Delimitation. Boundaries of time, place, or social structure that a researcher sets to keep a study within manageable parameters.

Democratic leadership. Sometimes referred to as participatory leadership; reflects a style that falls between the autocratic and laissez-faire styles. Characterized by a leader who is elected, who elicits input, and who then makes the decision.

Demyelinization. Loss of myelin, the fatty substance that encases nerve fibers

Denervated. A condition in which the nerve supply is removed or blocked.

Depolarization. A reduction in resting cell membrane electrical potential.

Descriptive research. Generally defined as describing the current state of the problem. Cause-and-effect conclusions should not be drawn from descriptive research.

Diabetes mellitus. A disease in which the body cannot produce insulin or cannot use insulin properly, resulting in an elevation of blood glucose.

Diabetic ketoacidosis. A condition caused by a lack of insulin, resulting in marked elevation of blood glucose and ketone bodies and a reduction of blood pH.

Diastole. The period of relaxation in the heart cycle.

Diastolic blood pressure. The point of lowest pressure in the arterial vascular system.

Dietary Reference Intake. DRI; has replaced RDA. The new standards for nutrient recommendations used to plan and assess diets for healthy individuals. There are four subcategories: Estimated Average Requirement (EAR), Recommended Dietary Allowance (RDA), Adequate Intake (AI), and Tolerable Upper Intake Level (UL).

Dislocations. Disruptions of the joint such that two or more bones become separated.

Distal attachments. The attachments of muscles that are farthest from the root of the limb.

Diuretics. Substances that result in water loss (increased urination).

Dose-response. Effects of an increasingly more intense exercise bout.

Double product. A parameter used to monitor myocardial oxygen demands obtained by multiplying heart rate times systolic blood pressure.

Duration. The length of time that information can be held in that memory store.

Dynamical systems theory. Theory that views changes in motor patterns as occurring as a result of the complex and dynamic nature of human behavior and influenced by multiple internal and external factors.

Dynamics. The study of motion in which changes in velocity are experienced by the body.

Dyspnea. Difficult or labored breathing.

Dysrhythmias. Abnormal heart rhythms.

Eccentric contraction. A muscle action in which the load exceeds the muscle force and the muscle lengthens.

Educational pyramid. A system of education adopted by institutions of higher learning whereby undergraduate students receive a broad-based experience (breadth) with little depth and the graduate student receives great depth with little breadth.

Elastic. Property of a material that allows it to return to its original size and shape after being deformed.

Electrocardiogram. A record of the electrical activity of the heart.

Electrolytes. A chemical substance which, when dissolved in water or melted, dissociates into electrically charged particles (ions), and thus is capable of conducting an electric current. Examples: sodium, chloride, and potassium; all are involved in fluid balance in the body, among other important functions.

Electron-transport chain. The final metabolic pathway that phosphorylates ADP to form ATP; water is produced as a by-product.

Emergency care plan. Plan to be executed when a severe or catastrophic injury occurs.

Empirical. Based on observation.

Encroachment. The act of working outside the established role of an occupation.

Endorphins. Hormones released in response to stressors; they act as painkillers

Endurance exercise. Exercise that can be performed with a steady-state oxygen consumption for long periods of time.

Epidemiology. The study of the distribution and determinants of health-related states or events in specified populations; the results are used to control health problems.

Equivocal. Mixed or uncertain; e.g., to say that a study showed equivocal results means that the results were mixed; some tests may have been found positive results, others negative results, and others no change.

Ergogenic aids. Ergogenic means "work enhancing"; thus ergogenic aids are substances that enhance exercise performance.

Essential amino acids. The amino acids that must be obtained by the diet. For humans, there are nine essential amino acids.

Evaluation. A process whereby the worth of a product, service, experience, person, or concept is determined and established.

Evaluation. Assessment of the nature and severity of an injury; information is transmitted to a physician who issues a diagnosis.

Exercise and sports psychology. Application of the principle of psychology to sports and exercise.

Exercise leader. According to the ACSM guidelines, a certification that "provides recognition for the professional involved in 'on-the-floor' exercise leadership; uses hands-on techniques to teach and demonstrate safe and effective methods of exercise by applying the fundamental principles of exercise science based on the results of fitness tests."

Exercise physiology. The study of how our bodies' structures and functions are altered when we are exposed to acute and chronic exercise.

Exercise prescription. A plan for physical activity formulated to achieve specific outcomes of exercise.

Exercise protocols. Method used for conducting an exercise test.

Exercise science. Any aspect of science applied to the phenomenon of exercise.

Exercise specialist. According the ACSM guidelines, "provides recognition of professionals who demonstrate competence in graded exercise testing (GXT), exercise prescription, exercise leadership, emergency procedures, and patient counseling/education for individuals with cardiovascular, pulmonary, and metabolic diseases."

Exercise. Any movement, but more commonly gross rather than fine motor activity.

Experience qualities. Aspects of the service or event that can be evaluated after the experience is over.

Experimental research. Generally defined as manipulating a variable or variables to investigate their effect on some outcome.

Experimental study. The investigator randomly assigns varying levels of the risk factor of interest to individuals without the disease and then follows those individuals to compare the development of the disease.

External respiration. An exchange of gases between the atmosphere and the lungs, and then the lungs and the blood.

Extroversion–introversion. Personality dimension characterized by relative levels of being sociable and outgoing vs. being shy and inhibited.

Fading knowledge of results. A method of providing KR whereby the frequency of the KR is faded or decreased throughout practice.

Fats. Class of energy nutrient that contains twice as much energy as glucose. Their structure is very concentrated, and they have a higher ratio of hydrogen to carbon than do carbohydrates.

Fluid intelligence. Reasoning and abstract thought, such as mental rotation. Learning is considered a mechanism of fluid intelligence. Fluid intelligence is generally considered to reach a peak in the mid-30s.

Force. The action of one object on another; a push or pull. An entity that causes an object to accelerate or deform.

Fractures. Disruptions in the continuity of a bone or bones.

Free energy. Form of energy that is "free" to do various kinds of cellular operations. The form of energy that powers muscle contraction.

Functional progression. Stage of sports-specific activity an athlete is at during a rehabilitation program.

Generalist. An academician capable of teaching in a number of the subdisciplines of exercise science.

Gerontology. The study of older adults, generally 50 years of age or older; researchers may focus on psychology, sociology, health care, biology, economics, etc.

Glycogen stores. Found in the liver and muscles; stored carbohydrates.

Glycolysis. The process whereby glucose is broken down to pyruvic acid or lactic acid.

Goals. Desired organizational and personal destinations. Goals tend to be broad, general, long-term indicators of desired outcomes; whereas objectives tend to be specific, short-term, measurable indicators of desired outcomes. Usually objectives represent stepping-stones on the path to the goal. Goals may be strategic, tactical, or operational. Operational goals are commonly referred to as objectives.

Ground reaction forces. Forces applied to the ground by a body are returned to the body in equal magnitude but an opposite direction, as explained by Newton's law of action–reaction.

Habit. Most well-learned way of responding to a stimulus

Health/Fitness Director. According to the ACSM guidelines, a certification that "provides recognition of professionals as an administrative leader of a health and fitness program in corporate, clinical, commercial, or community settings in which apparently healthy individuals participate in health promotion and fitness-related activities having advanced knowledge of applied exercise physiology and health-related issues, program administration, staff training and supervision, as well as overall facility and program management."

Health/Fitness Instructor. According to the ACSM guidelines a certification that "provides recognition of professionals qualified to assess, design, and implement individual and group exercise and fitness programs for apparently healthy individuals and individuals with controlled disease; is skilled in evaluating health behaviors and risk factors, conducting fitness assessments, writing appropriate exercise prescriptions, and motivating individuals to modify negative health habits and maintain positive lifestyle behaviors for health promotion."

Healthcare administration. Facility, financial, and personnel management, including minimizing exposure to the legal system

Heart rate. The frequency of cardiac contractions, measured in beats per minute.

Heat illness. Encompasses several disorders involving some degree of overload on thermoregulation; symptoms range from mild to severe cardiovascular and central nervous system distress.

Heat stroke. Life-threatening medical emergency in which the body's cooling system shuts down.

Hegemony. Power or dominance of an idea, ideal, or value over other ideas, ideals or values. Usually the power is hidden, subtle, and assumed to be the natural and received way things are done.

High-density lipoprotein cholesterol. HDL-C; the good cholesterol in your blood. It helps rid the body of bad cholesterol and can be increased through exercise, maintaining a healthy body weight, and quitting smoking.

Historiography. The methodologic process of producing historical accounts of the past through analyzing not only facts but also the assumptions and values of society and its people.

History of sports. The accumulative body of knowledge that recounts past practices and purposes of sport, games, athletics, leisure pursuits, and exercise through the ages.

History. The study that gives meaning and life to what people of the world have done, said, and thought in the past.

Homeostasis. The tendency of various control systems in the body to regulate physiologic processes within narrow limits. For instance, blood glucose levels, blood pH, and body temperature are all tightly controlled by homeostatic mechanisms.

Homeothermic. Same body temperature. Mammals maintain body temperatures within narrow limits, regardless of the external environmental conditions.

Hyperglycemic hyperosmolar nonketotic syndrome. Condition characterized by high blood glucose, lack of ketones, severe hyperosmolality, and marked dehydration.

Hypohydrated. Low body water content.

Hyponatremia. Below normal levels of sodium in the blood. Normal levels of sodium in the blood range from 135 to 145 mEq/L.

Hypoxemia. Insufficient oxygenation of the blood.

Incidence rates. Measured by the number of new cases of a disease in a specified time period divided by the population at risk of developing that disease over a given time period.

Inductive. Logical reasoning that proceeds from the level of facts generated by empirical observation to a more general description of phenomena. Reasoning from specifics to the generals.

Inflammation. Response of tissue to biologic insult.

Injury history. What, when, where, why, and how an injury happened, including whether the part had been injured before and what the outcome was.

Injury prevention. Stopping an injury before it occurs.

Insulin resistance. A condition in which the tissues of the body fail to respond normally to insulin.

Intangibility. Individuals cannot see, touch, or inspect the service before they use it.

Integrated marketing communications. Suggest that all promotional information present a clear image with one voice.

Interactionist theories. Ways to study meaning, identity, and social relationships, based on the assumption that there are choices in our behavior based on meanings we create as we interact with others.

Isoinertial. Special term for a muscle action in which the load on the muscle is constant.

Isokinetics. Special term used for muscle action when the rate of shortening or lengthening of the muscle is constant.

Isometric. Muscle action in which the muscle force equals the load and the total muscle does not change in length.

Jim Crow laws. The systematic practice of segregating and suppressing blacks in the United States.

Job description. A concise summation of the responsibilities, duties, and expectations for a specific employment position.

Job titles. Designated name for a particular occupation.

Kilocalories. kcal; equal to Calories (with a capital C); 1 kcal = 1000 calories (lower case c). The word *calorie* is commonly and incorrectly used for *kilocalorie*.

Kinematics. The study of motion in which temporal and spatial variables (displacement, velocity and acceleration) are considered.

Kinesiology. Study of human movement. Also the discipline that deals with human movement.

Kinetics. The study of motion in which force variables (force and torque) are considered.

Knickerbockers. A social club begun in the 1840s in New York that organized the first sports club (baseball) in the United States.

Knowledge of results. KR; defined as postresponse, augmented, error information. This means that KR is information given to learners about the success of the response. This information is not something learners would necessarily know by themselves. Telling a pitcher he or she threw a strike would be providing KR.

Krebs cycle. Cyclic reactions in the mitochondria that metabolize pyruvic acid and acetyl CoA; CO_2, NADH, and $FADH_2$ are the chief by-products.

Lactic acid. The by-product of anaerobic glycolysis.

Laissez-faire leadership. Reflects a style that is hands off, slow, flexible, and creative. Group input and decision making are valued in this style of leadership

Leadership power. Represents the degree of influence that the leader possesses. Power may be categorized as legitimate, expert, referent, reward, or coercive. These types of power are not mutually exclusive.

Leadership. May be thought of as the ability of an individual to influence others to facilitate his or her achievement of individual or organizational goals.

Learning. Defined as a relatively permanent change in behavior that results from practice or experience

Legal liability. Responsibilities and duties that exist among socially interacting people that are enforceable by law. For leisure, sports, and fitness leaders, certain legal responsibilities and duties exist regarding actions involving clients and players. If these responsibilities are not fulfilled, then legal action may result.

Leverage. The consideration of torques applied on levers based on the position of the axis of rotation to the point on the lever where the force is applied (lever arm).

Licensure. Granting of permission by a competent authority (usually a government agency) to an organization or individual to engage in a practice or activity that would otherwise be illegal.

Limitations. Factors that may affect a study over which the researcher has no control.

Linear motion. Movement of a body from point to point in space as measured in a straight line within a Cartesian coordinate system.

Lipolysis. The breakdown of triglycerides.

Load. An outside force acting externally on an object.

Longitudinal method. The study of motor development over time to see the effect of time on the subjects.

Macronutrients. Nutrients needed by the body in large quantities; e.g., carbohydrates, fats, and proteins.

Major minerals. An essential mineral needed in the diet in amounts greater than 100 mg/day.

Management. The art and science of facilitating the effective and efficient achievement of organizational goals; involves planning, organizing, leading, and controlling.

Marketing mix. The product or service, promotion, pricing, and distribution elements of the marketing strategy.

Marketing strategy. Contains five basic components: target market, product and service offering, promotion, pricing, and distribution.

Mass. That characteristic of matter which gives it inertia. The resistance of an object to motion.

Mechanical fatigue. Repetitive loading of a material that causes the material to fail or break.

Media. Forms of communication of information; e.g., electronic (radio, televisions, films, and cyberspace) and print (newspapers and magazines).

Metabolic capacity. The ability of a metabolic pathway to produce ATP. Great capacity refers to the ability to make large quantities of ATP with respect to pathways with less capacity.

Metabolic pathways. A sequence of enzyme-mediated chemical reactions resulting in specific product(s).

Metabolic power. The rapidity with which a metabolic pathway produces ATP.

Metabolism. The sum total of all the chemical reactions in the body.

Micronutrients. Nutrients needed by the body in small quantities; e.g., vitamins and minerals.

Mission statement. The broadest of all goals; a manifestation of the philosophy of the organization, it tells us why the organization exists.

Mitochondria. Specialized cellular structures responsible for producing ATP during aerobic metabolism.

Moment. The result of a force acting on an object at a distance from its axis; it tends to rotate the object.

Morbidity. Any departure, subjective or objective, from a state of physiologic or psychological well-being.

Mortality rates. The ratio of total number of deaths to the total number of individuals in the population.

Motivation. Energy thought to drive an individual; composed of direction, intensity, and persistence.

Motor behavior. Application of psychology to movement; includes control, development, and learning.

Motor control. Concerned with understanding the mechanisms by which the neural and muscular systems orchestrate the myriad movements made by the organism and the manner in which these mechanisms are constrained.

Motor development. Concerned with understanding the change in movement orchestration that results more from system maturation than practice or experience.

Motor learning. Concerned with understanding the mechanisms of the relatively permanent change in behavior resulting from practice or experience that manifests itself in a more efficient orchestration of movements.

Motor unit. The motor nerve and all the muscle fibers that it innervates.

Negligence. A type of tort that involves the commission or omission of a legally required act that causes an injury to occur.

Neurons. Nerve cells that send or receive messages throughout the CNS.

Neuroticism–stability. Personality dimension characterized by relative levels of being even-tempered and easygoing vs. anxious and moody

Nonessential amino acids. Amino acids that can be made in the body. Humans have 11 nonessential amino acids.

Observation. Visually inspecting an injury site, general body language, and facial expressions.

Observational study. The investigator observes the occurrence of the disease or condition in individuals who differ by the risk factor of interest.

Open loop. A system in which one does not receive feedback on line (i.e., during the movement). Instead, the movement is completely preplanned.

Organizational triad. Represents the three most essential areas of an organization: leadership, facilities and equipment, and programs.

Oscilloscope. An instrument that makes the presence, nature, and form of the cardiac electric current visible.

Osteophytes. Bones spur at the edges of joints, typically seen in osteoarthritis.

Overuse injuries. Any of a number of injuries occurring as a result of repetitive microtrauma.

Oxygen consumption. $\dot{V}O_2$max; the rate at which oxygen is used in the body; usually measured as liters per minute or milliliters per kilogram of body weight per minute.

p value. A statistic that quantifies the degree to which chance may account for an association observed in a particular study

Palpation. Placing hands on an injury site to feel for deformities, temperature changes, blood flow changes, and range of motion assessment

Parabolic path. The trajectory or curvilinear path of motion of a projectile when no air frictional forces are present.

Paradigm: A pattern, archetype, or set of rules, especially as related to a set way of viewing or doing things within one's worldview.

Pastiche. Composed of old and new and of images that would not normally be placed side by side.

Patriarchy. Political and social control of women by men in which the subordination of women is implicit.

Perceived value. What one gives for what one gets.

Performance. Observable behavior.

Perishability of inventory. The inventory of sports and fitness operators includes time and space, which cannot be stored for future use.

Personnel management. Hiring and assigning people (i.e., athletic trainers) to job sites

Pharmacokinetics. Study of the action of drugs with particular emphasis on time required for absorption, duration of action, distribution in the body, and method of excretion.

Phosphagen system. The metabolic pathway using creatine phosphate as the substrate that donates a phosphate group to ADP in the anaerobic formation of ATP. Used primarily during very intense exercise lasting a few seconds.

Phospholipids. Substances made up of phosphorus, lipids, and a nitrogen base.

Phosphorylation. Chemical process whereby a phosphate group is added to a molecule.

Physical activity epidemiology. Involves the specific investigation of the relationship between physical activity (and/or exercise) and health and diseases within a population.

Physical activity survey. A method of quantifying the amount of physical activity in which an individual engages, often during a specific time period (e.g., weekly).

Physical education. Discipline and/or profession that deals with education about physical activity and education through physical activity.

Picolinate. A substance chelated (or combined) with such minerals as chromium; it is thought to enhance the absorption of the mineral to which it has been chelated.

Postmodernism. A broad, vague label for a time period, literary form, or artistic style. The label is used to refer to changed contemporary society.

Potential energy. The energy stored in energy nutrients.

Practice–learning distinction. Sometimes known as the practice–learning paradox because it has been demonstrated that one's performance during practice is not necessarily an index of learning.

Preparatory period. Period of time encompassing the few seconds before beginning a response.

Presentism. Applying present-day standards, values, or beliefs to events or happenings of former periods.

Prevalence rates. Measure the number of existing cases of a disease divided by the total population at a point in time or over a given time period.

Primary sources. Works written at or near the time something occurred and usually by a party who was present to observe the occurrence.

Primary survey. Part of an evaluation that checks life-threatening situations.

Prime movers. Muscle that are directly responsible for producing particular movements.

Primitive reflexes. Associated with infants' basic needs, such as nourishment and security.

Profession. An occupation requiring detailed knowledge in a course of study, accompanied by advanced education and training involving intellectual skills.

Professional organizations. Associations of individuals formed for the purpose of self-regulating and advancing common goals and interests.

Program development cycle. A paradigm that depicts the flow of organizational operation. First a mission statement is established, then a comprehensive needs assessment is conducted, goals and objectives are engendered to address the needs and weaknesses, plans are formulated to effectively and efficiently meet the goals and objectives, the plans are implemented, and the program is evaluated. Because the process is cyclical, programs are evaluated in light of the mission statement, new needs are identified, and thus the process continues.

Program directors. According to the ACSM guidelines, a certification that "is directed toward professionals whose primary responsibilities are developing and directing safe and effective clinical exercise programs."

Program/Facility Certification. Certification of a program that meets specific criteria related to staff and facility requirements

Projectile. An object or body that is traveling through the air free of external forces, with the exception of gravity and air resistance.

Proprioception. The process of sensing, through organs such as the vestibular apparatus, muscle spindles, and Golgi tendon organs, the state and position of the body.

Prospective study. Identifies and follows individuals initially free of the health outcome of interest and seeks to establish if initial or subsequent physical activity levels differentiate those who do and do not develop the disease.

Proximal attachments. The attachment of the muscle that is closest to the root of the limb.

Psychological well-being. Amount of positive emotion relative to negative emotion.

Psychomotor function. The ability to integrate cognition with motor abilities, such as communication and locomotion.

Psychoticism–superego. Personality dimension characterized by relative levels of being impulsive and egocentric vs. cooperative and caring

Public health. The study and implementation of programs designed to inform the public about disease identification and prevention.

Quackery. A misrepresentation of the facts to deceive the consumer.

Qualitative analysis. The description of human motion without the benefit of quantitative instrumentation; one's ability to make unmeasured judgments is essential. The typical means by which coaches, physical education teachers, and fitness professionals assess the performance of athletes, students, and exercisers.

Qualitative research. Examines meanings, concepts, characteristics, definitions, symbols, and descriptions of things; conclusions from this research are most often drawn from analysis of descriptive data rather than from mathematical treatment of data.

Quantitative analysis. The description of human motion with the benefit of quantitative instrumentation to measure the kinematics and/or kinetics of the performance. The typical means by which a biomechanist assesses human motion for the purposes of performing research or providing information to improve performance or prevent injury.

Quantitative research. Refers to counts and measures of things; a collection of data that can be tested through statistical means in order to draw conclusions.

Range of motion. Normal arc that a joint moves through.

Rate. Number of cases or deaths divided by the population at risk in a given time period.

Rating of perceived exertion. Rating of an individual's perception of exercise intensity.

Reaction time. The time between stimulus onset and the initiation of a movement.

Recommended Dietary Allowances. RDA; the recommended levels of intake for essential nutrients for healthy individuals.

Registration. Recording of professional qualification information relevant to government licensing regulations

Registry. List of healthcare professionals who are registered with an agency or organization; provides information to employers and the public about the qualifications of individuals.

Regression. In the domain of motor development refers to a decrease in performance from peak and is generally associated with older adulthood.

Rehabilitation. Restoring normal strength and function

Relationship marketing. Focuses on making and keeping relationships with customers over the long term.

Relative task difficulty. Defined as the difficulty of the motor problem one must resolve to successfully complete a task relative to the performer completing the task.

Reliability. Precision; the degree to which the results obtained by a measurement procedure (e.g., physical activity questionnaire) can be repeated by retesting under the same conditions.

Repair. Phase of rehabilitation dealing with scar tissue formation.

Representations. Abstractions existing outside of the mind that are represented in ways that are thought to be accurate and true. Sometimes representations are actual objects; sometimes representations are ideas. Representations can be ephemeral (short lived) or of long endurance. Consumptivity plays a role in creating influential representations that we come to desire and purchase.

Resistance exercise. Form of exercise in which muscles are contracting at large percentages of their maximal voluntary contraction capability. Results in a distinctly different hemodynamic and metabolic pattern of responses compared to endurance forms. Weightlifting is the prime example of a resistance exercise.

Resolution. The process of separating a force into two perpendicular components.

Resultant. The force obtained by combining two or more forces.

Risk factor. Biologic, environmental, and behavioral variables (factors) that interact to cause disease in a population.

Risk management. Involves a systematic approach to minimizing the possibility of being successfully sued by players and clients for alleged torts such as negligence.

Role delineation. A study of the specific responsibilities of an occupation based on the knowledge, skills, and abilities expected of that professional.

Rotational inertia. The resistance a lever offers to a change in its state of angular motion in which the mass, length, and distribution of the mass along the lever are important.

Scalar. A quantity for which only its magnitude is of consideration.

Search qualities. Aspects of a service or event that can be examined before a client uses the service or attends the event.

Secondary services. Services that participants use while they are participating or using the primary service.

Secondary sources. Works based on primary sources; books, journal articles, newspaper articles, and other material written about a subject years after the event and by a person who was not an eyewitness to the occurrence.

Secondary survey. Part of an evaluation assessing the nature and severity of an injury.

Selective attention. A process whereby one actively chooses a single unit of information to pay attention to at a time.

Self-concept. Core of personality containing our values, interests, beliefs, worldview, and perceptions of self.

Self-confidence. Perception of ability.

Self-efficacy. Perception of ability to perform a specific task at a particular time; situation-specific self-confidence

Sensory neurons. Afferent neurons; signals from the senses to the CNS.

Sequential kinetic link principle. The production of velocity of the body (or an object) by virtue of a pattern of muscular forces that accelerate and decelerate the body segments in a sequential manner. The flow of energy is typically from proximal to distal segments or from the most massive (i.e., trunk) to the least massive (i.e., foot or hand) segments. This pattern is typically used when the mass of the object to be moved is small.

Sequential method. Combines longitudinal and cross-sectional methods. The method involves studying several different samples (cross-sectional) over a number of years (longitudinal).

Serotonin. 5-Hydroxytryptamine (5-HT); a neurotransmitter in the brain.

Service qualities. Relates to how well the service meets or exceeds customers' expectations.

Servicescape. The ambient and design factors that make up the facility environment.

Shear. Process in which two forces act in the same plane but not collinear in opposite directions toward each other.

Signs. Objective, quantifiable information about an athlete.

Simultaneous kinetic link principle. The production of velocity of the body (or an object) by virtue of a pattern of muscular forces that accelerate and decelerate the body segments in a simultaneous manner. This pattern is typically used when the mass of the body or object to be moved is great.

Skills. Learned movements; consist of the ability to bring about some end result with maximum certainty and minimum outlay of energy.

Sociology. The study of human behavior and social interactions as they occur in social and cultural settings.

Specialists. Academicians who teach in a specific subdiscipline of exercise science.

Sports biomechanics. Application of mathematics and principles of physics to specific sports.

Sports history. A scholarly field concerned with the historical study of sports; encompasses the practices and meanings of exercise, recreational pastimes, play, games, and athletics from the past.

Sports marketing. The development and management of the primary and secondary service offerings via promotion, pricing, and distribution aimed at satisfying viable target markets.

Sports medicine. Science applied to the individual in sports and exercise, with special attention to environment, psychological aspects, drugs, prevention and treatment of injuries, rehabilitation, and safety.

Sports nutrition. Principles of nutrition applied to individuals in sports and exercise.

Sports pedagogy. The discipline concerned with understanding and optimizing the process of teaching movement skills

Sports sociology. A subdiscipline of exercise science focusing on sports as a part of social and cultural life.

Sprains. Abnormal stretch to a ligament

Stacking. The over- or underrepresentation of certain racial or ethnic groups in central leadership or strategy positions in team sports.

States. Temporary thoughts or feelings; easily changeable.

Statics. The study of systems that are stationary or moving without acceleration.

Statistically significant. Indicates that the results of a particular study were not caused by chance occurrence or some other random variable.

Strain. The change of dimensions of a material when forces are applied to it.

Strains. Abnormal stretch of a muscle or tendon

Strategic goals. Very broad indicators of organizational or personal destinations usually set by high-level administrators or owners.

Stress fracture. Nondisplaced fracture of gradual onset with no specific cause.

Stress. The process of a material resisting the deformation caused by forces applied to it.

Stressor. Something that requires an individual to adapt.

Stride length. The distance measured along the ground between sequential foot positions of the same foot taken either at takeoff or initial contact during walking or running.

Stride rate. The number of strides (foot contact to foot contact of same foot) taken per unit of time during walking or running.

Stroke volume. The amount of blood pumped by the heart per beat.

Structural functionalism. A theoretical approach based on society's system needs of pattern maintenance and tension management, integration, goal setting, and adaptation. This theory contends that sports is an inspiration.

Subcultures. Subunit of culture that have different values from the larger culture; may be represented by concepts such as age, gender, religion, race, ethnicity, social class, physical ability, and sexual orientation.

Subluxation. Partial dislocation, in which the bones spontaneously return to normal alignment

Summary knowledge of results. A method of providing KR that requires the subject to complete several trials of a simple motor task without receiving KR.

Support phase. The time during which a part of the body is in contact with the ground (floor or apparatus), such as when the foot is on the ground to apply forces for the purpose of increasing or decreasing the body's velocity during sprinting.

Swing phase. The time during which a body or body segment is repositioning itself in an effort to perform additional work after the primary work or acceleration phase of the activity.

Symptoms. Subjective information obtained from an injured athlete.

Systole. The period of the heart cycle in which the heart is in contraction.

Systolic blood pressure. The highest blood pressure in the arterial vascular system, occurring during contraction of the ventricles.

Tactical goals. Destinations set by midlevel managers and supervisors that support the realization of strategic goals. Thus tactical goals are more specific than strategic goals but are less specific than operational goals (objectives).

Target market. Consists of consumers who have similar characteristics and needs that can be best met by the coordinated efforts of the organization.

Task difficulty. The difficulty of the motor problem one must resolve to successfully complete a task.

Tension. Process in which two forces act along the same line in opposite directions away from each other. The forces tend to pull the object apart.

Therapeutic modalities. Physical, thermal, and chemical agents used to modify the inflammatory response or speed the restoration of function after an athletic injury.

Title IX. The Educational Amendment of 1972 to the 1964 Civil Rights Act that stated: "No person in the United States shall on the basis of sex be excluded from participation in, be denied the benefits of, or be subjected to discrimination under any educational program or activity receiving Federal financial assistance."

Torques. The result of force being applied at a distance from the axis of rotation.

Torsion. The twisting of a rod around its axis caused by torque.

Torts. Civil wrongdoings (not crimes) that may result in lawsuits.

Total energy expenditure. Consists of physical activity or exercise, basal metabolic rate (which typically encompasses 50 to 70% of total energy expended), and the thermic effect of food (which accounts for another 7 to 10%).

Trace minerals. Essential minerals needed in the diet in amounts less than 100 mg/day.

Traits. More permanent ways of thinking or feeling; not easily changeable.

Transaminated. Transfer of an amino group from one compound to another.

Type 1 diabetes. Form of diabetes caused when the immune system attacks the beta cells of the islands of Langerhans so they can no longer produce insulin.

Type 2 diabetes. Form of diabetes characterized by insulin resistance and a relative, rather than absolute, insulin deficiency.

Valence. Degree to which something is rated as positive or negative or good or bad

Validity. Accuracy; the degree to which a measurement measures what it is intended to measure as determined by a gold standard measure.

Values. Socially determined and shared ideas regarding what is good, right, and desirable.

Vectors. Quantity having magnitude and direction values.

Verbal learning. The learning of such areas as history, mathematics, and learning about motor learning.

Viscoelastic. The property that combines the elasticity and damping that allow a material to return to its original size and shape at a controlled rate after the material has been deformed.

Whatever. From the philosopher Agamben: "precisely that which is neither particular nor general, neither individual nor generic." Associated with the theoretical idea "in the act of becoming" at any one time, it is difficult to fully articulate accurately the motivations, values, and inspirations of a minute exercise segment of society.

Wolff's law. Bone responds to the loads placed on it by increasing its mass under greater loads and decreasing its mass under low loads.

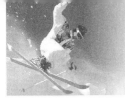

INDEX

Page numbers in *italics* denote figures; those followed by a "t" denote tables; and those followed by a "b" denote boxes.